An Introduction to Pet Dental Care

For Veterinary Technicians and Nurses

An Introduction to Pet Dental Care

For Veterinary Technicians and Nurses

Kathy Istace

RVT, VTS (Dentistry)

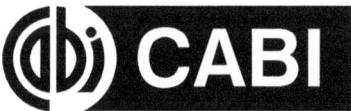

CABI

CABI is a trading name of CAB International

CABI
Nosworthy Way
Wallingford
Oxfordshire OX10 8DE
UK

CABI
WeWork
One Lincoln St
24th Floor
Boston, MA 02111
USA

Tel: +44 (0)1491 832111
Fax: +44 (0)1491 833508
E-mail: info@cabi.org
Website: www.cabi.org

T: +1 (617)682-9015
E-mail: cabi-nao@cabi.org

A catalogue record for this book is available from the British Library, London, UK.

Library of Congress Control Number: 2021939369

References to Internet websites (URLs) were accurate at the time of writing. All photos and diagrams are the author's own.

ISBN-13:   9781789248869   (paperback)
           9781789248876   (ePDF)
           9781789248883   (ePub)

DOI: 10.1079/9781789248869.0000

Commissioning Editor: Alexandra Lainsbury
Editorial Assistant: Lauren Davies / Alison Thompson
Production Editor: Tim Kapp

Typeset by Exeter Premedia Services Pvt Ltd, Chennai, India

Contents

Introduction

Dental diseases play a significant role in the lives of our companion animals. For example, periodontal disease – disease of the tissues surrounding the teeth – is the most prevalent type of oral disorder and one of the most common diseases observed by small animal practitioners (Gorrel, 2003). It is preventable by good dental hygiene, and dental hygiene is usually the responsibility of the veterinary nurse[1] (Bellows *et al.*, 2019). Other oral conditions commonly seen in veterinary medicine include tooth resorption, fractured teeth, persistent deciduous (baby) teeth, and dental malocclusions that can cause tissue trauma and pain. Less common – but often more serious – oral diseases include cancers, jaw fractures and inflammatory disorders such as stomatitis. Each of these conditions must be recognized and properly treated to ensure the health and quality of life of our patients.

In many veterinary practices it is not uncommon for the veterinary nurse to be the first professional to evaluate the patient's mouth after admittance. But, in contrast to the training for dental hygienists, who receive nearly 300 hours of specialized dental instruction prior to cleaning their human patients' teeth (Gingerich, 2012), dental-specific training for veterinary nurses is often limited to a lecture on veterinary dentistry and perhaps a single hands-on laboratory session. Veterinary nurses are nonetheless expected to provide oral health examinations and perform dental hygiene on various species, take dental radiographs, understand oral disease processes, assist with dental procedures and surgeries, maintain dental machines and instruments, and educate our clients (Woodward, 2004).

This book aims to bridge the gap that exists between current training for veterinary nurses in veterinary dentistry and what is required of us in practice, by providing instruction in essential skills such as dental cleaning, charting, radiography and equipment maintenance. It also

---

[1] The profession of veterinary nurse in the UK, Australia and New Zealand is known as 'veterinary technician' in the United States and 'veterinary technologist' in Canada. This book uses the term 'veterinary nurse' throughout.

contains information about more advanced skills, including administration of regional nerve blocks and periodontal treatments, as well as details of the aetiology and treatment of common oral conditions.

Improving competence in veterinary dental skills benefits veterinary nurses in a number of ways: it increases confidence, job satisfaction, employment opportunities and professional value. Benefits to the veterinary practice include increasing the quality of medicine offered and the number and range of billable procedures performed (Berg, 2020). A higher quality of dental medicine also has immeasurable benefits for our patients, in terms of better recognition and treatment of dental pain and infection, and thus improvement in their quality of life (Bellows *et al.*, 2019).

In addition to the information contained in this text, veterinary nurses can develop their knowledge of veterinary dentistry by attending lectures and laboratory events offered by veterinary dental conferences, both local and international, such as the Veterinary Dental Forum (VDF, 2021) and the European Veterinary Dental Forum (EVDF, 2021).

References

Bellows, J., Berg, M., Dennis, S., Harvey, R., Lobprise, H.B. *et al.* (2019) 2019 AAHA Dental Care Guidelines for Dogs and Cats. American Animal Hospital Association. Available at: https://www.aaha.org/globalassets/02-guidelines/dental/aaha_dental_guidelines.pdf (accessed 10 September 2020).

Berg, M. (2020) Dentistry Education for Patients and Practices. Today's Veterinary Nurse. Available at: https://todaysveterinarynurse.com/articles/dentistry-education-for-patients-and-practices (accessed 1 February 2021).

EVDF (2021) European Veterinary Dental Forum. Available at: https://www.evdf.org (accessed 9 March 2021).

Gingerich, W. (2012) Periodontal Cleaning and Non-Surgical Treatment. In: *Proceedings of the 26th Annual Veterinary Dental Forum.* Omnipress, Madison, Wisconsin, (CD Rom).

Gorrel, C. (2003) Periodontal Disease. *World Small Animal Veterinary Association World Congress Proceedings, 2003.* Available at: https://www.vin.com/apputil/content/defaultadv1.aspx?meta=Generic&pId=8768&id=3850088 (accessed April 16, 2021).

VDF (2021) Veterinary Dental Forum. Available at: https://www.veterinarydental-forum.org (accessed 9 March 2021).

Woodward, T.M. (2004) Blowing the Top Off Your Dental Department: A Guide for the General Practitioner. In: *Proceedings of the 18th Annual Veterinary Dental Forum.* Omnipress, Madison, Wisconsin, pp. 225–236.

More than Just Bad Breath: Periodontal Disease

1

'Doggy breath' (and kitty breath, too) is such a common problem that most pet owners accept it as normal. It isn't! Bad breath is usually the first sign of one of the most common preventable diseases afflicting pets today: periodontal disease (Perrone *et al.*, 2020). By 2 years of age, 80% of adult dogs and 70% of adult cats have periodontal disease (Niemiec *et al.*, 2020), which means that nearly every patient seen in a veterinary practice needs dental care. Periodontal disease is a progressive condition that can be prevented with proper dental homecare and regular professional dental cleanings, but once a patient develops the disease, it can often only be managed, not cured (Bellows *et al.*, 2019). The American Animal Hospital Association recommends annual dental cleanings starting at 1 year of age for cats and small-breed dogs, and starting at 2 years of age for large-breed dogs (Bellows *et al.*, 2019).

1.1 Dental Anatomy and Periodontal Disease

We divide teeth into two parts: the crown, which is the portion of tooth above the gumline which functions to hold, tear, and chew; and the root, which anchors the tooth into the surrounding bone (Holzman, 2020). The crown is covered with a thin (<0.03–0.6 mm) layer of enamel (see Fig. 1.1): a hard, non-porous substance composed primarily of the mineral hydroxyapatite (Hale, 1997). The root is covered by a hard tissue called cementum. The crown and root meet at the cementoenamel junction (CEJ), commonly called the 'neck' of the tooth (Holzman, 2020). Beneath both the enamel and cementum is dentin, which contains more organic material than enamel and is porous, with hollow channels called dentinal tubules that provide the dentin with nutrients from the pulp. Dentin is continually produced by cells called odontoblasts throughout an animal's life. As an animal matures, more dentin is produced. This causes the pulp chamber, an area of nerves and blood vessels contained in the crown, to

© CAB International 2022. *An Introduction to Pet Dental Care: For Veterinary Technicians and Nurses* (K. Istace)
DOI: 10.1079/9781789248869.0001

narrow and the tooth to become stronger. Gradual tooth wear can stimulate the formation of reparative dentin to protect the tooth from pulp
exposure (Hale, 1997).

At the centre of the tooth is the endodontic system, which contains the
tooth's blood supply and nerves, and enters the tooth through the apex
(base) of the root. The endodontic system is also divided into two parts:
the pulp chamber within the crown, and the pulp canals within the root
(Holzman, 2020).

Periodontal disease is the inflammation and infection of the periodontium: the tissues surrounding the teeth (Harvey, 2005). This inflammation
and infection leads to tooth loss. There are four types of periodontal tissues
(Hale, 1997; Stepaniuk, 2006; Holzman, 2020):

1. Gingiva (gums): soft tissue surrounding the teeth. It is the periodontium's first line of defence against harmful pathogens. It is comprised
   of the free gingiva, which is not attached to the tooth, and the attached
   gingiva, which is attached to the CEJ. The space between the free gingiva
   and the tooth is known as the gingival sulcus, containing sulcar fluid
   that includes antibodies and white blood cells. The gingiva is connected
   to the looser alveolar mucosa at the mucogingival junction.
2. Cementum: tissue similar to bone that covers the tooth roots, serving as
   a point of attachment for periodontal ligament fibres. It is continually
   deposited and resorbed throughout an animal's life.

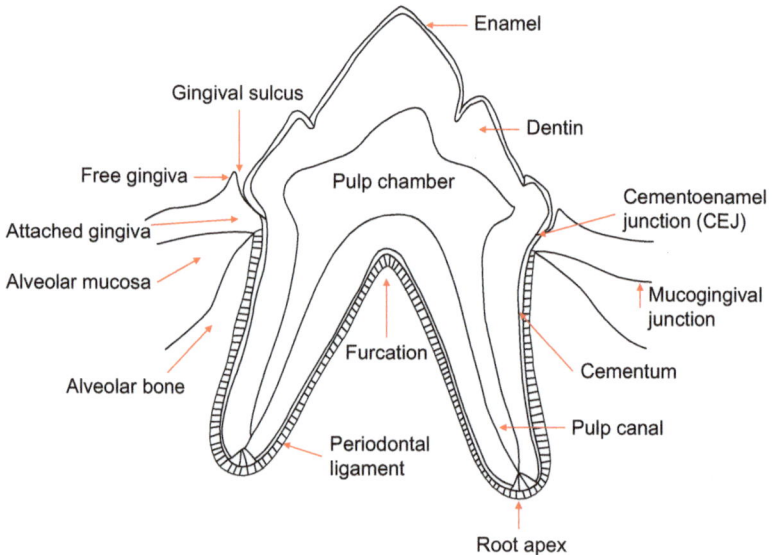

Fig. 1.1. Dental anatomy.

3. Periodontal ligament: holds the tooth within its socket and acts a as shock absorber during chewing.

4. Alveolar bone: surrounds a tooth's roots, and contains blood vessels, nerves and lymphatic vessels.

1.1.1 Pathophysiology of periodontal disease

Periodontal disease begins with plaque (Barthel, 2006). Plaque development occurs similarly in humans and other mammals (Gorrel, 2004). Saliva, a liquid secreted by the salivary glands to lubricate the mouth and aid in digestion, forms a coating on the teeth called the pellicle (Harvey, 2005). Within a few hours, several hundred strains of bacteria normally present within the oral cavity, such as *Actinomyces* and *Streptococcus* species (Eisner, 2006), start to colonize the pellicle, feeding on amino acids, proteins and glycoproteins within the saliva (Niemiec *et al.*, 2020). This bacteria-laden coating is known as dental plaque: a soft, sticky biofilm that adheres tenaciously to the tooth's surface (Perrone *et al.*, 2020). In addition to bacteria, plaque is composed of epithelial cells, white blood cells, macrophages, and salivary glycoproteins (Gorham, 2006). Plaque is usually invisible, but heavy plaque deposits may appear as a grey or white soft material on the tooth's surface. Once attached, plaque can only be removed from the teeth by mechanical scrubbing such as brushing, abrasive diets, or professional dental cleanings (Perrone *et al.*, 2020).

At first, plaque is confined to the tooth's crown, and contains predominantly non-motile, aerobic cocci (Lobprise and Wiggs, 2000a). When these cocci contact the gingiva, they stimulate an inflammatory response (Holmstrom *et al.*, 2000). White blood cells engulf the bacteria and burst when full, releasing toxins and enzymes that irritate the animal's periodontal tissues, causing an inflammation of the gums called gingivitis. The gingiva reddens and swells as it increases its blood supply in an attempt to fight off the invading bacteria. As the gum tissue swells, it loses its ability to cling tightly to the tooth's surface, creating a space between the tooth and the gingiva known as a periodontal pocket. Periodontal disease is considered to be present when pocket depths are greater than 3 mm in dogs and 1mm in cats. Plaque can now begin to creep beneath the gumline, and bacteria can freely attack the tissues that hold the tooth in the mouth (Holmstrom *et al.*, 2000). The bacteria also secrete substances that improve the biofilm's adhesion to the tooth and protect the bacteria from antimicrobial agents; bacteria found within plaque can be more than 1000 times more resistant to antiseptics and antibiotics than the same bacteria would be by itself (DuPont, 1997).

Once oxygen is no longer able to reach the deepest layers of this thick matrix, the bacterial population begins to shift, with anaerobic, mobile bacilli and filamentous organisms such as *Porphyromonas*, *Prevotella*, *Bacteroides*, *Fusobacterium* and *Treponema* taking over (Gingerich, 2012;

Niemiec *et al.*, 2020). These anaerobes produce endotoxins which, along with the patient's own defence mechanisms, lead to soft tissue loss (Lobprise and Wiggs, 2000a; Perrone *et al.*, 2020) or, sometimes, gingival hyperplasia, an overgrowth of gum tissue that occurs secondary to chronic inflammation (Barnette, 2020).

If plaque is not removed, within 24–72 hours calcium carbonate and calcium phosphate salts within the saliva begin to mineralize into a hard substance called calculus or tartar (Clarke, 1999; Perrone *et al.*, 2020). Calculus itself doesn't cause periodontal disease, but it is thick, rough, and porous, allowing bacteria to proliferate within and beneath it (Gorrel, 1998). It is firmly attached to the tooth and can only be removed by mechanical means such as dental scaling with hand instruments or ultrasonic scalers (Perrone *et al.*, 2020). Calculus deposits can become so large that they displace and damage the gingiva.

As the gum tissue is destroyed, it begins to recede, exposing the tooth root. The infection can create periodontal pockets so deep that the ligament holding the tooth within its socket, and even the bone of the socket itself, are also destroyed (Bellows *et al.*, 2019; Niemiec *et al.*, 2020).

1.1.2 Health problems associated with periodontal disease

Oral pain, bleeding gums and tooth loss are obvious consequences of untreated periodontal disease (Holmstrom *et al.*, 2000). Less obvious, though serious, consequences also exist.

- Oronasal fistulas occur when severe periodontal disease affects the upper canine teeth, whose roots are separated from the nasal cavity by only a thin shelf of bone that is easily destroyed by infection. This leads to communication between the oral and nasal cavities and results in sinusitis (Lobprise and Wiggs, 2000a). This is very common in older, small-breed dogs such as miniature Dachshunds (Perrone *et al.*, 2020).
- Pathologic jaw fractures can be caused by severe bone loss due to periodontal disease in the lower jaw, most commonly around the roots of the lower first molar in small-breed dogs. In these cases, dogs have been known to fracture their jaws while eating, playing with toys or other dogs, or while having diseased teeth extracted (Niemiec *et al.*, 2020).
- Osteomyelitis, an area of dead, infected bone, can also be a result of severe periodontal disease (Niemiec, 2004). Osteomyelitis typically does not respond well to antibiotic therapy and may require surgical removal of part or the entire upper or lower jaw. Septicaemia, commonly known as blood poisoning, may occur secondarily to osteomyelitis.
- Alveolar bone expansion, a thickening of the alveolar bone due to chronic inflammation caused by periodontal disease in cats, presents as a bulging appearance of the bone, usually around the maxillary canine teeth (Lobprise and Wiggs, 2000b; American Veterinary Dental College

(AVDC), 2021). Maxillary canine tooth extrusion in cats can also be seen in response to periodontal disease.

- Class II perio-endo lesions occur in multi-rooted teeth when infection progresses down through the alveolar bone and around the apex of one root, allowing bacteria to gain access to the tooth's endodontic system and infecting the tooth itself (Niemiec, 2012a).
- Periodontal disease can lead to infections of organs such as the kidneys, liver and heart (Pavlica *et al.*, 2008). The risk of heart disease (endocarditis and cardiomyopathy) has been shown to be higher for dogs with moderate to severe periodontal disease than for dogs without periodontal disease (Fitzgerald, 2008). Each time a pet with periodontal disease chews, tiny abrasions occur in its fragile, infected periodontal tissues (Niemiec, 2012b). Capillaries in these abrasions rupture, allowing bacteria to enter the bloodstream and settle in other organs. This is especially dangerous in patients whose health is already compromised, such as diabetics, the immunosuppressed, or pets in poor body condition (Reiter, 2013). Preventing or controlling periodontal disease may play a role in reducing the severity or development of other health conditions (Niemiec, 2012a).

1.1.3 Contributors to periodontal disease

- Crowded teeth allow food and bacteria to become trapped between teeth more easily, causing more plaque accumulation (Bellows *et al.*, 2019). Tooth crowding is common in smaller and brachycephalic breeds, and can also be caused by persistent deciduous (baby) teeth, dental or jaw malocclusions, and the presence of supernumerary (extra) teeth (Kangas, 2019).
- Fractured, painful (Lewis, 2017), or missing (Hale, 2004) teeth can also contribute to the development of periodontal disease. If an animal cannot chew properly on one side of its mouth due to pain or missing teeth, it will chew on the opposite side. The side of the mouth not used for chewing will develop more plaque due to the lack of self-cleaning that occurs with chewing (Lewis, 2017).
- Enamel hypocalcification, areas of rough or missing enamel, which possibly occur as a result of high fever or illness in very young patients, increases the ability of plaque to attach to a tooth (Niemiec, 2014).
- Malnutrition and physical or psychological stress can weaken a patient's immune defences (Reiter, 2013), while some conditions, such as diabetes, can decrease peripheral circulation, reducing the immune response in the gingiva (Niemiec, 2012c). Untreated periodontal disease has also been correlated with poor blood-glucose control in diabetics, so managing periodontal disease often helps in the successful treatment of diabetes (Van Nice, 2006).

- Excessive levels of corticosteroids, either from medications or health conditions, can decrease the immune response by suppressing the numbers and activity of white blood cells. They may also cause osteoporosis of the alveolar bone, degradation of gingival collagen, and destruction of periodontal tissues (Niemiec, 2012c).
- Other factors, such as poor chewing habits, abnormal oral anatomy, poor saliva quality or conditions which can reduce saliva output, such as kerato-conjunctivitis sicca (KCS) and chronic renal failure, can all affect the efficacy of the mouth's self-cleaning during chewing (Gingerich, 2012).

1.1.4   Clinical signs of periodontal disease

Pet owners are often unaware of the existence or extent of their pet's periodontal disease (Niemiec, 2012a). Most periodontal disease is discovered during routine annual examinations or during a visit for unrelated health issues (Berg, 2020). Some clinical signs that owners may or may not notice include bad breath (halitosis), which is the most common reason pet owners present their animals for oral examination (Holmstrom *et al.*, 2000). Red, inflamed gingiva (gingivitis) is also a typical sign of periodontal disease, but is less often noticed by owners (Berg, 2020). Increased drooling or blood in the saliva is less commonly seen (Holmstrom *et al.*, 2000), but some owners may see blood left on toys or rawhide chews. Head shyness is uncommon, though can be noticed by owners who try to brush the teeth or handle the mouths of pets afflicted with periodontal disease (Carey, 2021). Pawing at the mouth is rare, but can be seen in patients with loose teeth or severe oral pain (Holmstrom *et al.*, 2000). Difficulty eating is also rare, though some animals will prefer soft food. Pet owners often claim that their pet's mouth must be healthy or else they would stop eating, but this is not the case (Lewis, 2017). The drive to eat to survive surpasses most oral pain, except for severe pain caused by conditions such as stomatitis and some oral cancers (Rancilio *et al.*, 2016).

Exam room findings may also include gingival recession, purulent discharge, facial swellings (particularly beneath the eye, caused by abscessing of the upper fourth premolar), draining tracts, and nasal discharge (Gingerich, 2012).

1.1.5   Periodontal disease affects the human–animal bond

Bad breath, or halitosis, is a significant cause of tension in the human–animal bond (Rawlings and Culham, 1998a). In pets, halitosis is most commonly caused by the microbial metabolism of rotting periodontal tissues, which produces volatile sulphur compounds (VSCs) such as hydrogen sulphide and methyl mercaptan (Culham and Rawlings, 1998). These volatile sulphur compounds are what give bad breath its offensive odour.

A pet's bad breath can cause owners to avoid close contact (Rawlings and Culham, 1998b). Since halitosis is usually the first clinical sign of periodontal disease in pets, we can see how periodontal disease can have an adverse effect on the human–animal bond, and how preventing, or treating, periodontal disease can improve the quality of life for both pets and pet owners.

1.2 Diagnosis of Periodontal Disease

The severity of periodontal disease is scored by the amount of tissue and bone loss, which together are known as attachment loss (Juriga, 2008). Attachment loss is determined by measuring periodontal pocket depth in millimetres from the CEJ to the bottom of the pocket with an instrument called a periodontal probe (Hale, 2004), and assessing the percentage of bone loss with dental X-rays (Gorham, 2006). Patients who have no supragingival (above the gumline) signs of periodontal disease can have disease subgingivally (below the gumline) (Bellows *et al.*, 2019). Because it is impossible to see beneath the gumline, the only way periodontal disease can be accurately scored and treated is with the use of dental radiographs (Beckman, 2004), so full mouth dental X-rays should be performed on every dental patient (Bellows *et al.*, 2019). There may be, and usually are, teeth with different periodontal indices within the same mouth (Gorham, 2006).

1.2.1 Stages of periodontal disease

The following characteristics are as described by the American Veterinary Dental College (AVDC, 2021).

PD0: Normal (see Fig. 1.2)

- Attachment loss is 0%.
- No inflammation of the gingiva: it is pink, smooth, and lies flat against the teeth.
- No treatment required, but dental homecare should be initiated to maintain oral health.
- Usually only seen in very young patients.

PD1: Gingivitis (see Fig. 1.3)

- Attachment loss is 0%.
- Gingivitis is now present.

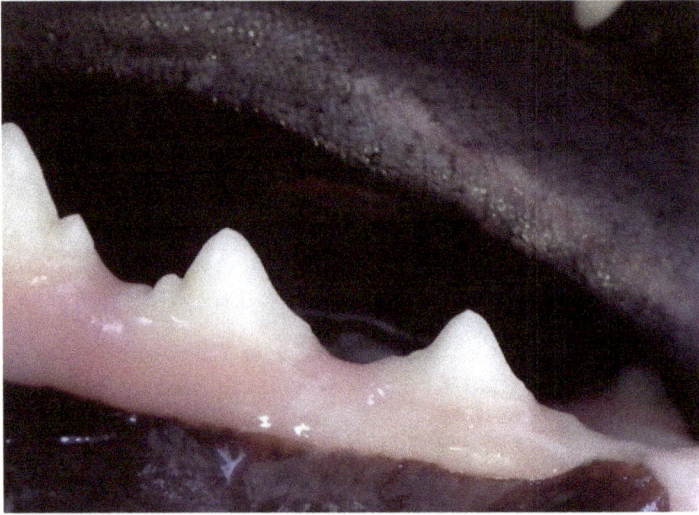

Fig. 1.2. PD0: Normal.

- There may be a slight increase in sulcus depth because of gingival swelling (this is called a pseudopocket), though no attachment loss has yet occurred.
- Plaque bacteria are aerobic, non-motile cocci.
- Treatment: COHAT (Comprehensive Oral Health Assessment and Treatment) including teeth cleaning under general anaesthesia to remove all biofilm and reverse inflammation; dental homecare (Bellows *et al.*, 2019).

Note: this is the only stage of periodontal disease that is reversible!

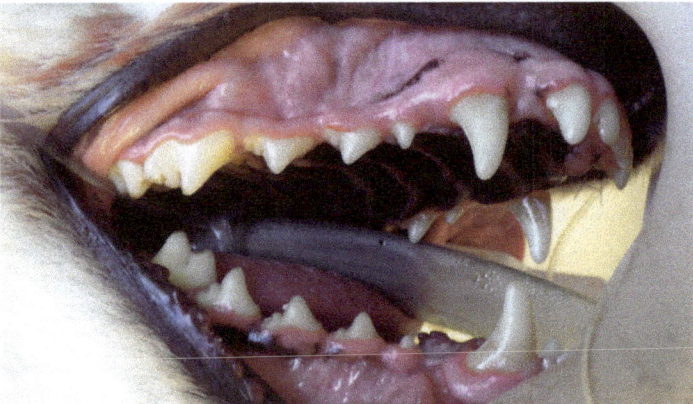

Fig. 1.3. PD1: Gingivitis.

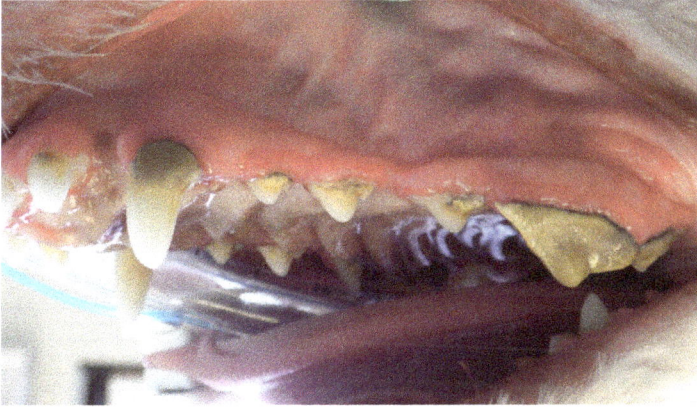

Fig. 1.4. PD2: Early periodontitis.

PD2: Early periodontitis (see Fig. 1.4)

- Attachment loss is < 25%.
- Bacteria in subgingival regions are anaerobic, motile rods and filamentous organisms.
- Pocket depth increases due to attachment loss.
- Bone around the neck of the tooth starts to deteriorate.
- Treatment: COHAT and closed root planing +/- perioceutic (antibiotic gel) placement (Bellows *et al.*, 2019) to re-establish soft tissue attachments and reduce pocket depths. Dental homecare.

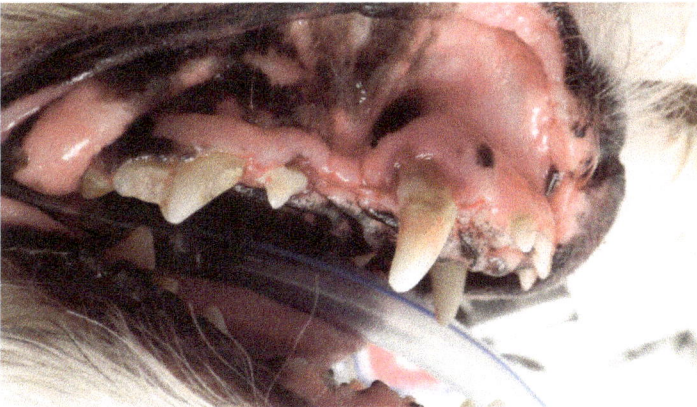

Fig. 1.5. PD3: Moderate periodontitis.

PD3: Moderate periodontitis (see Fig. 1.5)

- Attachment loss is 25–50%.
- Plaque bacterial population is almost entirely anaerobic.
- Bone surrounding the roots of the teeth starts to deteriorate; tooth roots may be exposed; possible furcation exposure (loss of bone where the roots of multi-rooted teeth meet). Alveolitis (inflammation of the alveolus) or osteomyelitis may occur.
- Treatment: frequent COHATs and periodontal therapy including closed or open root planing +/- perioceutic application; guided tissue regeneration; extraction of affected teeth if owner is unable or uninterested in performing dental homecare or frequent COHATs (Bellows *et al.*, 2019). Dental homecare.

PD4: Severe periodontitis (see Fig. 1.6)

- Attachment loss is > 50%.
- Plaque bacterial population similar to PD3.
- Tooth roots and root furcations are exposed.
- Teeth may be loose; some held in place only by calculus or granulation tissue.
- Teeth with more than 50% attachment loss may not be possible to salvage.
- Treatment: extraction or guided tissue regeneration, possible periodontal splinting of mobile teeth. Frequent COHATs (Bellows *et al.*, 2019). Dental homecare.

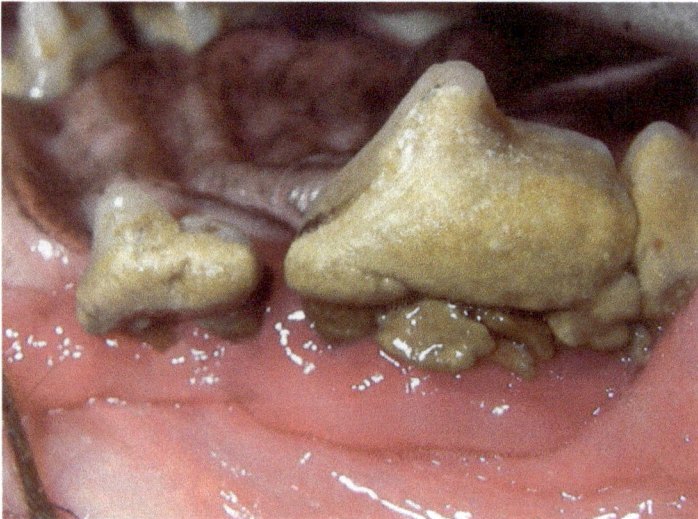

Fig. 1.6. PD4: Severe periodontitis.

Without intervention, periodontal disease will progress until the teeth fall out (exfoliate) (Niemiec, 2013). During this time, the patient suffers with chronic infection, oral pain and possible damage to other vital organs (Niemiec *et al.*, 2020). In small-breed dogs, the bone of the jaw can become so infected that normal chewing may cause it to fracture (Niemiec, 2012a).

References

AVDC (2021) AVDC nomenclature. American Veterinary Dental College. Available at: https://avdc.org/avdc-nomenclature/ (accessed 3 February 2021).

Barnette, C. (2020) Gingival hyperplasia in dogs: causes, symptoms, and treatment, 28 July. Dispomed. Available at: https://www.dispomed.com/gingival-hyper-plasia-in-dogs-causes-symptoms-and-treatment/ (accessed 1 February 2021).

Barthel, R. (2006) Veterinary dentist at work – treatment of vertical bone loss in a dog. *Journal of Veterinary Dentistry* 23(4), 237–242.

Beckman, B. (2004) Treatment of an infrabony pocket in an American Eskimo dog. *Journal of Veterinary Dentistry* 21(3), 159–163. DOI: 10.1177/089875640402100303.

Bellows, J., Berg, M., Dennis, S., Harvey, R. and Lobprise, H.B. (2019) 2019 AAHA dental care guidelines for dogs and cats. American Animal Hospital Association. Available at: https://www.aaha.org/globalassets/02-guidelines/dental/aaha_dental_guidelines.pdf (accessed 10 September 2020).

Berg, M. (2020) The examination room and the dental patient. In: Perrone, J. (ed.) *Small Animal Dental Procedures for Veterinary Technicians and Nurses.* Wiley Blackwell, Hoboken, New Jersey, pp. 21–28.

Carey, S. (2021) Oral health affects all aspects of pet wellbeing, UF Veterinarians Say. College of Veterinary Medicine, University of Florida. Available at: https://www.vetmed.ufl.edu/2021/02/02/oral-health-affects-all-aspects-of-pet-wellness-uf-veterinarians-say/ (accessed 5 February 2021).

Clarke, D.E. (1999) The crystalline components of dental calculus in the domestic cat. *Journal of Veterinary Dentistry* 16(4), 165–168. DOI: 10.1177/089875649901600402.

Culham, N. and Rawlings, J.M. (1998) Oral Malodor and its relevance to periodontal disease in the dog. *Journal of Veterinary Dentistry* 15(4), 165–168. DOI: 10.1177/089875649801500401.

DuPont, G.A. (1997) Understanding dental plaque; biofilm dynamics. *Journal of Veterinary Dentistry* 14(3), 91–94. DOI: 10.1177/089875649701400301.

Eisner, E. (2006) Identification and treatment of early stage periodontal disease. In: *Proceedings of the 20th Annual Veterinary Dental Forum.* Omnipress, Madison, Wisconsin, pp. 371–375.

Fitzgerald, W. (2008) Periodontal disease management and homecare. In: *Proceedings of the 22nd Annual Veterinary Dental Forum.* Omnipress, Madison, Wisconsin, pp. 57–59.

Gingerich, W. (2012) Periodontal disease: pathophysiology, recognition, and diagnosis. In: *Proceedings of the 26th Annual Veterinary Dental Forum.* Omnipress, Madison, Wisconsin (CD Rom).

Gorham, M. (2006) Recognizing periodontal disease. In: *Proceedings of the 20th Annual Veterinary Dental Forum.* Omnipress, Madison, Wisconsin, pp. 389–393.

Gorrel, C. (1998) Periodontal disease and diet in domestic pets. *The Journal of Nutrition* 128(12), 2712S–2714S. Available at: https://doi.org/10.1093/jn/128.12.2712S (accessed 23 January 2021).

Gorrel, C. (2004) A Practical approach to managing periodontal disease. In: *Proceedings of the 18th Annual Veterinary Dental Forum.* Omnipress, Madison, Wisconsin, pp. 101–102.

Hale, F. (1997) The tooth. Hale Veterinary Clinic. Available at: http://www.toothvet.ca/PDFfiles/tooth.pdf (accessed 28 January 2021).

Hale, F. (2004) Periodontal disease. Hale Veterinary Clinic. Available at: http://www.toothvet.ca/VSTEP/m%20-%20%20Perio%20and%20Homecare.pdf (accessed 28 January 2021).

Harvey, C.E. (2005) Management of periodontal disease: understanding the options. *Veterinary Clinics of North America: Small Animal Practice* 35(4), 819–836. DOI: 10.1016/j.cvsm.2005.03.002.

Holmstrom, S., Holmstrom, L.A., McGrath, C.J., Richey, M.T. and Wiggs, R.B. (2000) Pathogenesis of periodontal disease. In: Holmstrom, S. (ed.) *Veterinary Dentistry for the Technician & Office Staff.* Saunders, Philadelphia, Pennsylvania, pp. 149–157.

Holzman, G. (2020) The basics. In: Perrone, J. (ed.) *Small Animal Dental Procedures for Veterinary Technicians and Nurses.* Wiley Blackwell, Hoboken, New Jersey, pp. 1–20.

Juriga, S. (2008) Periodontal disease: recognition, etiology and compliance strategies. In: *Proceedings of the 22nd Annual Veterinary Dental Forum.* Omnipress, Madison, Winsconsin, pp. 251–255.

Kangas, K.B. (2019) Are small dogs more prone to dental problems? Animal Wellness. Available at: https://animalwellnessmagazine.com/small-dogs-dental-problems/ (accessed 27 January 2021).

Lewis, J. (2017) How to spot signs of oral pain in your pet patients. Veterinary Practice News. Available at: https://www.veterinarypracticenews.com/how-to-spot-signs-of-oral-pain-in-your-pet-patients/ (accessed 27 January 2021).

Lobprise, H.B. and Wiggs, R.B. (2000a) Periodontal disease. In: Lobprise, H.B. and Wiggs, R.B. (eds) *The Veterinarian's Companion for Common Dental Procedures.* AAHA Press, Lakewood, Colorado, pp. 39–70.

Lobprise, H.B. and Wiggs, R.B. (2000b) Feline oral and dental disease. In: Lobprise, H.B. and Wiggs, R.B. (eds) *The Veterinarian's Companion for Common Dental Procedures.* AAHA Press, Lakewood, Colorado, pp. 137–148.

Niemiec, B.A. (2004) Severe local effects of periodontal disease. In: *Proceedings of the 18th Annual Veterinary Dental Forum.* Omnipress, Madison, Wisconsin, pp. 57–60.

Niemiec, B.A. (2012a) Periodontal disease: utilizing current information to improve client compliance. Today's Veterinary Practice. Available at: https://todaysveterinarypractice.com/practical-dentistry-periodontal-disease-utilizing-current-information-to-improve-client-compliance/ (accessed 26 January 2021).

Niemiec, B.A. (2012b) Treating and preventing dental disease in geriatric pets. Veterinary Practice News. Available at: https://www.veterinarypracticenews.

com/treating-and-preventing-dental-disease-in-geriatric-pets/ (accessed 26 January 2021).

Niemiec, B.A. (2012c) Updates on periodontology. In: *Proceedings of the 24th Annual Veterinary Dental Forum.* Omnipress, Madison, Wisconsin (CD Rom).

Niemiec, B.A. (2013) Periodontal disease of the mandible. Today's Veterinary Practice. Available at: https://todaysveterinarypractice.com/dental-diagnosis-periodontal-disease-of-the-mandible/ (accessed 3 February 2021).

Niemiec, B.A. (2014) Disorders of dental hard tissues in dogs. Today's Veterinary Practice. Available at: https://todaysveterinarypractice.com/disorders-of-dental-hard-tissues-in-dogs/ (accessed 27 January 2021).

Niemiec, B., Gawor, J., Nemec, A., Clarke, D., McLeod, K. *et al.* (2020) World Small Animal Veterinary Association global dental guidelines. *Journal of Small Animal Practice* 61(7), E36–E161. Available at: https://onlinelibrary.wiley.com/doi/10.1111/jsap.13132 (accessed 21 September 2020).

Pavlica, Z., Petelin, M., Juntes, P., Erzen, D., Crossley, D.A. *et al.* (2008) Periodontal disease burden and pathological changes in organs of dogs. *Journal of Veterinary Dentistry* 25(2), 97–105. DOI: 10.1177/089875640802500210.

Perrone, J., Sharp, S. and March, P. (2020) Common dental conditions and treatments. In: Perrone, J. (ed.) *Small Animal Dental Procedures for Veterinary Technicians and Nurses.* Wiley Blackwell, Hoboken, NJ, pp. 131–168.

Rancilio, N., Ko, J. and Fulkerson, C.M. (2016) Strategies for managing cancer pain in dogs and cats, part 2: definitive and palliative management of cancer pain. Today's Veterinary Practice. Available at: https://todaysveterinarypractice.com/elements-oncologystrategies-managing-cancer-pain-dogs-catspart-2-definitive-palliative-management-cancer-pain/ (accessed 5 February 2021).

Rawlings, J.M. and Culham, N. (1998a) Studies of oral malodor in the dog. *Journal of Veterinary Dentistry* 15(4), 169–173. DOI: 10.1177/089875649801500402.

Rawlings, J.M. and Culham, N. (1998b) Halitosis in dogs and the effect of periodontal therapy. *The Journal of Nutrition* 128(12), 2715S–2716S. Available at: https://doi.org/10.1093/jn/128.12.2715S (accessed 27 January 2021).

Reiter, A.M. (2013) Periodontal disease in small animals. MSD Veterinary Manual. Available at: https://www.merckvetmanual.com/digestive-system/dentistry/periodontal-disease-in-small-animals (accessed 26 January 2021).

Stepaniuk, K. (2006) Understanding periodontal disease: pathophysiology, clinical significance, and treatment options in your general practice. In: *Proceedings of the 20th Annual Veterinary Dental Forum.* Omnipress, Madison, Wisconsin, pp. 243–245.

Van Nice, E. (2006) Management of multiple dental infections in a dog with diabetes mellitus. *Journal of Veterinary Dentistry* 23(1), 18–25. DOI: 10.1177/089875640602300103.

Comprehensive Oral Health Assessment and Treatment (COHAT); Dental Instrument Use and Maintenance

2

2.1 Treatment of Periodontal Disease

Once a patient has red or bleeding gums, tartar build-up or loose teeth, a Comprehensive Oral Health Assessment and Treatment (COHAT) under general anaesthesia (Niemiec, 2003) must be performed to remove plaque and tartar from both the tooth crown and the gingival sulcus, and to diagnose and treat problem areas such as periodontal pockets (Perrone *et al.*, 2020). This procedure was once referred to as a dental prophylaxis, or 'prophy', but since the word prophylaxis means 'to prevent', and the majority of our patients already have existing periodontal disease, this terminology was updated to better describe the procedure (American Animal Hospital Association (AAHA), 2021). We are treating existing periodontal disease (Crocker, 2010), not preventing periodontal disease. Ideally, veterinarians and nurses will become better at promoting routine preventative dental cleanings and homecare for young patients not already affected by periodontal disease, and one day we may be able to return to using the term 'dental prophy'!

2.1.1 Preanaesthetic considerations

Before the COHAT, a full physical examination must be performed by the veterinarian to determine the animal's overall health status prior to general anaesthesia (Mills, 2020). Obtaining a thorough patient history from the pet owner is essential, including any signs of oral problems noted at home, current and past health or behavioural issues, and any complications during or upon recovery from previous anaesthetic procedures. Information about chewing and eating habits (e.g. the dog chews tennis balls or kennel bars; the cat has refused to eat hard food during the past few months) is important: pet owners may not volunteer this without prompting, but will report if questioned (Berg, 2020).

© CAB International 2022. *An Introduction to Pet Dental Care: For Veterinary Technicians and Nurses* (K. Istace)
DOI: 10.1079/9781789248869.0002

Oral examinations are usually limited in the conscious patient (Nemec *et al.*, 2019) because our patients are often uncooperative and unused to having their mouths opened and their lips pulled back. When experiencing oral pain, this reluctance to have their mouths examined only increases (American Veterinary Medical Association (AVMA), 2021). The client should be made aware that, during anaesthesia, a more thorough examination including periodontal probing and dental radiographs will provide a better idea of the treatment required (Bellows *et al.*, 2019). Conscious oral examinations can be useful to evaluate asymmetries of the face and head, extra-oral swellings, enlarged lymph nodes, areas of calculus accumulation, gingivitis, gingival recession, oral masses, fractured teeth, tooth resorption observable above the gumline, and malocclusions of individual teeth or jaws (Miller, 2006).

Preanaesthetic labwork, including a complete blood count, chemistry panel and urinalysis are recommended prior to anaesthesia to rule out any major organ dysfunction (Mills, 2020). Depending upon the age and health status of the pet, chest X-rays and a preoperative ECG or cardiac ultrasound may be performed.

An anaesthetic risk score is assigned to the patient based upon physical examination findings, laboratory results and medical history (Zeltzman, 2016). Veterinary patients are assessed on a 1–5 score adapted from that used in human medicine, developed by the American Society of Anesthesiologists (ASA, 2020). An ASA score helps the veterinarian determine a patient's prognosis, decide which pre-medication and anaesthetic drugs can be safely administered, and influences how the nurse handles the patient's induction, anaesthetic monitoring and recovery. Patients with higher ASA scores will need a more thorough preanaesthetic work-up, and very high-risk patients should be referred to a veterinary anaesthesiologist (Zeltzman, 2016).

2.1.2 ASA classifications

The following classifications are as described by Zeltzman (2016).

ASA Class 1: Minimal risk

Healthy patient with no underlying disease conditions.

ASA Class 2: Slight risk

Patient with slight or mild systemic disease, e.g. neonatal, geriatric or obese animals.

ASA Class 3: Moderate risk

Patient with moderate systemic disease. Examples include animals with anaemia, fever, low-grade heart murmur or cardiac disease, or brachycephalic syndrome.

ASA Class 4: High risk

Patient with severe, systemic, and life-threatening disease. Examples include animals with severe dehydration, uraemia, toxaemia, shock, high fever, pulmonary disease, uncompensated heart disease, uncontrolled diabetes or emaciation.

ASA Class 5: Extreme risk

Moribund patient who may die with or without surgery. Includes animals with advanced liver, kidney, or endocrine disease, severe shock or trauma, pulmonary embolus or terminal malignant cancer.

2.2   Anaesthetic Monitoring, Patient and Nurse Positioning, and Protection During COHATs

Once the patient has been fully evaluated, safe anaesthesia (see Chapter 12, this volume) for dental COHATs includes (Mills, 2020):

- placement of a cuffed endotracheal tube to prevent the patient from inhaling fluids, debris, and aerosolized bacteria
- intravenous fluids
- a warming device such as a forced-air blanket, resistive heating system, or circulating water blanket to maintain body temperature while under general anaesthetic
- a multiparameter monitor including heart rate, ECG, arterial oxyhaemoglobin saturation (pulse oximetry), respiratory rate, end tidal CO_2, blood pressure and body temperature.

Place the patient in either dorsal or lateral recumbency with the head positioned lower than the body so fluids don't accumulate in the throat (Altier, 2020). This can be achieved by laying the pet on thick towels or blankets, or on a tilting table. Using dental suction (Bellows, 2019) and/or packing the back of the mouth with gauze (Gingerich, 2012a) also reduces the risk that any fluid or debris can be aspirated by the pet (Niemiec *et al.*, 2020). If a gauze pack is used, it should be noted on the patient's chart and ideally tied to the endotracheal tube (McMahon, 2020) to prevent it accidentally being left behind after the patient is extubated, causing asphyxiation.

Sit on an adjustable, wheeled chair, stool or saddle seat (DeForge, 2002). Adjust the seat's height so your feet rest flat on the floor, with knees slightly below your hips, and shoulders relaxed (Holmstrom *et al.*, 2000a).

A wheeled seat allows you to change position around the patient's head during the procedure to access hard-to-reach areas within the mouth. An adjustable dental table which raises or lowers the patient also allows for more flexibility and minimizes lifting of heavy patients. The working height (in this case, the patient's mouth) should be at a height between your elbow and shoulder (Cherry, 2010). Your back should be straight, not slumped, with your neck tilted not more than 15 degrees forward.

The scaling movements should be performed as much as possible with the wrist and shoulder, not the fingers, to prevent repetitive motion injuries such as carpal tunnel syndrome (Aller, 2005). Other symptoms of poor technique or positioning may include stiffness (especially in the neck and shoulders), hand and finger fatigue, headaches or tendonitis (Hernandez, 2006). This can often be prevented by using thicker instrument handle sizes, hollow handles (which are light and provide better tactile sensation) or textured-grip handles (which are easier to hold) (Ericsson, 2020). Wearing gloves fitted specifically for right and left hands may relieve hand pain better than ambidextrous gloves, which can cause hand fatigue by pulling the thumb out of a neutral position (Cherry, 2010).

Stretch during and between dental procedures. Consider avoiding scheduling consecutive large-breed dental patients or multiple procedures requiring extensive extractions on the same day, to reduce unnecessary physical strain on both the nurse and veterinarian (Cherry, 2010).

A good light source such as an adjustable overhead lamp or headlamp is essential (DeForge, 2002). Using dental mirrors, retractors and gentle mouth gags (non-metal, non-spring-type) (Bellows *et al.*, 2019) will aid access to and proper visualization of the oral cavity. Gentle, flexible mouth gags can be easily fashioned by cutting old endotracheal tubes in a variety of lengths, or using red rubber Kong toys in larger dogs. Magnifying loupes are also helpful to maintain proper neck posture while still being able to assess small defects and pathologies, and to identify areas of missed plaque and calculus (DeForge, 2002).

Any staff within 1 m of the dental patient, such as the dental and anaesthesia nurses, should wear surgical masks to prevent bacterial inhalation and infections of the face, and protective eyewear to shield the eyes from bacteria as well as from water spray, flying debris such as calculus or sectioned teeth, broken or loose burs, etc. (Holmstrom *et al.*, 2000a). Wear examination gloves to protect the skin from infectious or chemical agents and prevent cross-contamination between patients (Altier, 2020). A surgical cap and gown are also recommended to stop the patient's oral bacteria from contaminating staff and being carried to other areas of the veterinary hospital.

2.3 The Dental Equipment Arsenal

Several different types of instruments are necessary to properly perform a COHAT.

2.3.1 Periodontal instruments

Dental mirror

This allows visualization of hard-to-see areas, such as tooth surfaces facing towards the back of the mouth; illuminates dark areas by reflecting light from the dental operatory's overhead lamp; provides retraction to prevent damage to the mucosa, tongue and lips (McMahon, 2020) while cleaning teeth; and helps prevent operator neck and back strain by maintaining proper ergonomics. Mirrors range in sizes from the small #3 to the large #6 (Miller, 2012). The heads often come separately from the handle so that multiple sizes of mirror can be screwed onto a single handle.

Explorer

This is a sharp, fine-tipped instrument designed to examine the tooth's surface by allowing the nurse to feel vibrations carried through the tip. The vibrations are caused by encountering irregularities such as calculus, tooth resorption, and caries (Crocker, 2010). Types of explorers include Shepherd's Hook (curved), Pig's Tail (extremely curved) and Orban (very short) (Holmstrom *et al.*, 2000b; Miller, 2006).

Periodontal probe

This is used to measure periodontal pocket depth, gingival recession, gingival hyperplasia, tooth mobility (by rocking the tooth) and furcation exposure (by sliding the probe into the root furcation) (McMahon, 2020). Probes can be round or flat, and have measurement markings which vary depending on the type of probe. Common probes include the Michigan 'O' probe with Williams markings, which is notched at 1, 2, 3, 5, 7, 8, 9 and 10 mm (Miller, 2006, 2012) and is especially useful for feline patients, because any pocket depths over 1 mm are an indicator of periodontal disease in cats (McMahon, 2020); and the Marquis probe, which is marked at 3, 6, 9 and 12 mm (Gingerich, 2012b). The Marquis probe is useful for canine patients, whose periodontal disease begins with pocket depths over 3 mm, but is not as suitable for use in cats (Miller, 2012).

Calculus (tartar) removal forceps

Similar to extraction forceps, these have a curved 'beak' which allows for rapid removal of large areas of calculus (Holmstrom *et al.*, 2000b).

Ultrasonic scaler

This performs the majority of plaque and tartar removal. Piezoelectric scalers are the most common type of ultrasonic scaler in veterinary clinics.

These operate with a linear tip oscillation in 25,000–45,000 cycles per second (Altier, 2020), and generate a moderate amount of heat (Verez-Fraguela *et al.*, 2000). The tip must be kept in constant motion, and water irrigation must be provided to prevent thermal damage to the tooth (Brine *et al.*, 2000). Place the side of the tip against the tooth, parallel to the tooth surface, using a light touch. Using heavy force will result in less cleaning action and potential tooth death from heat build-up, since the oscillations will be suppressed (Brine *et al.*, 2000). Directing the tip at the tooth can result in tooth damage, as the oscillating tip can penetrate the enamel or any exposed dentin (Gingerich, 2012a). Many ultrasonic tips can be used both supragingivally (above the gumline) and subgingivally (below the gumline) (Niemiec, 2004).

Hand scaler

This is used only for supragingival scaling (Crocker, 2010). Hand scalers are particularly useful for removing calculus in small grooves such as those found buccally (towards the cheek) on the upper fourth premolars of both dogs and cats, and on the canine teeth of cats (McMahon, 2020). Hand scalers are triangular in cross section and have two cutting edges and a sharp point (see Fig. 2.2), which will cause tissue damage if used subgingivally (Gingerich, 2012a). They are used in vertical pull strokes away from the gingiva. Common types include Jacquette scalers, with straight working ends, and Sickle scalers, with curved working ends. A particularly useful scaler is the Morse 0/00 miniature scaler (Holmstrom *et al.*, 2000b), which is small enough to be used in all sizes of patient. Scalers should be held in the modified pen grasp, i.e. with the instrument between the index finger and thumb on the handle close to the working end, while the middle finger is placed near the shank to stabilize the instrument and provide control (Gingerich, 2012a).

Curette

This can be used both supragingivally and subgingivally (Holmstrom *et al.*, 2000b), following ultrasonic scaling to ensure all calculus is removed from the tooth's crown and subgingival areas (Niemiec, 2004). Curettes have either one or two cutting edges and a rounded toe on the working end (Holmstrom *et al.*, 2000b), and are used in overlapping vertical and horizontal pull strokes away from the gingiva. Longer-bladed curettes are used for larger patients, and short 'mini' blades are available for cats and small dogs (Miller, 2012). Currettes are numbered for the teeth they were designed to be used on in humans (Gingerich, 2012a). In veterinary medicine, these numbers do not correspond exactly to our patients' teeth, but in general, small-numbered curettes have less shank angulation and are useful on anterior teeth such as incisors and canines, and large-numbered

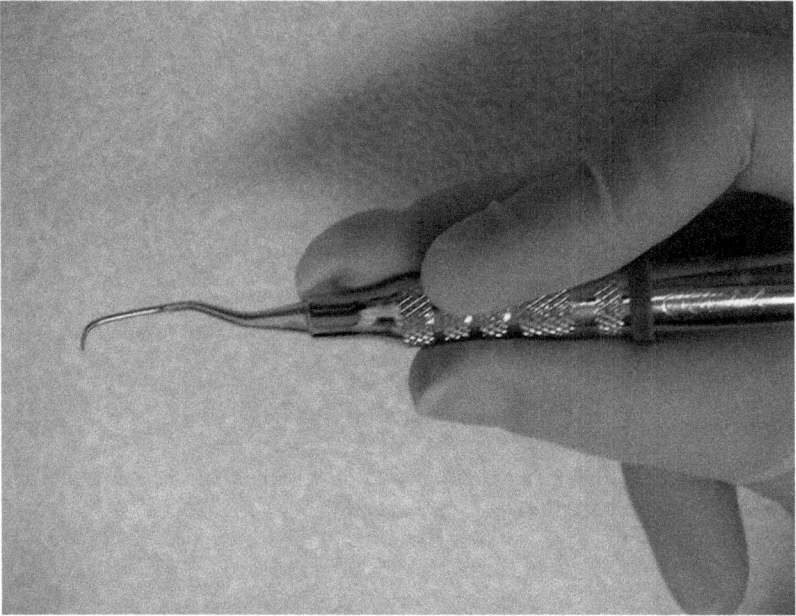

Fig. 2.1. Modified pen grasp.

curettes have increased shank angulation and are more useful for reaching around posterior teeth such as premolars and molars (Gingerich, 2012a). All curettes are held in the modified pen grasp (as described for the hand scaler; see also Fig. 2.1).

Curettes come in two types:

- Universal curettes. The face of the working end of universal curettes is positioned at 90 degrees to the terminal shank (Gingerich, 2012a), providing two cutting blades on each working end of the instrument, and can be used on all tooth surfaces. The terminal shank is held at an angle that will engage the blade with plaque and calculus (McMahon, 2020). This angle must be created by the fingers and wrist, and poor angulation can lead to burnishing the calculus onto the tooth instead of removing it (Wanless, 2017).
- Gracey curettes. The Gracey curette is an area-specific instrument, which means each blade is not appropriate for all areas of a tooth's surface (Gingerich, 2012a). The face of the working end is offset at 70 degrees to the terminal shank on one end of the instrument, causing one cutting blade at that end to be lower than the other. This lower blade is placed in contact with the tooth to remove plaque and calculus. The blade on the opposite end of the instrument is its mirror image (LeVan, 2013),

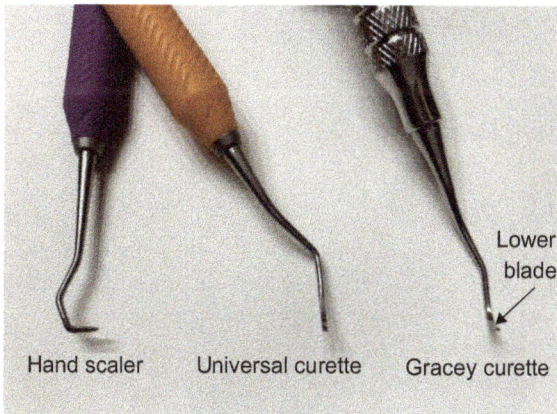

Fig. 2.2. Hand scaler, universal curette, Gracey curette.

so that by using either one end or the other, the instrument can clean a surface of any angle. The terminal shank (see Fig. 2.3) is held parallel to the root or tooth surface (Gingerich, 2012a), automatically creating the proper angle to engage plaque and tartar.

Prophy angle

This attaches to a low-speed handpiece and has a rotating cup that holds polish (prophy paste) for polishing teeth (Holmstrom *et al.*, 2000b). Prophy angles can be disposable (plastic) or reusable (metal, requiring the use of disposable rubber cups). Some are available in reciprocating (back

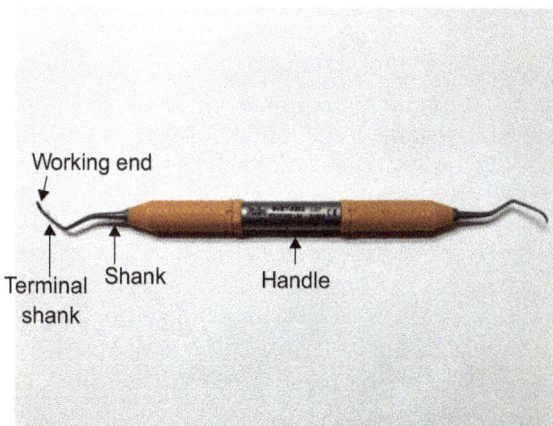

Fig. 2.3. The parts of a hand instrument; in this case a universal curette.

and forth) motion (McMahon, 2020), which prevents a patient's fur being caught around the prophy angle during polishing.

2.3.2 Surgical instruments

High-speed handpiece

This operates at over 100,000 rpm, ideally at 300,000 rpm (Holmstrom *et al.*, 2000b), and accommodates burs (see below) for sectioning teeth, bone removal, endodontic access, finishing restoratives, cavity preparations (Holmstrom *et al.*, 2000c) and gingivectomies (Lewis, 2016). It requires water spray for cooling and irrigation.

Low-speed handpiece

This operates at 1000–25,000 rpm and is used primarily for polishing, but also accommodates low-speed burs for crown reduction in lagomorphs and rodents (Kolb, 2017), Gates Glidden drills for endodontic access (Caiafa, 2013) and reduction angles for spiral fillers to carry sealants into a tooth during endodontic procedures (Altier, 2020).

Burs

These are rotary dental instruments with cutting blades or abrasive surfaces; they are mainly used for sectioning teeth, bone smoothing and removal, and endodontic access. Burs are classified by shape (round, pear, tapered fissure, flame, inverted cone), blade type (non-crosscut vs crosscut), material (carbide, diamond), length (standard: S vs surgical length: SL), and attachment type (friction grip: FG; right angle: RA; Doriot/large type: HP) (Holmstrom *et al.*, 2000b). General practices should have on hand the following types of carbide burs: tapered-fissure crosscut (e.g. #701, for cutting through large teeth to separate roots), pear (e.g. #330, an all-purpose bur for cutting through small-to-medium-sized teeth, bone smoothing and bone removal), and round (e.g. #½, 2 and 4, for sectioning teeth and removing bone) (Lewis, 2015). Diamond burs are encrusted with diamond dust and act like sandpaper to finish restorations, remove enamel to prepare a tooth to accept prosthodontics, smooth bone, or perform odontoplasty (Eubanks and Gilbo, 2006). Burs come in different shank types depending on their intended use and the type of handpiece or contra angle to which they attach (Holmstrom *et al.*, 2000b).

Luxators (elevators)

These instruments are used to extract teeth, and are available in various sizes and curvatures to match the different sizes and shapes of teeth

(Holmstrom *et al.*, 2000e). The luxator blade is inserted between the tooth and the alveolar crest, with steady pressure applied apically to stretch and tear the periodontal ligament, loosening the tooth from the alveolus (Carmichael, 2006).

Periosteal elevators

These are sharp-tipped, flat or curved elevators designed to lift tissue flaps off from bone (O'Morrow, 2007), providing increased visualization and access to oral structures during periodontal surgeries, including surgical extractions. Examples include the commonly used EX9 and EX7 periosteal elevators.

Scalpel blades

Small scalpel blades such as the #15 are often preferred when working in tight spaces such as the oral cavity (O'Morrow, 2007). These can be used on a standard scalpel handle, but round scalpel handles are easier to manoeuvre around curved teeth and oral structures (LeVan, 2013).

2.3.3   Miscellaneous instruments

Mouth gags

These improve visualization and access to the oral cavity, but come with the risks of myalgia, neuralgia and temporomandibular joint (TMJ) trauma (Bellows *at al.*, 2019). Do not use metal, spring-type mouth gags, as they force the jaw open too wide, increasing these risks. Short gags, such as needle caps or endotracheal tubes cut at 20–30 mm lengths are preferred (Berg, 2015). These are placed between the upper and lower teeth, and should be short enough that the jaw is opened as minimally as possible to complete the procedure. Remove mouth gags as soon as possible.

Air-water syringe

This is a three-way syringe that provides irrigation, rinsing and air-drying by pressing the water button, air button or both (Holmstrom *et al.*, 2000b). Irrigation of the gingival sulcus is necessary after cleaning and polishing to ensure no debris or polish is left behind to cause a foreign-body reaction or trauma to the gingiva. Air-drying is useful for detecting areas of missed plaque after scaling (Gingerich, 2012a) or to dry teeth prior to fluoride application (Niemiec, 2004), and is necessary for the use of most dental adhesives (Holmstrom *et al.*, 2000c).

2.4   The Comprehensive Oral Health Assessment and Treatment (COHAT) in 10 steps

The veterinary nurse is usually responsible for performing dental hygiene (Bellows *et al.*, 2019). Completing the following steps ensures that the patient receives a consistent and thorough COHAT. Consider taking high-resolution photos of the patient's oral cavity prior to and following the COHAT, to show the client. This gives them a unique opportunity to understand any problem areas in their pet's mouth, and also helps them to appreciate the quality of service you provide.

The order of the following steps can, to some extent, be altered depending upon personal preference or situation – for example, radiographs can be performed prior to cleaning – as long as all steps are completed in a logical order (e.g. polishing is followed by irrigation to remove polishing paste from the gingival sulci).

2.4.1   Step One: chlorhexidine rinse

Ultrasonic scalers aerosolize billions of bacteria as teeth are cleaned (Bellows *et al.*, 2019). These bacteria settle onto counters, tables, walls, etc., within 1 m of the patient, as well as on the face, hair and clothing of veterinary staff (Niemiec *et al.*, 2020). This can cause skin and eye infections, and, if inhaled, can cause nasal, throat and lung infections (Dias and Delgado, 2020). The risks of this bacterial aerosolization can be minimized by rinsing the patient's mouth with chlorhexidine gluconate 0.1% prior to cleaning (Niemiec, 2003). Chlorhexidine kills much of the surface bacteria, reducing the bacterial load introduced into the patient's bloodstream during the procedure and the number of bacteria that can drift through the dental operatory (Bowersock *et al.*, 2000).

2.4.2   Step Two: supragingival scaling

Supragingival scaling involves the removal of plaque and calculus from tooth crowns, i.e. above the gumline (Niemiec, 2003). This can be done manually with calculus removal forceps and hand scalers, or by ultrasonic scalers (see Fig. 2.4).

Calculus removal forceps are used to remove heavy calculus deposits from teeth by placing the hooked beak at the top of a calculus deposit, being careful not to damage the gingiva, with the other blade placed upon the lingual surface (towards the tongue) of the tooth (McMahon, 2020). The forceps are gently squeezed, then pulled or rolled coronally (toward the cusp of the tooth crown) to dislodge a large chunk of tartar. Removing large areas of tartar in chunks speeds up the cleaning process, decreases wear and tear on more delicate hand instruments and ultrasonic instrument tips, and decreases the aerosolization of bacteria (Niemiec *et al.*, 2020).

Once any large calculus deposits have been removed, an ultrasonic scaler is used to remove the remaining tartar. Ultrasonic scalers are recognized as the preferred method of disrupting plaque biofilm (Cox, 2015). They vibrate at high frequencies and generate heat, therefore a steady stream of water is used to cool the tip (Verez-Fraguela *et al.*, 2000). The side of the tip is placed in contact with the tooth (McMahon, 2020), and calculus is removed by mechanical kick (metal tip vibrating against calculus) and cavitation (energized water spray) (Brine *et al.*, 2000). The tip should not be held in contact with the tooth for more than 15 seconds at a time, to prevent thermal damage and tooth death (Crocker, 2010). If a tooth cannot be completely cleaned before the tip becomes hot, move on to the next tooth and return to complete cleaning the first one later. See also 'Ulstrasonic scaler', p. 18.

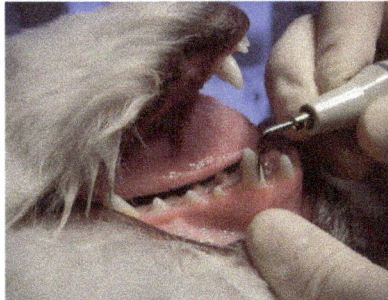

After most of the plaque and tartar is removed with calculus forceps and the ultrasonic scaler, any missed areas can be addressed with hand instruments. Hand scalers must be used only supragingivally, as their pointed tips will damage soft tissues below the gumline (Gingerich, 2012a). They are used on the tooth's crown in a push or pull stroke away from the gingiva (McMahon, 2020). Curettes may also be used in this way to clean the crowns of teeth. Both hand scalers and curettes are held in the modified pen grasp, between the thumb, index and middle fingers (Gingerich, 2012a). The ring finger rests on an adjacent tooth or structure in the same quadrant to stabilize the hand, and the wrist is rotated to pull plaque and calculus from the tooth.

Once the supragingival surfaces have been cleaned, it is important to ensure that all plaque has been removed, as plaque is often not apparent to the naked eye. Two methods may be used to detect missed plaque. The teeth can be dried using an air-water syringe, and areas of missed plaque will become visible as a chalky substance (Gingerich, 2012a). Alternatively, commercial plaque-revealing products, which are brightly staining liquids, can be painted onto the teeth with a cotton swab (Holmstrom *et al.*, 2000d).

Calculus removal forceps   Ultrasonic scaler

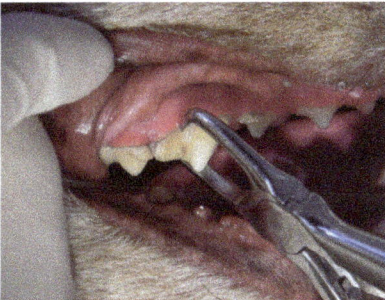

Fig. 2.4. Supragingival scaling.

The mouth is rinsed with water, and any stains remaining on the teeth indicate areas of missed plaque. Plaque-revealing products can also stain the patient's fur, so take care when applying and rinsing them off.

2.4.3   Step Three: subgingival scaling

Subgingival scaling involves removing plaque and calculus from the gingival sulcus: the space between the surface of the tooth and the surrounding gum tissue (Niemiec, 2003). Curettes and some piezoelectric ultrasonic scaler tips can be used for this (see Fig. 2.5) (Niemiec, 2004). To be used subgingivally, ultrasonic tips must be thin enough not to cause gingival trauma when introduced to the sulcus, and water must flow to the end of the tip to cool it (Gorham, 2006; Miller, 2008). When using a curette, hold it in the modified pen grasp and gently introduce it into the sulcus, then angle it to bring the blade into contact with the tooth surface. Use a pull stroke (either vertical, horizontal or oblique) to dislodge calculus and debris and remove it. Continue until the surface of the tooth looks and feels smooth. Verify this by using an air-water syringe to gently blow open the gingival sulcus for visual examination, or by tactile examination with a dental explorer: if the explorer encounters no rough areas, the subgingival portion of the tooth is clean (Gingerich, 2012a).

2.4.4   Step Four: oral examination and charting

Evaluate the head, face and oral cavity including throat, tonsils, soft and hard palate, tongue, mucosa and gingiva for any abnormalities, including asymmetry, ocular or nasal discharge, swellings, stomatitis, lacerations, granulomas, foreign bodies, etc. (McMahon, 2020). Then, beginning in quadrant 100 (upper right) and continuing through each quadrant, evaluate each tooth and record any pathology on the patient's dental chart. (See Chapter 3 for an explanation of dental charting.)

Use a periodontal probe to measure periodontal pockets and gingival recession (Gorham, 2006; Crocker, 2010). Move the probe gently up and down in at least four locations on each tooth (McMahon, 2020) – buccal (towards the check), lingual/palatal (towards the tongue and palate), mesial (towards the midline of the oral cavity) and distal (away from the midline of the oral cavity) – and record the measurements for each site. Measure periodontal pocket depth from the free gingival margin to the bottom of the sulcus (Vall, 2012). Dogs should have no more than 3 mm of free gingiva and cats should have no more than 1 mm (McMahon, 2020), so any measurements deeper than this (in the absence of gingival overgrowth or hyperplasia) are true periodontal pockets. Measure gingival recession from the cementoenamel junction (CEJ) to the gingival margin. Other abnormalities to note include tooth wear (attrition: tooth-on-tooth contact; abrasion: tooth wear from an extra-oral source, such as ball or

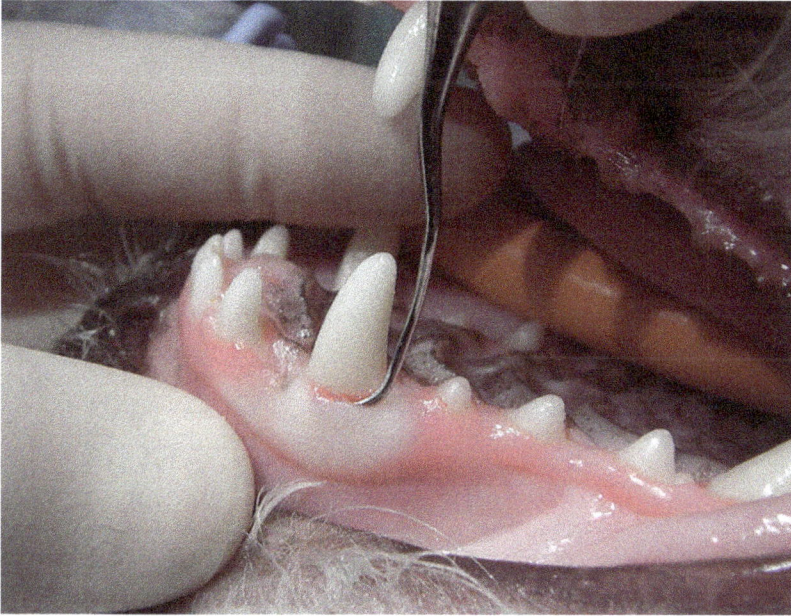

Fig. 2.5. Subgingival scaling.

cage chewing), tooth mobility, malocclusions (of jaws or individual teeth), fractures, resorption, caries, missing or supernumerary teeth, gingivitis, gingival hyperplasia (overgrowth), oral masses, granulomas, lesions or fistulas (Crocker, 2010; McMahon, 2020; Perrone *et al.*, 2020). See Chapter 3, this volume for more information about dental charting.

2.4.5   Step Five: polishing

Scaling the teeth with hand and power instruments causes micro-etches in the enamel and the cementum (Brine *et al.*, 2000), creating a rough surface that can attract plaque. Smoothing the tooth surfaces by polishing removes these microscopic grooves (Gingerich, 2012a). Use a fine polishing paste (O'Morrow, 2007) in a polishing cup on a prophy angle attached to a low-speed handpiece. A light hand during polishing decreases heat production from the polishing cup, which can cause thermal damage and even death of the tooth (McMahon, 2020). Keep the speed of the handpiece even throughout polishing by maintaining steady pressure on the pedal of the machine. The handpiece speed should be kept at 2000–4000 rpm (McMahon, 2020). Keep the prophy cup full of prophy paste at all times, in constant motion over the tooth, and pressed just hard enough that the cup lip flares beneath the gumline (Crocker, 2010). A reciprocating prophy angle, which rotates back and forth rather than spins, helps prevent the patient's facial fur from becoming entangled during polishing. Many polishing pastes contain fluoride, which can interfere with bonding agents, so should not be used on teeth that are receiving restorations (McMahon, 2020).

2.4.6   Step Six: irrigation

Irrigation flushes tooth surfaces and pockets to remove all loose debris and polishing paste. Any material left behind can cause a foreign-body reaction, resulting in inflammation or abscesses of the gingiva (Gingerich, 2012a). Air-water syringes are most commonly used for irrigation in veterinary dentistry (Crocker, 2010), but a blunt-tipped needle or urinary catheter on a large syringe, or a curved-tipped syringe filled with water, saline or chlorhexidine rinse can also be used (McMahon, 2020).

2.4.7   Step Seven: dental radiography

Full-mouth dental radiography (see Chapter 3, this volume) will often reveal pathologies hidden beneath the gumline (Bannon, 2008), such as bone loss, root resorption, root fracture, tooth impaction, dentigerous cysts, retained root tips, etc.

2.4.8   Step Eight: additional procedures including periodontal therapies (as required)

Veterinary nurses can place regional nerve blocks (see Chapter 3, this volume) (Mills, 2020). The veterinarian then performs any required oral surgery or additional procedures with the assistance of the nurse. The nurse records these treatments on the dental chart (Crocker, 2010). Additional procedures include extraction or endodontic treatment (see Chapter 4, this volume), orthodontic treatment (see Chapter 6, this volume), biopsy of oral masses (see Chapter 7, this volume) or periodontal therapies to treat periodontitis (Shourky *et al.*, 2007). Examples of periodontal therapies include root planing, subgingival curettage, perioceutic application, open root planing, guided tissue regeneration, periodontal splinting and gingivectomy. Nurses may perform closed root planing, subgingival curettage and perioceutic application, while all other periodontal therapies are surgeries that must be performed by a veterinarian (Holzman, 2006).

Closed root planing and subgingival curettage

Root planing is performed when normal gingival attachment has been lost and the tooth roots must be cleaned of calculus and debris to stimulate gingival reattachment (Gingerich, 2012a). Root planing is similar to subgingival scaling, but involves using a curette to clean the surface of the root in a deep periodontal pocket (Beckman, 2010). Closed root planing is performed on teeth with periodontal pockets of less than 6 mm (Gorham, 2006). Introduce a curette into the sulcus and bring the cutting blade into contact with the root. Use the curette subgingivally in crosshatch pull strokes until the root surface feels smooth (Eisner, 2006).

Subgingival curettage is performed after closed root planing to clean the soft tissue of the sulcus in periodontal pockets, removing diseased and/or necrotic tissue, bacteria and debris (Eisner, 2006). Introduce a curette into the sulcus and bring the cutting blade into contact with the soft tissue lining the periodontal pocket. Gently pull the curette along the soft tissue, using a finger to apply light pressure upon the outer surface of the gingiva to ensure the curette does not perforate the delicate tissue (Gingerich, 2012a).

Perioceutic application

Perioceutics are products typically consisting of a biodegradable gel that acts as a carrier for antibiotics such as doxycycline or clindamycin (Berg, 2012). These are instilled into a periodontal pocket after root planing and subgingival curettage to aid in gingival reattachment (see Fig. 2.6) (Gingerich, 2012a). The gel releases antibiotics into the pocket at much higher levels than can be achieved with systemic antibiotics (Zetner and Rothmueller, 2019), and occupies the periodontal pocket space to prevent plaque deposition so gingival reattachment can occur. Perioceutics typically dissolve within 2 weeks. They are not to be used in oronasal fistulas, periapical abscesses, or to treat teeth with mobility, furcation exposure or other cases of severe periodontal disease (Zoetis, 2021).

Depending upon the product, perioceutic gels may need to be kept refrigerated and mixed before use (Zoetis, 2021). Follow the manufacturer's instructions for mixing and storing. Inject the gel into the bottom of the periodontal pocket using a blunt-tipped cannula or needle. Once solidified (a few drops of cold water can speed up this process) (Holzman, 2006), pack the gel into the pocket with a plastic or metal packing instrument, a curette, or a periodontal probe until the pocket is filled to a normal sulcar depth. Instruct the owner not to brush the teeth for 14 days after placement, to avoid dislodging the gel (Zoetis, 2021). Oral rinses or water additives can be used during this time to prevent plaque build-up (Holzman, 2006).

Open root planing

Open root planing is performed to salvage teeth with periodontal pockets of 6 mm or greater (Gorham, 2006). To reach this depth requires the creation of a gingival flap to allow access to the diseased area; therefore

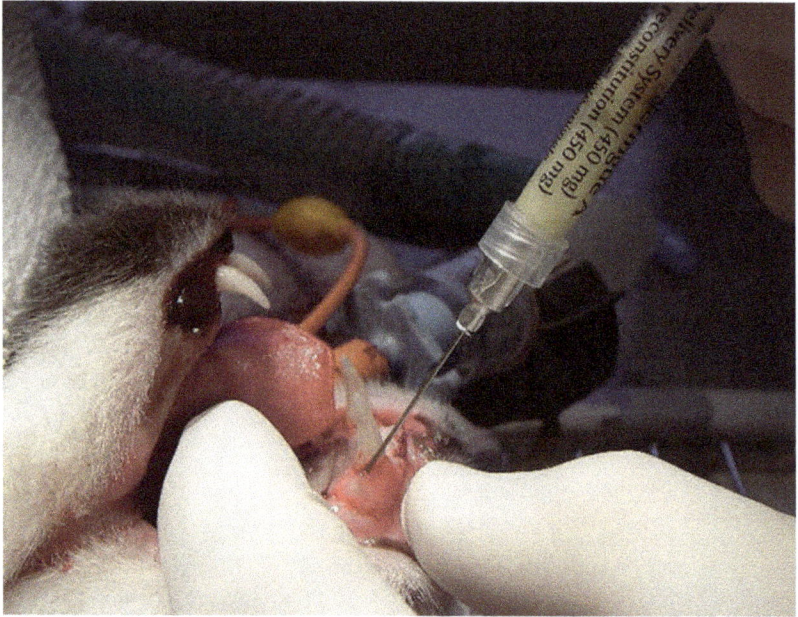

Fig. 2.6. Perioceutic application.

this is a surgical procedure that must be performed by a veterinarian. Once the flap is created, the root and subgingival tissues are cleaned as in closed root planing, then the flap is sutured closed to prevent bleeding and further infection (Perrone, 2016). Patients should receive pain medication for several days postoperatively (Gorham, 2006). Instruct the owner to feed soft food, restrict access to hard treats and toys, and use oral rinses twice daily until recheck in 14 days (Niemiec, 2010), at which time tooth brushing can commence.

Guided tissue regeneration

After open root planing, tissue graft materials can be placed into some infrabony defects prior to suturing to treat bone loss by preventing faster-growing gingival soft tissues from filling the defect, thus allowing time for regrowth of the slower-growing periodontal ligament and bone (Barthel, 2006). Various products, such as resorbable membranes and bone graft materials including allografts (demineralized, freeze-dried bone), calcium phosphate and bioactive glass can be used (Beckman, 2004; Perrone, 2016). Guided tissue regeneration is not suitable for resorbing or severely mobile teeth, or in cases where owners cannot commit to frequent COHATs and daily tooth brushing, which are required for the success of this procedure (Niemiec, 2010).

Periodontal splinting

This is the temporary splinting of mildly or moderately mobile teeth after a guided tissue regeneration procedure to stabilize the teeth during bone healing (Perrone, 2016). Once regenerative material has been placed and the tissues sutured, cold-curing dental acrylic (see Chapter 9, this volume) is placed around the mobile teeth and at least one stable tooth on either side (Gingerich, 2012a). Oral rinses must be used twice daily to keep the splint and oral tissues clean, and the pet must eat soft food and have no access to hard food or toys while the splint is in place. Recheck radiographs are taken in 3 months to assess bone healing, after which the splint is removed (Perrone, 2016).

Gingivectomy (gingivoplasty)

This is surgery to excise or recontour gingival tissue, often used in cases of gingival hyperplasia to re-establish normal pocket depths (Eisner, 2006). The pocket depths are measured with a periodontal probe, then the probe is held against the outer surface of the gingiva to show the depth of the pocket (Holmstrom *et al.*, 2000c). Marks called bleeding points are made by pressing the tip of the probe around the circumference of the tooth at 2–3 mm (normal pocket depth) from the base of the pocket, and a bevelled incision is made along the bleeding points by cutting at 45 degrees toward the tooth crown (Eisner, 2006) using a scalpel blade, electrocautery or CO_2 laser (Hale, 2012). Haemorrhage is controlled with gauze and digital pressure (Holmstrom *et al.*, 2000c). Patients should eat soft food and receive pain medications for several days postoperatively (Eisner, 2006). Oral rinses are used to clean the area twice daily until recheck in 14 days, at which time tooth brushing can commence.

2.4.9   Step Nine: fluoride application (optional)

In humans, fluoride is used to kill oral bacteria, prevent tooth sensitivity, and strengthen teeth by encouraging enamel and dentin remineralization (Gingerich, 2012a). Many veterinary dentists also choose to use it, due to the similarities of tooth structure and composition across species. Veterinary patients often have areas of gum recession or exposed dentin, both of which can cause tooth sensitivity. Fluoride can help to desensitize these areas. The effects of topical fluoride treatment last approximately 6 weeks (Eisner, 2006).

Fluoride solutions come in foams, liquids, or gels. Dry the teeth with an air syringe or gauze (Niemiec, 2004). Apply the fluoride directly to the teeth using a gloved finger or gauze, and leave it on the teeth for the amount of time recommended by the manufacturer (usually 1–3 minutes). Wipe off the fluoride thoroughly so none remains to be swallowed by the patient. Because fluoride is very acidic, it can cause gastric upset and oesophageal irritation if not completely removed (Eisner, 2006). Do not rinse the fluoride with water, as this will interfere with the fluoride's action (Niemiec, 2004). For this reason, fluoride application should only be performed after any surgical or endodontic procedures where water will be used in the mouth. Fluoride may interfere with the adhesion of dental bonding agents, so do not use it on teeth requiring restorations (McMahon, 2020).

2.4.10 Step Ten: suctioning of the oral cavity and/or removing of any packing material from the throat

Remove all debris, chunks of tartar, tooth or bone remnants and gauze from the oral cavity, to prevent asphyxiation during recovery from anaesthesia (Gingerich, 2012a). Blood-soaked gauze from extractions or other oral surgery can blend in with oral tissues and are easy to overlook.

2.5 Dental Machine Maintenance

Well-maintained dental equipment is essential to the ease and efficiency of dental cleanings and oral surgeries. Poorly maintained equipment can cause sluggish performance, especially of dental handpieces and ultrasonic scalers, increasing the time required for hygiene and surgical processes. In some cases the instruments can overheat, causing burns to patients' oral tissues.

2.5.1 Handpiece maintenance

Unless otherwise stated in the instruction manual, lubricate both low- and high-speed handpieces after each use. Remove the handpiece from the dental unit, then wipe clean (do not submerge in water) and sterilize it in an autoclave (Miller, 2004). Do not run bleach through the high-speed handpiece when shocking the waterlines (see Section 2.5.4, this volume), as this may damage it (Altier, 2020). Drip or spray handpiece lubricating oil (available through dental suppliers) into the smaller of the two large metal holes at the base of each handpiece (see Fig. 2.7) (Altier, 2020). Wipe away any excess oil. Replace the handpieces on the dental machine and run them for approximately 10 seconds to distribute the oil throughout the handpiece, making sure to place a bur or blank into the high-speed handpiece before running it (Holmstrom, 2019). Lubricate low-speed handpieces around the metal band that twists to lock prophy angles, contra angles and HP burs into place (Miller, 2004).

High-speed handpieces have a small hole in the head where water spray exits. To ensure no minerals or debris clog this hole, insert a small-gauge wire into this hole on a daily basis to remove any plugs (Johnson-Promident, 2021).

Inspect the O-rings (rubber or plastic washers) if your handpiece has them, checking for cracks or hardening. The O-rings are used to create a watertight seal (Holmstrom *et al.*, 2000b). These are inexpensive and easy to replace if any defects are discovered.

Running a high-speed handpiece without a bur or blank inserted can cause the turbine to permanently clamp shut, ruining the turbine (Holmstrom, 2019). Always place a bur or blank in the high-speed handpiece before running it, to prevent seizing of the turbine. Be alert for increased noise, vibration, or failure of the handpiece chuck to completely tighten. Any of these indicate that the turbine needs professional maintenance or replacing (Holmstrom *et al.*, 2000b). Before replacing the turbine, turn off the dental unit, then loosen the cap at the back of the handpiece head (it may unscrew by hand or require a small wrench), and press on the inserted bur or blank to remove the turbine cartridge. Insert the new turbine and screw the cap back into place. If the turbine housing has been damaged (usually from dropping the handpiece), the entire handpiece may need replacing.

2.5.2   Ultrasonic scaler maintenance

Clean and sterilize ultrasonic scaler tips after each use (Altier, 2020). Remove the scaler tip with the wrench provided by the manufacturer and autoclave in a cassette or sterilization pouch.

Ultrasonic scaler tip wear occurs gradually. If it is taking longer than usual to remove tartar with the ultrasonic scaler, this may indicate that the scaler tip has become fatigued and needs replacement (Holmstrom, 2019). Weakened tips may break during use, so always keep a spare on hand. Some dental companies offer tip wear guides, or you can easily create your own

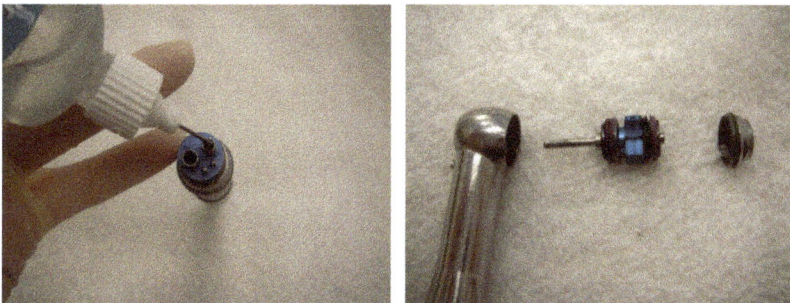

Fig. 2.7. Handpiece maintenance: oiling; changing the turbine.

by measuring the length of a new tip and drawing a line of this length on a piece of paper. Place a tip suspected of wear over the line. If there is a 2-mm reduction in tip length, this reduces scaling efficiency by 50% (Altier, 2020), and it is time to replace the tip.

2.5.3 Dental compressor maintenance

Follow the manufacturer's maintenance instructions carefully to maximize the life and performance of the dental compressor. If the instruction manual has been lost, these are often available online or by contacting the manufacturer.

Maintenance of oil-cooled dental compressor motors includes regular checking of the oil levels, periodical topping-up of the compressor oil, and yearly oil changes (Miller, 2004). Air-cooled dental compressor motors require less maintenance (Altier, 2020). For both types of compressors, as well as nitrogen-gas-driven compressors, check daily to ensure the unit is able to reach and maintain a minimum pressure of 30–40 psi, drain water from the handpiece tubes at the end of the day by flushing them with air, and decompress the machine at the end of each day (Holmstrom, 2019).

2.5.4 Dental waterline maintenance

Prior to use each day, flush the dental unit waterlines with air or water for at least 2 minutes prior to attaching handpieces, scalers, air-water syringe tips or other devices. Between patients, flush dental waterlines and devices with water for at least 20 seconds (Wirthlin *et al.*, 2003).

Dental waterline contamination with bacterial biofilm is inevitable (Partridge, 2019). Shocking the waterlines periodically kills these bacteria, while continuous waterline treatment prevents large numbers of bacteria from growing within the lines between shock treatments. Shocking is generally recommended every 1–3 months, or when waterline testing reveals microbial counts of greater than 500 cfu/ml (colony-forming units per millilitre) (Fritz, 2019), which is the Centers for Disease Control and Prevention (CDC) guideline for safe water.

To shock waterlines, fill each dental machine water bottle with a solution of one part household bleach (sodium hypochlorite) to ten parts distilled water, and reattach the bottles to the unit (Patterson Dental, 2021). Run the bleach solution through the air-water syringe, the ultrasonic scaler and the waterline of the high-speed handpiece (do not attach the high-speed handpiece to the line, as bleach may damage the handpiece) over a sink or into a draining tray for 10 seconds each (Fritz, 2019). Leave the bleach solution in the lines and bottles for 10 minutes before disconnecting the water bottles and discarding the remaining diluted bleach solution (Patterson Dental, 2021). Refill the water bottles with distilled water and flush through the air-water syringe, the ultrasonic scaler and the line of the high-speed handpiece for 3 minutes each or until the bleach odour disappears (Fritz, 2019). Do not leave the diluted bleach solution in the waterlines for longer than 10 minutes, as this may damage the lines.

Continuous waterline treatments are available as tablets, liquids or cartridges placed within dental water bottles to reduce bacterial growth on a daily basis. Continuous waterline treatment on its own without periodic shocking treatments is ineffective (Fritz, 2019).

Over 30% of all treated dental waterlines fail to meet the CDC guideline of less than 500 cfu/ml (CDC, 2018; Fritz, 2019). Testing helps to ensure the waterline treatment protocol is working. Waterline testing can be done in-office or at a laboratory. In-office tests are convenient and easy to use, but are less accurate than lab tests, which must be shipped to the lab for incubation. Both types of testing are available through dental supply companies.

Test waterlines monthly after establishing a treatment protocol, until all lines grow less than 500 cfu/ml for 2 months in a row (Fritz, 2019). After that, test every 3 months. Return to monthly testing if the lines grow more than 500 cfu/ml.

2.6   Hand Instrument Maintenance

The time taken to perform a COHAT increases as the sharpness of dental instruments decreases. Improperly sharpened instruments lose their angles and become inefficient (Holmstrom *et al.*, 2000b), possibly damaging the root and soft tissues. Dull instruments skim over calculus, burnishing it instead of removing it (Wanless, 2017). Dull instruments also put stress on the nurse's hands, wrists, arms and shoulders, because greater force is required to remove calculus, leading to repetitive injuries (Cherry, 2010).

2.6.1   Dental instrument sharpening materials

Sharpening stones

Sharpening stones sharpen instruments by removing metal from them (Scaramucci, 2007). They come in a variety of shapes and grits. Use fine-grit stones to sharpen instruments that are only slightly dull, or to freshen an instrument's blade between procedures. These remove only a very small amount of metal with each stroke. Use medium-grit stones on very dull instruments to restore their blades (McMahon, 2020). These remove a greater amount of metal with each stroke. Common stone types are Arkansas (fine grit), Ceramic (fine grit) and India (medium grit). Sharpening stones come in various shapes, such as rectangular, wedge-shaped and conical. Instruments should be clean and disinfected prior to sharpening, to prevent bacteria from transferring to the stone. Wash dirty or clogged stones with warm water and soap (Serona, 2018).

Sharpening oil

Sharpening oil lubricates the stone's surface and carries away the small metal shavings created while sharpening instruments. Ceramic stones use water for lubrication, while Arkansas and India stones use oil (Lowe, 2010). Sharpening oil is available from dental supply companies.

Test sticks

Test sticks are thin, round acrylic sticks used to determine the sharpness of dental instruments. Sharp instruments will catch or remove a fine strip of acrylic from the test stick, while dull instruments will skim over the stick (Holmstrom *et al.*, 2000b).

2.6.2   Hand instrument sharpening techniques

There are many different sharpening techniques, all of which work equally well so long as the operator performs the technique properly, maintaining the correct angles. The techniques described below for sharpening scalers and curettes are 'moving stone' methods, and the techniques for sharpening luxators and periosteal elevators are 'stationary stone' methods. For different techniques, including dental instrument sharpening machines, contact your dental instrument supplier.

Sharpening scalers and curettes

The following guidance is [taken from] Scaramucci (2007) and Serona (2018).

1. Place a drop or two of oil on a rectangular or wedge-shaped stone and smooth it across the sharpening stone with a lens-cleaning wipe or tissue.
2. Stand in front of a clock (with an analogue clock face) or kneel at the edge of a counter in front of a small, portable clock, and stabilize the handle of the instrument against the counter.
3. Hold the instrument in your non-dominant hand, with the terminal shank perpendicular to the floor and the working end pointing toward you at eye level. For double-ended instruments, you will first be sharpening the working end closest to the floor, so make sure this end is at eye level.

Sharpening scalers and universal curettes

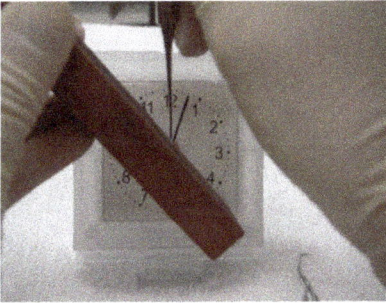

Sharpening Gracey curettes

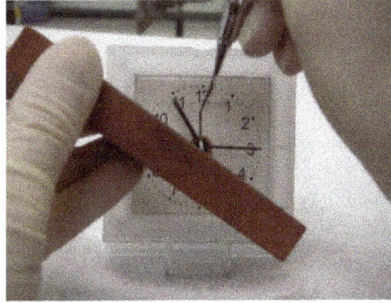

Fig. 2.8. Sharpening scalers and curettes.

4. Hold the oiled stone in your dominant hand and bring the stone into contact with one of the blades of your instrument, making sure that the stone is flat against the entire length of the blade.

5. Angle the stone at 110° to the face of the blade. For scalers and universal curettes this is between 12 and 1 on the clock for the right-sided blade, and between 11 and 12 on the clock for the left-sided blade. For Gracey curettes (you will be sharpening the lower blade only) this is between 1 and 2 on the clock if sharpening the right blade, or between 10 and 11 on the clock if sharpening the left blade (see Fig. 2.8).

6. Maintain this angle and move the stone up and down with smooth strokes, keeping the stone flat against the blade. Always finish on a down stroke, to prevent curls of metal from building up on the face of the instrument. Use only the minimum number of strokes required to sharpen the instrument, as sharpening removes metal, so over-sharpening can cause unnecessary thinning of the blade. If the instrument is not very dull, use only one to three up-and-down strokes, then test the instrument for sharpness.

7. Test for sharpness by scraping the instrument's blade along a test stick as though removing calculus from a tooth. If the instrument pulls up a curl of acrylic, it is sufficiently sharp. If the instrument slides along the stick or only catches without removing a strip of acrylic, it requires further sharpening.

8. Once both blades on one working end are sharp (or the lowest blade of a Gracey curette), flip the instrument upside-down to sharpen the opposite end.

9. Place a drop of oil on a fine-grit conical stone. Holding the widest end of the stone in your dominant hand, roll the stone over the face of each blade from the terminal shank to the tip or toe. This will ensure that there are no tiny curls of metal on the instrument's face.

10. Wipe the oil from the instrument with a tissue or paper towel.

Sharpening luxators   Sharpening periosteal
                                              elevators

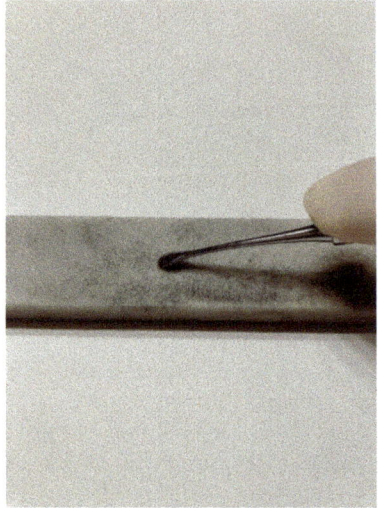

Fig. 2.9. Sharpening luxators and periosteal elevators.

Sharpening luxators

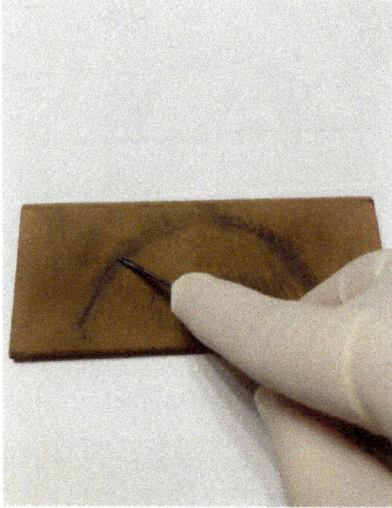

The following guidance is as described by Issuu (2014) and Serona (2018).

1. Place a drop or two of oil on a wide rectangular or wedge-shaped sharpening stone (5-cm width works well) and smooth it across the stone with a lens-cleaning wipe or tissue.
2. Place the stone horizontally on a counter. If using a wedge-shaped stone, place the narrower edge toward you.
3. Grasp the luxator handle in your palm with the blade facing up ('U'-shape).
4. Place your index finger at the end of the terminal shank and drag the blade back and forth in an arc at a 45-degree angle across the stone, rocking your wrist so the entire blade eventually comes into contact with the stone (see Fig. 2.9).
5. Test the luxator for sharpness by pushing it against a test stick. If it sticks, it is sufficiently sharp. If not, repeat Step 4.
6. Place a drop of oil on the narrow end of a fine-grit conical stone. Roll the tip of the stone back and forth along the inner curve of the blade to remove any rough spots or nicks.
7. Wipe the oil from the instrument with a tissue or paper towel.

Sharpening periosteal elevators

The following guidance is as described by Beckman, 2021.

1. Place a drop or two of oil on a rectangular or wedge-shaped stone and smooth it across the stone with a lens-cleaning wipe or tissue.
2. Place the stone horizontally on a counter.
3. Hold the periosteal elevator in the modified pen grasp and push the blade back and forth against the stone in short strokes, making sure to sharpen all surfaces of the blade.
4. Test the elevator for sharpness by pushing it against a test stick. If it sticks, it is sufficiently sharp. If not, repeat Step 3.
5. Examine the blade to make sure any nicks or rough spots have been removed.

2.6.3 When enough is enough

Instruments, no matter how well-maintained, have a finite lifespan. Continued use and sharpening will eventually remove so much metal that the blade becomes thin and weak (Scaramucci, 2007). Instruments can also drop on the floor and break, luxator blades can bend, extraction forceps may no longer meet, and periosteal elevators can develop nicks or notches.

If a dental tray is full of bent, broken or unidentifiable instruments, buy new ones! If your dental budget is tight, purchase one instrument a month until you have a full set – or, better yet, educate your practice manager about how having properly maintained dental instruments will result in more efficient, faster dental procedures, allowing your practice to perform more COHATs and thus generating more income. Make an appointment with a veterinary dental instrument representative or visit an instrument booth at a dental conference to become familiar with instrument options such as handle length and width. Many veterinary dental instrument suppliers offer sets of instruments for canine and feline dental hygiene. These are often less expensive than purchasing each instrument separately. Additional instruments can be added later if desired.

2.6.4 Instrument sterilization

Sterilize dental instruments in the same manner as general surgical instruments. Clean blood and debris from the instrument using a brush and surgical-instrument cleaning fluid in water, then place the instrument in an ultrasonic cleaner for at least 10 minutes to remove any microscopic debris (Fuchs *et al.*, 2006). Rinse and dry the instrument. Place the instruments in an autoclave basket, cassette, disposable plastic sterilization package or pack wrap. Autoclave dental instruments at the same temperature and for the same length of time as a general surgical instrument pack (Holmstrom *et al.*, 2000b; Fuchs *et al.*, 2006).

References

AAHA (2021) AAHA guidelines, dental anatomy & pathology definitions. American Animal Hospital Association. Available at: https://www.aaha.org/aaha-guidelines/dental-care/anatomy-pathology/definitions/ (accessed 3 February 2021).

Aller, M.S. (2005) Personal safety and ergonomics in the dental operatory. *Journal of Veterinary Dentistry* 22(2), 124–131.

Altier, B. (2020) Components of the dental operatory. In: Perrone, J. (ed.) *Small Animal Dental Procedures for Veterinary Technicians and Nurses*. Wiley Blackwell, Hoboken, New Jersey, pp. 29–49.

ASA (2020) ASA physical status classification system. American Society of Anesthesiologists. Available at: https://www.asahq.org/standards-and-guidelines/asa-physical-status-classification-system (accessed 5 February 2021).

AVMA (2021) Pet dental care. American Veterinary Medical Association. Available at: https://www.avma.org/resources-tools/pet-owners/petcare/pet-dental-care (accessed 3 February 2021).

Bannon, K. (2008) Secrets to dental success using the AAHA guidelines. In: *Proceedings of the 22nd Annual Veterinary Dental Forum*. Omnipress, Madison, Wisconsin, pp. 175–176.

Barthel, R. (2006) Treatment of vertical bone loss in a dog. *Journal of Veterinary Dentistry* 23(4), 237–242. DOI: 10.1177/089875640602300407.

Beckman, B. (2004) Treatment of an infrabony pocket in an American Eskimo dog. *Journal of Veterinary Dentistry* 21(3), 159–163. DOI: 10.1177/089875640402100303.

Beckman, B. (2010) The technician's role in stage II periodontal disease. In: *Proceedings of the 24th Annual Veterinary Dental Forum*. Omnipress, Madison, Wisconsin (CD Rom).

Beckman, B. (2021) Veterinary dental hand instrument sharpening. Webinar. International Veterinary Dental Institute. Available at: https://veterinarydentistry.net/veterinary-dental-hand-instrument-sharpening/ (accessed 10 February 2021).

Bellows, J. (2019) The dental operatory. In: *Small Animal Dental Equipment, Materials and Techniques: A Primer*, 2nd edn. Wiley Blackwell, Ames, Iowa, pp. 1–36.

Bellows, J., Berg, M., Dennis, S., Harvey, R. and Lobprise, H.B. (2019) 2019 AAHA dental care guidelines for dogs and cats. American Animal Hospital Association. Available at: https://www.aaha.org/globalassets/02-guidelines/dental/aaha_dental_guidelines.pdf (accessed 10 September 2020).

Berg, M. (2012) Why perioceutics – do they really decrease tooth loss? In: *Proceedings of the 26th Annual Veterinary Dental Forum*. Omnipress, Madison, Wisconsin (CD Rom).

Berg, M. (2015) Dental corner: to gag or not to gag – that is the question. Dvm360. Available at: https://www.dvm360.com/view/dental-corner-gag-or-not-gag-question (accessed 6 February 2021).

Berg, M. (2020) The examination room and the dental patient. In: Perrone, J. (ed.) *Small Animal Dental Procedures for Veterinary Technicians and Nurses*. Wiley Blackwell, Hoboken, New Jersey, pp. 21–28.

Bowersock, T., Wu, C.C., Inskeep, G. and Chester, T. (2000) Prevention of bacteremia in dogs undergoing dental scaling by prior administration of oral clindamycin or chlorhexidine oral rinse. *Journal of Veterinary Dentistry* 17(1), 11–16. DOI: 10.1177/089875640001700101.

Brine, E., Marretta, S., Pijanowski, G. and Siegel, A. (2000) Comparison of the effects of four different power scalers on enamel tooth surface in the dog. *Journal of Veterinary Dentistry* 17(1), 17–21. DOI: 10.1177/089875640001700102.

Caiafa, A. (2013) Endodontics: it's all about the pulp. In: *World Small Animal Veterinary Association World Congress Proceedings*. Available at: https://www.vin.com/apputil/content/defaultadv1.aspx?id=5709741&pid=11372&print=1 (accessed 6 February 2021).

Carmichael, D. (2006) Dental extraction. In: *Proceedings of the 20th Annual Veterinary Dental Forum*. Omnipress, Madison, Wisconsin, pp. 185–190.

CDC (2018) Dental unit waterline quality. Centers for Disease Control and Prevention. Available at: https://www.cdc.gov/oralhealth/infectioncontrol/summary-infection-prevention-practices/dental-unit-water-quality.html (accessed 10 February 2021).

Cherry, B. (2010) Ergonomics and safety for the dental technician. In: *Proceedings of the 24th Annual Veterinary Dental Forum*. Omnipress, Madison, Wisconsin (CD Rom).

Cox, R. (2015) Getting the most out of ultrasonic scaling: a guide to maximizing efficiency. Dentsply Sirona. Available at: https://www.dentsplysirona.com/content/dam/dentsply/microsites/cavitron_CA/GettingtheMostoutofUltrasonicScaling.pdf (accessed 10 February 2021).

Crocker, C. (2010) Dentistry techniques. In: *Proceedings of the 24th Annual Veterinary Dental Forum*. Omnipress, Madison, Wisconsin (CD Rom).

DeForge, D. (2002) Physical ergonomics in veterinary dentistry. *Journal of Veterinary Dentistry* 19(4), 196–200. DOI: 10.1177/089875640201900402.

Dias, I. and Delgado, E. (2020) Bacterial aerosols released during dental ultrasonic scaling in dogs. Science Repository. Available at: https://www.sciencerepository.org/bacterial-aerosols-released-during-dental-ultrasonic-scaling-in-dogs_DOBCR-2020-3-102 (accessed 6 February 2021).

Eisner, E. (2006) Identification and treatment of early stage periodontal disease. In: *Proceedings of the 20th Annual Veterinary Dental Forum*. Omnipress, Madison, Wisconsin, pp. 371–375.

Ericsson, I. (2020) Importance of ergonomics in dentistry work. Veterinary Ireland Journal. Available at: http://www.veterinaryirelandjournal.com/focus/221-importance-of-ergonomics-in-dentistry-work (accessed 7 February 2021).

Eubanks, D. and Gilbo, K. (2006) Bur basics. *Journal of Veterinary Dentistry* 23(3), 196–199. DOI: 10.1177/089875640602300312.

Fritz, C. (2019) How to shock your dental unit waterlines. ProEdge Dental Water Labs blog, 14 March. Available at: https://blog.proedgedental.com/blog/how-to-shock-your-dental-waterlines (accessed 10 February 2021).

Fuchs, W., Biering, H., Drouin, H.J., Henn, H. and Glasmacher, R. (2006) Proper maintenance of instruments in veterinary surgeries. Available at: https://8ad5d244-3245-4d36-bc7f-7e3589f4c29b.filesusr.com/ugd/e5e300_b38f0821c69e4a23a1f933fc85e84826.pdf?index=true (accessed 10 February 2021).

Gingerich, W. (2012a) Periodontal cleaning and non-surgical treatment. In: *Proceedings of the 26th Annual Veterinary Dental Forum*. Omnipress, Madison, Wisconsin (CD Rom).

Gingerich, W. (2012b) Periodontal disease: pathophysiology and diagnosis. In: *Proceedings of the 26th Annual Veterinary Dental Forum*. Omnipress, Madison, Wisconsin (CD Rom).

Gorham, M. (2006) Recognizing periodontal disease. In: *Proceedings of the 20th Annual Veterinary Dental Forum*. Omnipress, Madison, Wisconsin, pp. 389–393.

Hale, F. (2012) Surgical management of gingival hyperplasia. In: *Proceedings of the 26th Annual Veterinary Dental Forum*. Omnipress, Madison, Wisconsin (CD Rom).

Hernandez, J. (2006) My achy breaky hand. In: *Proceedings of the 20th Annual Veterinary Dental Forum*. Omnipress, Madison, Wisconsin, p. 383.

Holmstrom, S.E. (2019) Dental instruments and equipment. In: Holmstrom, S.E. (ed.) *Veterinary Dentistry: A Team Approach*, 3rd edn. Elsevier, St. Louis, Missouri, pp. 111–124.

Holmstrom, S., Holmstrom, L.A., McGrath, C.J., Richey, M.T. and Wiggs, R.B. (2000a) Personal safety and ergonomics. In: Holmstrom, S. (ed.) *Veterinary Dentistry for the Technician & Office Staff*. Saunders, Philadelphia, Pennsylvania, pp. 99–113.

Holmstrom, S., Holmstrom, L.A., McGrath, C.J., Richey, M.T. and Wiggs, R.B. (2000b) Dental instruments and equipment. In: Holmstrom, S. (ed.) *Veterinary Dentistry for the Technician & Office Staff*. Saunders, Philadelphia, Pennsylvania, pp. 65–98.

Holmstrom, S., Holmstrom, L.A., McGrath, C.J., Richey, M.T. and Wiggs, R.B. (2000c) Advanced veterinary dental procedures. In: Holmstrom, S. (ed.) *Veterinary Dentistry for the Technician & Office Staff*. Saunders, Philadelphia, Pennsylvania, pp. 247–282.

Holmstrom, S., Holmstrom, L.A., McGrath, C.J., Richey, M.T. and Wiggs, R.B. (2000d) The complete prophy. In: Holmstrom, S. (ed.) *Veterinary Dentistry for the Technician & Office Staff*. Saunders, Philadelphia, Pennsylvania, pp. 159–179.

Holmstrom, S., Holmstrom, L.A., McGrath, C.J., Richey, M.T. and Wiggs, R.B. (2000e) Exodontics (Extractions). In: Holmstrom, S. (ed.) *Veterinary Dentistry for the Technician & Office Staff*. Saunders, Philadelphia, Pennsylvania, pp. 205–222.

Holzman, G. (2006) Advanced periodontal therapy for the veterinary technician. In: *Proceedings of the 20th Annual Veterinary Dental Forum*. Omnipress, Madison, Wisconsin, pp. 399–401.

Issuu (2014) Dental instrument sharpening guide. Issuu. Available at: https://issuu.com/foschigroup/docs/ch13 (accessed 10 February 2021).

Johnson-Promident (2021) Handpiece maintenance instructions. Johnson-Promident. Available at: https://johnsonpromident.com/handpiece-maintenance-instructions/ (accessed 10 February 2021).

Kolb, S. (2017) Rabbit dentistry. Today's Veterinary Nurse. Available at: https://todaysveterinarynurse.com/articles/rabbit-dentistry/ (accessed 3 March 2021).

LeVan, L.M. (2013) Dentistry on a dime – part 2: basic dental instrumentation, use, and maintenance. Vet Folio. Available at: https://www.vetfolio.com/learn/article/dentistry-on-a-dime-part-2-basic-dental-instrumentation-use-and-maintenance (accessed 5 February 2021).

Lewis, J. (2015) A veterinary practitioner's guide to dental burs. Veterinary Practice News. Available at: https://www.veterinarypracticenews.com/a-veterinary-practitioners-guide-to-dental-burs/ (accessed 6 February 2021).

Lewis, J. (2016) How to treat gingival hyperplasia. Veterinary Practice News. Available at: https://www.veterinarypracticenews.com/how-to-treat-gingival-hyperplasia/ (accessed 6 February 2021).

Lowe, A. (2010) The cutting edge of dental instruments. Nature. Available at: https://www.nature.com/articles/vital1242.pdf?proof=t (accessed 10 February 2021).

McMahon, J. (2020) The dental cleaning. In: Perrone, J. (ed.) *Small Animal Dental Procedures for Veterinary Technicians and Nurses.* Wiley Blackwell, Hoboken, New Jersey, pp. 65–91.

Miller, B. (2004) TLC for your dental equipment. In: *Proceedings of the 18th Annual Veterinary Dental Forum.* Omnipress, Madison, Wisconsin, pp. 306–307.

Miller, B. (2006) Dental charting. In: *Proceedings of the 20th Annual Veterinary Dental Forum.* Omnipress, Madison, Wisconsin, pp. 181–183.

Miller, B. (2008) Good vibes for your patients: fundamentals of power scalers. In: *Proceedings of the 22nd Annual Veterinary Dental Forum.* Omnipress, Madison, Wisconsin, pp. 195–197.

Miller, B. (2012) Instrument choices for use during a professional dental cleaning: what do you need on your tray? In: *Proceedings of the 24th Annual Veterinary Dental Forum.* Omnipress, Madison, Wisconson (CD Rom).

Mills, A. (2020) Anesthesia and the dental patient. In: Perrone, J. (ed.) *Small Animal Dental Procedures for Veterinary Technicians and Nurses.* Wiley Blackwell, Hoboken, New Jersey, pp. 51–63.

Nemec, A., Jouppi, R., Niemiec, B.A. and Steagall, P.V. (2019) Limitations of oral examination in the conscious patient. Clinician's Brief. Available at: https://www.cliniciansbrief.com/article/limitations-oral-examination-conscious-patient (accessed 3 February 2021).

Niemiec, B.A. (2003) Professional teeth cleaning. *Journal of Veterinary Dentistry* 20(3), 175–180. DOI: 10.1177/089875640302000305.

Niemiec, B.A. (2004) Dental prophylaxis and home care. In: *Proceedings of the 18th Annual Veterinary Dental Forum.* Omnipress, Madison, Wisconsin, pp. 314–320.

Niemiec, B.A. (2010) Periodontal surgery. In: *Proceedings of the 24th Annual Veterinary Dental Forum.* Omnipress, Madison, Wisconsin (CD Rom).

Niemiec, B.A., Gawor, J., Nemec, A., Clarke, D. and Tutt, C. (2020) World small animal veterinary association global dental guidelines. Available at: https://wsava.org/wp-content/uploads/2020/01/Dental-Guidleines-for-endorsement_0.pdf (accessed 6 February 2021).

O'Morrow, C. (2007) Basic dental instruments. In: *Proceedings of the 21st Annual Veterinary Dental Forum.* Omnipress, Madison, Wisconsin, pp. 193–197.

Partridge, B. (2019) What dangers lie within your dental units? Veterinary Practice, 6 March. Available at: https://veterinary-practice.com/article/what-dangers-lie-within-your-dental-units (accessed 10 February 2021).

Patterson Dental (2021) How do I 'shock' treat the water bottles and lines with 5.25% sodium hypochlorite (household bleach)? Patterson Dental. Available at: https://content.pattersondental.com/items/PDFs/images/PDF_629069.pdf (accessed 10 February 2021).

Perrone, J.R. (2016) When extraction is not an option. Today's Veterinary Nurse. Available at: https://todaysveterinarynurse.com/articles/when-extraction-is-not-an-option/ (accessed 10 February 2021).

Perrone, J., Sharp, S. and March, P. (2020) Common dental conditions and treatments. In: Perrone, J. (ed.) *Small Animal Dental Procedures for Veterinary Technicians and Nurses.* Wiley Blackwell, Hoboken, New Jersey, pp. 131–168.

Scaramucci, M.K. (2007) Sharpening 101. Dimensions of Dental Hygiene. Available at: https://dimensionsofdentalhygiene.com/article/sharpening-101/ (accessed 11 February 2021).

Serona (2018) Dental instrument sharpening. Serona Animal Health blog, 8 may. Available at: https://serona.ca/blogs/news/dental-instrument-sharpening-101 (accessed 11 February 2021).

Shourky, M., Ali, L.B., Naby, M.A. and Soliman, A. (2007) Repair of Experimental Plaque-Induced Periodontal Disease in Dogs. *Journal of Veterinary Dentistry* 24(3), 152–165. DOI: 10.1177/089875640702400303.

Vall, P.R. (2012) Gingival physiology: what happens in the sulcus? In: *Proceedings of the 26th Annual Veterinary Dental Forum.* Omnipress, Madison, Wisconsin (CD Rom).

Verez-Fraguela, J.L., Valles, M. and Calvo, L.J. (2000) Effects of ultrasonic dental scaling on pulp vitality in dogs: an experimental study. *Journal of Veterinary Dentistry* 17(2), 75–79. DOI: 10.1177/089875640001700202.

Wanless, T. (2017) The role of hygienists in recognizing and healing supervised neglect related to burnished calculus. RDH. Available at: https://www.rdhmag.com/patient-care/article/16409765/the-role-of-hygienists-in-recognizing-and-healing-supervised-neglect-related-to-burnished-calculus (accessed 5 February 2021).

Wirthlin, R., Marshall, G.W. and Rowland, R.W. (2003) Formation and decontamination of biofilms in dental unit waterlines. *Journal of Periodontology* 74(11), 1595–1609. DOI: 10.1902/jop.2003.74.11.1595.

Zeltzman, P. (2016) How ASA scores help make anesthesia safer for your pet patients. Veterinary Practice News. Available at: https://www.veterinarypractice-news.com/how-asa-scores-help-make-anesthesia-safer-for-your-pet-patients/ (accessed 5 February 2021).

Zetner, K. and Rothmueller, G. (2019) Treatment of periodontal pockets with doxycycline in beagles. Vet Folio. Available at: https://www.vetfolio.com/learn/article/treatment-of-periodontal-pockets-with-doxycycline-in-beagles (accessed 10 February 2021).

Zoetis (2021) Doxirobe gel. Zoetis Inc. Available at: https://www.zoetisus.com/_locale-assets/mcm-portal-assets/msds_pi/pi/doxirobe-gel-marketing-package-insert.pdf (accessed 10 February 2021).

Dental Essentials: Dental Charting, Dental Radiography and Pain Management

3

3.1 Dental Charting

Dental charting includes not only the teeth but also all structures of the head, face and oral cavity (McMahon, 2020). Examples of dental charts and a continually updated list of dental pathologies and their abbreviations can be found on the website of the American Veterinary Dental College (AVDC, 2021a). The British Veterinary Dental Association website also offers downloadable dental charts (BVDA, 2021). Any abnormalities should be recorded on the patient's dental chart, including facial or jaw asymmetries and swellings; enlarged lymph nodes or tonsils; lesions or masses in the oral mucosa, gingiva or tongue; excessive or deficient saliva production; dental or jaw malocclusions; and any tooth or oral pathology. Refer to other chapters in this book for in-depth explanations of common oral pathologies.

3.1.1 Anatomical nomenclature

Anatomical nomenclature is the identification of teeth by type and number (McMahon, 2020). The convention when speaking or writing is to first describe whether the tooth is on the right or left side of the patient's mouth, then whether it is in the upper or lower jaw, the tooth number (counted rostrally to caudally – from the front of the mouth to the back – for each tooth type) and finally the type of the tooth (AVDC, 2021b). For example: left upper fourth premolar. The types of teeth (from the front to the back) are as follows.

- **Incisors:** small, front teeth used primarily for grooming, gnawing and tearing (RVC, 2002a). There are three incisors in each maxilla (right and left upper jaws) and mandible (right and left lower jaws) in dogs and cats. Each incisor has one root (Koenig, 2004).
- **Canines:** also known as 'fang' teeth, these are strategic teeth used for catching, holding and tearing prey, balls, toys and other objects (Koenig,

DOI: 10.1079/9781789248869.0003

2004). They also keep the lips and tongue in their proper positions (Holmstrom *et al.*, 2000a). There is one canine tooth in each maxilla and mandible of the dog and cat. Each canine tooth has one large root, about twice as long as the tooth's crown (Perrone, 2008).

- **Premolars:** teeth located behind the canine teeth, with pointed crowns which occlude or come together in a scissors-like fashion to hold and cut food (RVC, 2002a). Dogs have four premolars in each maxilla and mandible. Cats have three premolars in each maxilla and two in each mandible. Premolars in the maxilla can have one, two or three roots (Koenig, 2004; Holzman, 2020), while premolars in the mandible have only one or two roots. There are no teeth with three roots in the mandibles of cats and dogs (Holzman, 2020). 'Carnassial' is a term used to refer to the upper fourth premolar and lower first molar in both dogs and cats. These are large, strategic teeth used for shearing and chewing (Perrone, 2008).
- **Molars:** caudal teeth located behind the premolars. They have at least one flat occlusal surface for grinding food (Koenig, 2004). Dogs have two molars in each maxilla, each of which has three roots, and three molars in each mandible, each of which has two roots. Cats have one molar in each maxilla, which has one root, and one in each mandible, which have two roots.

To chart teeth using anatomical nomenclature, record the first letter of the tooth type (the exception being premolar, which is recorded as PM) – uppercase if the tooth is permanent; lowercase if the tooth is deciduous. Then count which tooth of its type it is, from rostral to caudal. If the tooth is in the maxilla, the number is written as a superscript. If the tooth is in the mandible, the number is written as a subscript. Place this number to either the left or the right side of the tooth-type letter depending on which side of the mouth the tooth is located (Holmstrom *et al.*, 2000b). For example:

- Left upper fourth premolar: ^{4}PM
- Right lower first incisor: I_{1}
- Right upper canine: C^{1}
- Left lower third molar: $_{3}M$
- Deciduous right upper second premolar: pm^{2}

3.1.2 Dental formulae of dogs and cats

The following formulae are as described by Holzman (2020).

Dental formulae are written as the number of each type of tooth in one side of the upper jaw over the number of each type of tooth in one side of the lower jaw, multiplied by two. Thus:

Dog: 2(I3/3, C1/1, PM4/4, M2/3) = 42
Cat: 2(I3/3, C1/1, PM3/2, M1/1) = 30

The anatomical system of nomenclature is intuitive and easy to learn, but is difficult to enter into computerized records (McMahon, 2020). Anatomical nomenclature is modified for computers by typing 'R' for right and 'L' for left; 'U' for Upper and 'L' for Lower. For example, the lower left first premolar is typed as LLPM1, while the upper right second incisor becomes RUI2.

3.1.3   The modified Triadan system

The Triadan system is a human-based dental charting system which assigns each tooth a three-digit number. Veterinary dentistry uses a modification of this system (AVDC, 2021b).

The first digit identifies in which quadrant of the mouth a tooth is located (Holmstrom *et al.*, 2000b; McMahon, 2020). There are four quadrants: the upper right, numbered quadrant 100; the upper left, numbered quadrant 200; the lower left, numbered quadrant 300; and the lower right, numbered quadrant 400 (AVDC, 2021b).

The last two digits identify the number of the tooth in the mouth as counted back from the midline (Holmstrom *et al.*, 2000b; McMahon, 2020). The central incisor is tooth 01, the middle incisor is tooth 02, the lateral incisor is tooth 03, the canine is tooth 04, the first premolar is tooth 05, and so on. For example:

- Upper left fourth premolar: 208
- Lower right first incisor: 401
- Upper right canine: 104
- Lower left third molar: 311

To differentiate between permanent and deciduous teeth, another four quadrant numbers have been added. The upper right deciduous quadrant is numbered quadrant 500, the upper left deciduous quadrant is numbered quadrant 600, the lower left deciduous quadrant is numbered quadrant 700, and the lower right deciduous quadrant is numbered quadrant 800 (AVDC, 2021b). For example:

- Deciduous upper right second premolar: 506
- Deciduous lower left canine: 704

The Triadan system is easy to record in computerized medical records and is very precise. Its biggest disadvantage is that it must be memorized and takes time to learn (Holmstrom *et al.*, 2000b).

3.1.4   Cats and their 'missing' teeth

The tooth identification systems used in small animal practice are based on dog oral anatomy. Because dogs have 42 teeth while cats only have 30, the numbering system for the cat assumes that it is 'missing' certain teeth.

The convention in veterinary dental nomenclature is that cats are missing the first maxillary premolar, the second maxillary molar, the first and second mandibular premolars, and the second and third mandibular molars (Domnick, 2012; AVDC, 2021b). For example, this means that the most rostral right maxillary premolar tooth present in the cat is numbered as the second right maxillary premolar (PM², 106), and the most rostral left mandibular premolar tooth present in the cat is numbered as the third left mandibular premolar (₃PM, 307).

Also, what is considered the cat's upper first molar is a tiny tooth tucked closely behind the upper fourth premolar. The cat's lower first molar does not have a flattened cusp and functions as a premolar.

3.1.5   The rule of fours and nines

This rule is a convenient way to quickly assign Triadan numbers to the teeth. In both dogs and cats, all canine teeth are numbered 04, and all first molars are numbered 09 (McMahon, 2020). Knowing this, it is an easy matter to identify the canine tooth and count rostrally (forwards) to obtain the number of the incisors: 03, 02, 01; or to identify the first molar and count rostrally to obtain the number of the premolars: 08, 07, 06, 05 in the dog; 08, 07, 06 in the cat maxilla, or 08 and 07 in the cat mandible. Remember: in veterinary dental nomenclature, the cat is 'missing' teeth. In the dog, there is also an upper second molar: 10, and lower second and third molars: 10 and 11.

3.1.6   Directional nomenclature

Directional nomenclature (see Fig. 3.1) makes it possible to accurately describe and record exactly where on or around a tooth or in the mouth a pathology or treatment is located (Holzman, 2020).

- Mesial: toward the midline.
- Distal: away from the midline.
- Apical: toward the root apex.
- Coronal: toward the crown.
- Cervical: toward the 'neck' of the tooth (the cementoenamel junction).
- Palatal: toward the palate.
- Lingual: toward the tongue.
- Buccal: toward the cheek.
- Labial: toward the lips.
- Vestibular: toward the vestibule (area of the oral cavity between the teeth and cheeks/lips). *Vestibular* can be used interchangeably with either *buccal* or *labial.*
- Line angles: corners of a tooth where two surfaces join, such as: mesiobuccal, distobuccal, distolingual and mesiolingual.

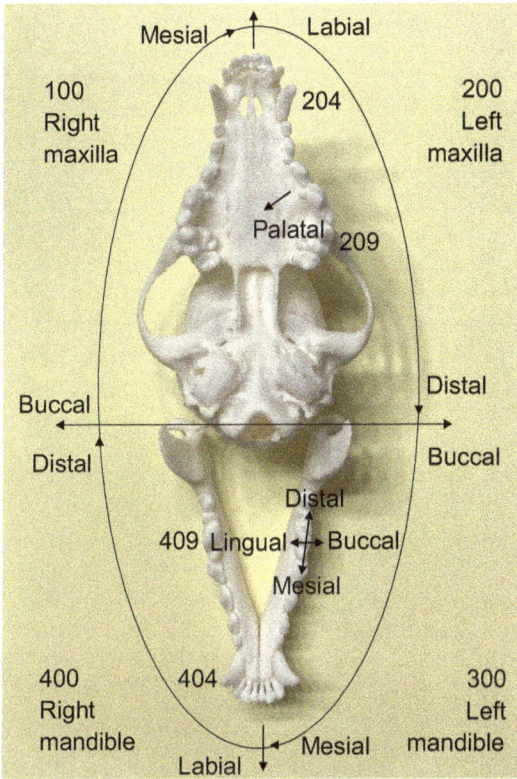

Fig. 3.1. Directional terminology.

- Facial: toward the front of the head.
- Occlusal: facing a tooth in the opposite jaw, or the chewing surface of a tooth.
- Interproximal: area between two adjacent teeth
- Extra-oral: outside of the mouth.
- Intra-oral: inside of the mouth.
- Periapical: around the apex of the tooth root.
- Sublingual: beneath the tongue.
- Subgingival: below the gumline.
- Supragingival: above the gumline.

3.2 Dental Radiography

Dental radiography is a vital tool in veterinary dentistry, assisting in diagnosis, treatment planning, and monitoring of oral diseases (DuPont and

DeBowes, 2009), as well as being an integral part of the medical record. It is not possible to give our patients proper dental care without dental radiographs, because most dental pathology lies below the gingival margin (Niemiec *et al.*, 2020).

Dental radiographs provide accurate diagnosis of periodontal and endodontic disease, enable visualization of the tooth root structure and periodontal tissues, aid in assessment of oral masses, allow evaluation of the mandibles and maxillae in cases of oral trauma, differentiate between missing vs unerupted teeth, help determine appropriate treatment(s), document the dental procedures performed, follow the progress of therapeutic programs, and aid in client education (Niemiec *et al.*, 2020).

All patients undergoing COHATs should receive full-mouth dental radiographs, since many problems beneath the gumline might otherwise go undiagnosed (Niemiec, 2011). Dental radiographs are essential in diagnosing pathology including periodontal disease, fractured teeth, non-vital teeth, tooth and root resorption, oral masses, facial swellings, draining tracts, painful or sensitive teeth, nasal discharge and/or epistaxis, jaw fractures, malocclusions or missing teeth. Radiographs should be taken of all teeth that are to be extracted for any reason (Holmstrom *et al.*, 2013).

Postoperative radiographs should be taken after any dental procedure, particularly extractions, to ensure no root remnants have been left behind and no iatrogenic trauma such as jaw fracture has occurred during extraction (Holmstrom *et al.*, 2013). Radiographic documentation of treatment is good medicine, and protects the veterinary practice from potential litigation by pet owners if complications occur postoperatively.

3.2.1 Dental radiography units

Dental radiography units can be wall-mounted or freestanding, often on wheels to allow for easy movement. Most dental radiography units have a fixed kVp (Kilovoltage peak: the maximum electron energy produced by the X-ray tube), usually 60–70 kVp; and a fixed mA (milliamperage: the amount of electrical current used to generate electrons), usually 6–8 mA; with only the exposure time being variable (Niemiec, 2010). Dental radiographs require shorter exposure times than standard radiographs, since oral tissues are much less dense than larger areas of the body such as the torso and abdomen; therefore leaded walls are generally not required in the dental operatory (Canadian Dental Association (CDA), 2014). Digital dental radiography reduces exposure time even further, resulting in approximately 70% less radiation than standard dental radiography (the Canadian Academy of Dental Health & Community Sciences (CADH), 2014). If using a digital radiography system, the dental radiography unit must be capable of achieving very low exposure times (0.01–0.08 seconds, depending upon the system and software used) (DuPont and DeBowes,

2009). Some dental radiography units require the operator to input the exposure time in seconds on the control panel; other units control exposure time via feline vs canine options and settings for the type of tooth being radiographed (DuPont and DeBowes, 2009).

Dental X-ray tube heads produce the X-rays. They are lead-lined, attached to an adjustable arm, and can aim in any direction. Most have angle-degree number markings to aid in positioning (Bird, 2020).

Position indicating devices (PIDs), also called tubes or cones, are attached to the X-ray tube head and come in different lengths (DuPont and DeBowes, 2009). A longer PID allows more parallel rays from the centre of the X-ray beam to strike the area of interest, which improves image sharpness by reducing magnification and distortion (Williamson, 2006). This also results in less radiation exposure to the patient. The length of the PID determines the source-to-film distance, which is the distance between the source of X-rays and the film, X-ray sensor, or plate (Shaw and Voglewede, 2018). A longer source-to-film distance will result in less image magnification (Williamson, 2006). Object–film distance is the distance between the tooth and the X-ray film. The shorter the object–film distance, the less image magnification will occur (Berry, 2010).

3.2.2   Types of dental radiography systems

Three main types of dental radiography systems are used in veterinary dentistry: manual films, digital sensors, and phosphor plates that are read by a computer scanner (DuPont and DeBowes, 2009).

Digital sensors and phosphor plates both have several advantages over manual film systems. Less radiation is used to produce digital X-rays, the X-rays appear on the computer screen very quickly, images are high-quality and can be enlarged or enhanced for better detail and visualization of pathology (Luechtefeld, 2012). Digital images are easily transferred into a patient's computerized medical record (Bird, 2020), can be shared with veterinary dental specialists for further evaluation, emailed or printed to show pet owners pre- and postoperatively, and require no harmful chemicals to produce (Luechtefeld, 2012).

The disadvantages of digital sensors and phosphor plate systems are that they are more expensive (Bird, 2020), require the use of a computer and software, and are not portable unless the software is installed on a laptop computer.

3.2.3   Manual dental radiography systems

Manual dental radiography systems commonly use D-speed X-ray films and developing chemicals (Niemiec, 2010). Paper and foil-lined packets protect the film, which must be removed without exposure to light prior to development. This is done in a standard darkroom or a chairside developer (Bird, 2020): a plastic box containing a transparent red lid; light-impermeable hand holes; and containers of developer, fixer, rinse water, and film clips. Films are available in small (Size 0 and 1 films), medium (Size 2 films), long (Size 3 films), and large (Size 4 films) (Holmstrom *et al.*, 2000c).

3.2.4 Digital radiography (DR) systems

A DR dental radiography system consists of a digital, wired X-ray sensor that connects to a computer via USB port and requires the use of software (Heflin, 2018). Most sensors are comparable to a Size 2 manual film, but are thicker due to their plastic casing and the attached wire (DuPont and DeBowes, 2009; Heflin, 2018).

The sensor is exposed using a dental X-ray unit, and the image appears almost instantly upon the computer screen (DuPont and DeBowes, 2009). Since sensor size is limited, more than one image may be required to visualize large teeth (Bird, 2020), and the thickness of the sensor can make obtaining views in small patients and tight spaces more challenging (Heflin, 2018). Sensors have a long lifespan, but cost thousands of dollars, so take care not to damage them. Inadequately sedated or anaesthetized patients can bite and ruin the sensor.

3.2.5 Computed radiography (CR) systems

CR dental radiography systems use phosphor plates similar in size and shape to manual X-ray films, but require the use of a computer and software.

The plate is placed within a plastic cover to protect it from fluids and debris within the patient's mouth during exposure. The plastic cover is opened and the plate is fed into a scanner that transfers the image to the computer and removes the image from the plate, allowing the plate to be used again (Woodward, 2020). Because of this extra scanning step, CR systems do not produce an image quite as quickly as DR systems; however, because of the variable sizes and thinness of the phosphor plates in comparison with DR sensors, they are easier to use (Heflin, 2018) and the time required to produce a set of full-mouth X-rays is often comparable.

Digital phosphor plates have a lifespan of approximately 300–600 uses unless they become bent or scratched, and are much less expensive to replace than DR sensors (Woodward, 2020).

3.2.6 Producing diagnostic dental radiographs

A diagnostic dental radiograph must display (Devulapalli, 2015; Tompe and Sargar, 2020):

- Good density and contrast.
- Sharp outlines.
- An image that is the same shape and size as the object of interest.

Density refers to the overall darkness of a dental radiograph (Dalgarno, 2014). Radiographs with correct density reveal air as black areas upon the radiograph, while enamel, dentin and bone appear white. Grey areas indicate soft tissue. Increasing the exposure time will increase the image density, making the image appear darker, while decreasing the exposure time will decrease the image density, making the image appear lighter.

Contrast refers to the difference in the degrees of darkness between adjacent areas on a dental radiograph (Dalgarno, 2014). A radiograph that contains both very light and very dark areas has high contrast, while a radiograph that contains many shades of grey has low contrast. Contrast is determined primarily by the kVp (Geha, 2019). A higher kVp produces images with low contrast, while a low kVp produces images with high contrast (Berry, 2010). Since the kVp of most dental radiography units is fixed, many digital dental radiography software packages allow the operator to manipulate an image's contrast once an image has been obtained. In digital radiography, contrast also depends upon the bit-depth of the sensor or plate (Geha, 2019). Bit-depth denotes the number of possible grey values that can be stored in an image. The higher the bit-depth, the more values can be stored. In manual film radiography, the concentration and temperature of the developing solution and the developing time influences contrast (Diagnostic Imaging Systems (DIS), 2021). Scatter radiation decreases both contrast and density (DIS, 2021). Reduce scatter radiation by placing the end of the PID as close as possible to the patient (Bird, 2020).

The sharpness of an image determines the amount of detail visible upon the dental X-ray. Source-to-film distance influences sharpness, with a longer PID reducing the penumbra (blurring at the edges of an object on the radiograph), resulting in a sharper image. Object–film distance also affects sharpness, with a greater distance between the tooth and the film resulting in a less sharp image (Berry, 2010). Movement of either the X-ray tube or the patient while the X-ray is taken will also produce a blurred, less sharp image (Holmstrom *et al.*, 2000c).

To reduce image magnification, place the film, sensor or plate as close as possible to the tooth or structure to be radiographed. Use positioning aids such as gauze squares and paper towel, etc. to keep the film in its proper place in the mouth (Beckman, 2012). Do not bend or curve the film to make it fit, as this will cause distortion of the image (Leary, 2017).

Place film, digital X-ray sensors or digital phosphor plates so the leaded or non-exposure side is away from the X-ray beam and the object of interest, otherwise the film will be improperly exposed (Williamson, 2020). Most have the reverse or 'back' side labelled.

3.2.7   Radiation safety

The operator should stand at least 2 m from the primary beam, preferably behind a wall, and maintain a 90–135-degree angle from the path of the beam (CDA, 2005). Leaded gowns are not required unless the operator is unable to maintain these minimums (CDA, 2005). Dosimeter badges should be worn by everyone in the area, and the radiography unit must be regularly inspected (usually yearly) for radiation leakage by a professional according to local regulatory guidelines.

Use shortest exposure time necessary to obtain a diagnostic image, and do not hold film in mouth with fingers while exposing (Bird, 2020). Instead, use gauze squares, paper towel, or other positioning devices to hold the film, sensor, or digital plate in place (Beckman, 2012). Do not touch the X-ray tube head or cone while exposing.

3.2.8   Dental radiography positioning

Dental X-ray images are usually taken with the film, sensor or phosphor plate placed intra-orally (within the mouth). The least amount of distortion results when the film is parallel to the tooth and the X-ray beam is directed perpendicular to both (Woodward, 2012). This is only possible in dogs and cats in the caudal mandible (DuPont and DeBowes, 2009), where the film can be placed between the tongue and mandible, directly behind the area of interest. Because veterinary patients have a flat palate and a long mandibular symphysis, with tooth roots that extend backward, not up-and-down, films cannot be placed parallel to the teeth in the maxilla or near the mandibular symphysis (Holmstrom *et al.*, 2000c). In these areas, a technique called bisecting angle technique is used, which adjusts the angle of the X-ray beam to capture an image of the proper proportions of the teeth (Bird, 2020).

3.2.9   Bisecting angle technique

Bisecting angle technique uses geometry to allow accurate radiographic representations of teeth in areas of the mouth where parallel technique cannot be performed due to the spatial limitations of oral anatomy (DuPont and DeBowes, 2009).

A useful analogy to visualize bisecting angle technique is that of a tree and its shadow (Woodward, 2012). In this analogy, the tree represents the tooth, the sun represents the X-ray beam, and the tree's shadow represents the tooth's image upon the radiograph. In the morning when the sun is

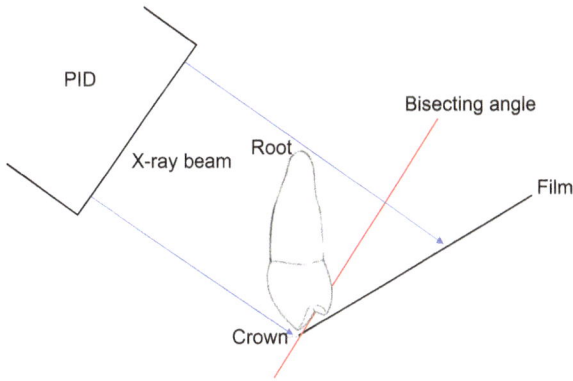

Fig. 3.2. Bisecting angle.

just rising, the shadow of the tree is longer than the tree itself. As the sun rises further, the shadow eventually becomes the same length as the tree. This is the bisecting angle. Eventually, the sun rises higher in the sky and the shadow becomes shorter than the tree.

Bisecting angle technique can take time to master, so practice on skull models or cadavers prior to attempting to obtain dental radiographs on live patients under general anaesthesia. Some distortion will inevitably occur at first, as accurately visualizing the correct angles can be challenging. When properly mastered, bisecting angle technique minimizes this distortion as much as possible.

1. Place the film, sensor or plate as close as possible to the tooth without bending the film. The cusp of the tooth's crown should be close to one edge of the film, with the rest of the film placed within the patient's mouth, sufficiently deep so the root tips and at least 2–3 mm of surrounding tissue can be captured upon the X-ray (Bird, 2020).
2. Visualize the angle created between the plane of the film and the long axis of the tooth (between the cusp of the crown and the root apex). Place cotton-tipped applicators or the handles of curettes or scalers along these lines to help visualize this angle (Bird, 2020).
3. Imagine a line that bisects this angle (cuts the angle into two equal halves) (DuPont and DeBowes, 2009).
4. Aim the X-ray beam perpendicular to this line (see Fig. 3.2) (DuPont and DeBowes, 2009).

Make a note of the angle degree on the X-ray tube head when taking dental radiographs. If you are consistent with placing each patient in the same recumbency for each radiograph (lateral, dorsal or sternal), you will find there are common degree angles for each view (Bird, 2020). The bisecting angles listed below apply to patients in lateral recumbency or in dorsal recumbency with the torso and head tilted laterally.

Bisecting angles for a patient in lateral recumbency (head parallel to table)

The following is as described by Bird (2020):

- Incisors: 0 degrees (PID is parallel to the table, aimed through rostral maxilla or mandible).
- Maxillary canines: 15–30 degrees (PID aimed down towards the table).
- Maxillary premolars and molars: 45 degrees (PID aimed down towards table).
- Mandibular canines: 0 degrees (PID parallel to the table, aiming through rostral mandible).
- Rostral mandible (first to third premolars): 45–55 degrees (film is placed across the mouth behind both mandibular canine teeth; PID aimed down towards table).

The exception to the bisecting angle technique is in the case of the caudal mandible (fourth premolars and molars). Here, the parallel technique is used (film placed directly behind teeth and the end of the PID is placed parallel to film).

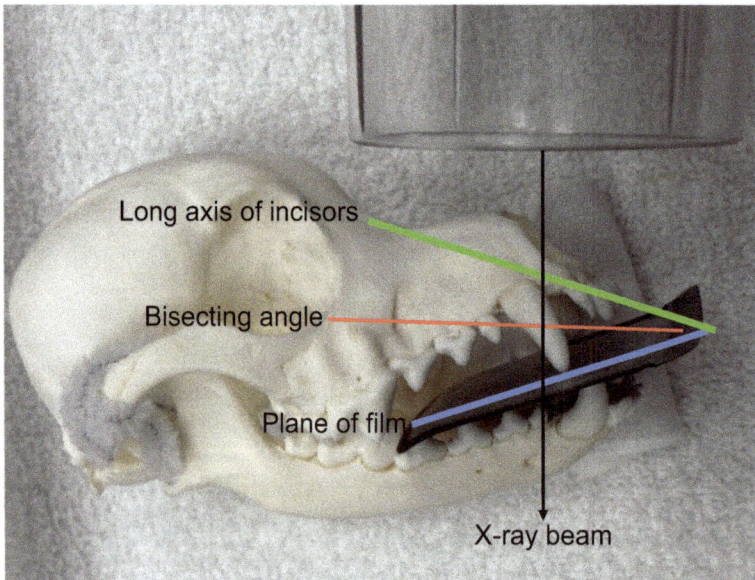

Fig. 3.3. Bisecting angle for incisors.

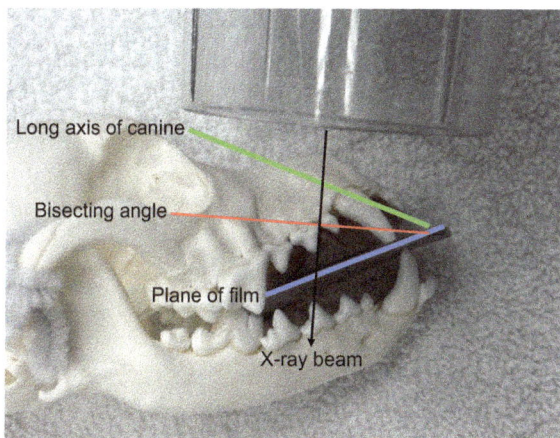

Fig. 3.4. Bisecting angle for maxillary canine (from side).

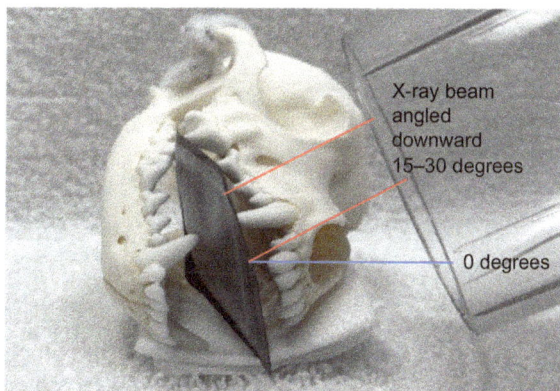

Fig. 3.5. Positioning shown in Fig. 3.4, for maxillary canine, from front.

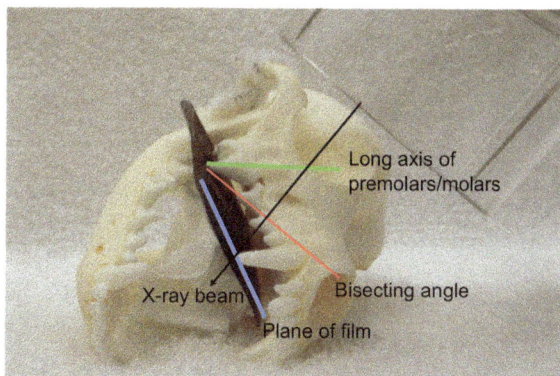

Fig. 3.6. Bisecting angle for maxillary premolars/molars.

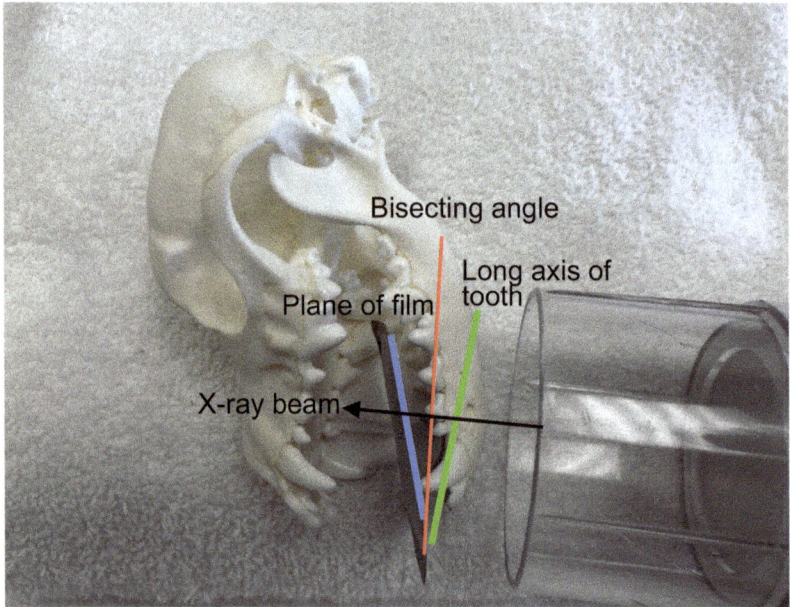

Fig. 3.7. Bisecting angle for mandibular canines and incisors.

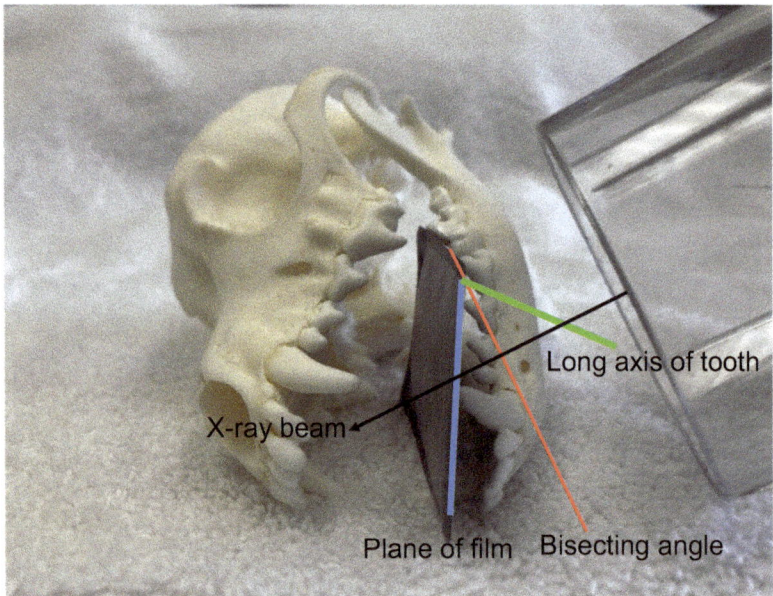

Fig. 3.8. Bisecting angle for rostral mandible.

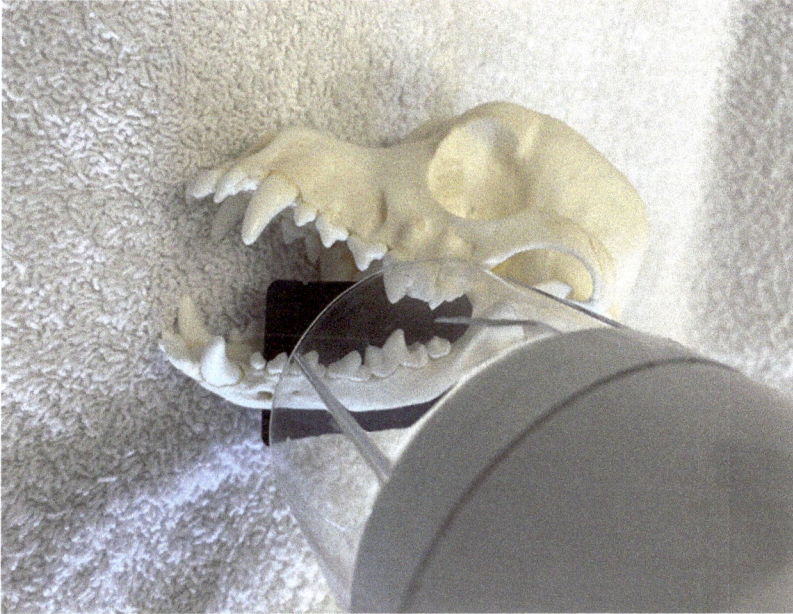

Fig. 3.9. Parallel technique for caudal mandible.

3.2.10 Troubleshooting dental radiograph positioning

Despite our best efforts, veterinary dental radiography takes time to learn and perfect. Knowing why mistakes occur and how to correct them reduces the number of retakes. Incorrect angles can produce artefacts that interfere with diagnosing oral pathologies, as follows:

- Lengthening: the tooth or object appears longer than the tooth is in reality. This happens when the X-ray beam is directed too perpendicular to the long axis of the tooth (DuPont and DeBowes, 2009). Remember the analogy about the sun and the tree casting a long shadow in the morning! Fix this problem by aiming the X-ray beam more parallel to the long axis of the tooth.
- Shortening: the tooth or object appears shorter on the film than it is in reality. This happens when the X-ray beam is directed too parallel to the long axis of the tooth (DuPont and DeBowes, 2009). Fix this problem by aiming the X-ray beam more perpendicular to the long axis of the tooth.

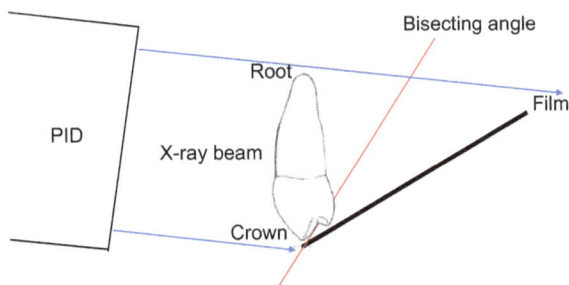

Fig. 3.10. 'Lengthening' artefact.

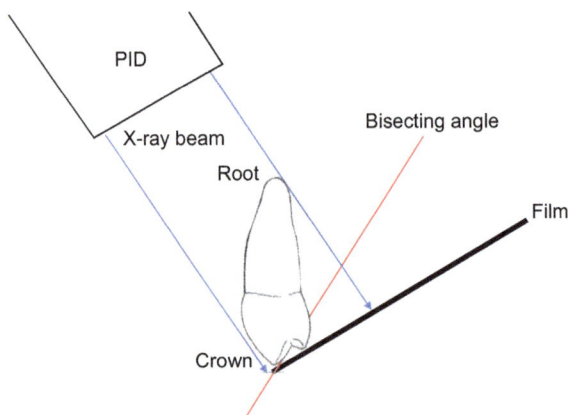

Fig. 3.11. 'Shortening' artefact.

- 'Cone cutting': a circular area of exposed film, while the rest of the film is blank (Bird, 2020). This is caused by improper positioning of the cone relative to the film. The area of interest may not be contained upon the exposed portion of the film. Fix this problem by ensuring the collimator tube head is positioned directly over the film, including the area of interest.
- Distortion: teeth or oral structures on the film appear larger, smaller, wider or otherwise distorted from reality (Williamson, 2020). Distortion is caused by curving or bending the film or phosphor plate to fit within the mouth, placing the film unevenly in the mouth (film is placed in contact with the crown of one tooth but further away from the crown of another) or improper beam angulation (aiming the X-ray beam on a slant rather than perpendicular to a tooth or group of teeth) (Williamson, 2020). Solve this problem by ensuring the film is not curved or bent within the mouth, by placing the film at an equal distance to all teeth being radiographed, and aiming the X-ray beam directly at the area of interest.

- Blurred image: caused by motion, either of the patient or the collimator (Holmstrom *et al.*, 2000c). Correct this problem by ensuring the patient remains in an appropriate plane of anaesthesia and that all screws in the adjustable arm of the dental X-ray unit are sufficiently tight, so the arm doesn't swing during exposure.

3.2.11 Extra-oral technique

Use this technique to prevent superimposition of the zygomatic arch upon the maxillary premolars in dental X-rays of the cat (Royal Veterinary College (RVC), 2002b). Extra-oral techniques are also used to X-ray the teeth of small mammals such as rabbits and guinea pigs when dental films are too large to fit in their mouths (see Chapter 10). Extra-oral technique may also be necessary in cases where a patient's mouth cannot be opened wide enough to insert a film or sensor, e.g. some temporomandibular joint (TMJ) conditions, craniomandibular osteopathy, and some oral tumours (Johnston, 2001).

When viewing extra-oral films, what appears to be a film taken of the left maxilla will actually be a film of the *right* maxilla, and vice versa. Most digital radiography software programs will allow you to flip the image horizontally (horizontal mirroring) to compensate for this, while other programs will allow notations of Triadan tooth numbers on the image.

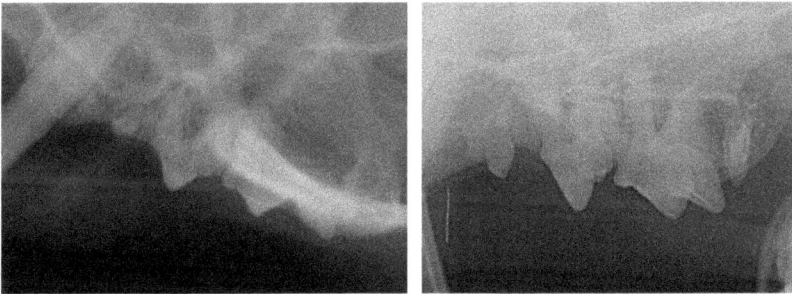

Fig. 3.12. Intra-oral (left) vs extra-oral (right) radiograph of cat maxilla.

Extra-oral technique for cat upper premolars

1. Place the cat in lateral recumbency. The image obtained will be of the maxilla that is facing down (closest to the table).
2. Use a radiolucent mouth gag between the upper and lower canine teeth to keep the mouth open. Syringe cases or cut endotracheal tubes are good for this.
3. Place a Size 2 or 4 film, sensor or digital plate on the table directly beneath the patient's maxilla. Ensure no other objects, i.e. ET tube, tube tie, mouth gag, etc. are over the area of interest.

4. Aim the X-ray beam through the patient's open mouth at approximately 65 degrees (refer to the degree marker on the X-ray tube head) (RVC, 2002b). The exposure time may need to be increased as there is a greater distance between the tube head and the area of interest.

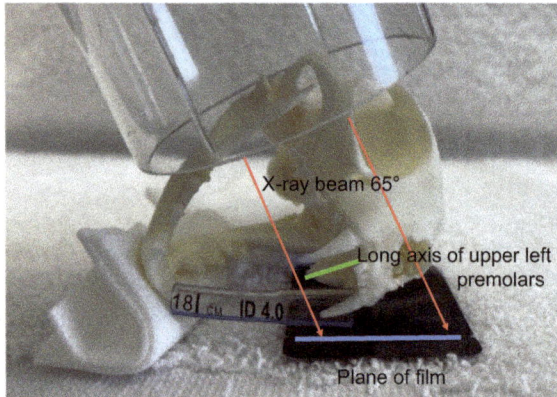

Fig. 3.13. Extra-oral technique.

3.2.12   Localizing techniques

Localizing techniques are useful because radiographs can provide only two-dimensional images, while oral structures are three-dimensional. Two-dimensional images do not permit differentiation between buccal and lingual planes (Holmstrom *et al.*, 2000c). This is usually not a problem, as most teeth in the mouth have only one or two roots in the same horizontal plane, which do not overlap on dental films. However, when dealing with three-rooted teeth, distinguishing between overlapping roots in buccal and palatal planes on dental radiographs is essential in order to accurately diagnose and treat dental pathologies.

One common localizing technique is known as the tube shift technique (Bird, 2020). Use this technique to distinguish between the mesiobuccal and mesiopalatal (referred to as 'lingual' in this technique) roots of upper fourth premolars. This is also known as the SLOB rule ('same lingual, opposite buccal') (Holmstrom *et al.*, 2000c).

The tube head is moved either mesially or distally in the horizontal plane while not changing the bisecting angle. For example, if the tube is moved mesially (the X-ray beam is no longer perpendicular to the tooth, but aimed from rostral to caudal), then the mesial root that appears more rostrally on the film is the mesiopalatal (lingual) root, and the mesial root that appears more distally on the film is the mesiobuccal root. If the tube head is moved distally (the X-ray beam is aimed from caudal to rostral), then the mesial root that appears more distally on the film is the mesiopalatal (lingual) root, and the mesial root that appears more rostrally on the film is the mesiobuccal root (Holmstrom *et al.*, 2000c; Bird, 2020).

3.2.13 Orienting dental radiographs

The following is as described by Gawor (2018) and Bird (2020).

- Always rotate radiographs so maxillary roots point up and man-dibular roots point down. To determine which views are maxillary vs mandibular, use the following anatomical references. Maxillary views will include dark, paired palatine fissures on images taken of the incisor and canine teeth, with a white line (alveolar process) above the roots of the maxillary premolars. Mandibular views will include the mandibular symphysis as a dark line bisecting the bone on incisor/canine views, and the wide mandibular canal below the mandibular premolars.
- Digital radiographs taken of the left side of the mouth will appear on the right side of the computer screen and vice versa, as though the patient is facing you. This is known as labial orientation (see Fig. 3.14).
- When orienting manual films, place the raised dot toward you. Rotate the film so the maxillary roots are up and the mandibular roots are down. Imagine the patient is facing you. If the more mesial teeth are towards the right side of the film, that is the right side of the patient, and vice versa.

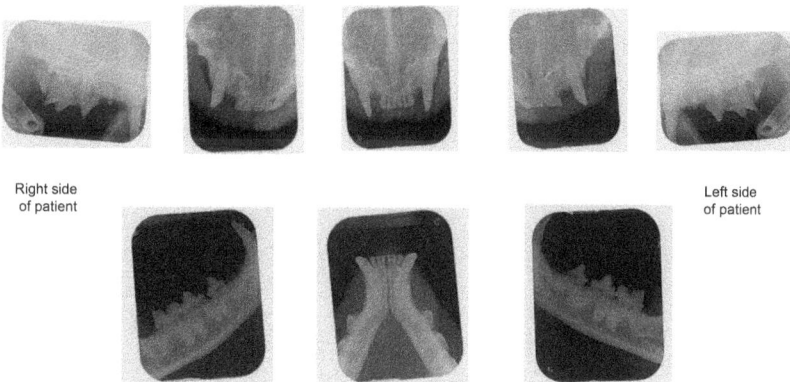

Right side
of patient

Left side
of patient

Fig. 3.14. Labial orientation of full-mouth radiographs.

3.2.14 Distinguishing normal vs abnormal from dental radiographs

Diagnosing pathology on dental radiographs is the responsibility of the veterinarian, not the veterinary nurse. However, it is useful to know what normal vs abnormal radiographs look like, in order to be better able to obtain diagnostic-quality dental radiographs, to understand how dental pathologies progress, and to explain pathology and procedures to pet owners.

Normal dental radiographic anatomy

Most dental radiographs are obtained to assess the tooth and supporting tissues below the gumline. The following describes the appearance of normal, healthy periodontium on radiographs (Niemiec, 2007; Peralta, 2017a; Bird, 2020).

- Bone: should appear slightly more radiopaque than the tooth roots. Normal bone appears mottled and relatively uniform throughout. Bone should fill the furcation (area between the roots), and rise to the cementoenamel junction or 'neck' of the tooth.
- Root canals/pulp chambers: the canals of a patient's contralateral teeth (i.e. both upper canines, or both lower carnassials) should be the same width.
- Periodontal ligament space: a uniform, thin, dark line should be seen around each tooth root.
- Mandibular symphysis: should appear as a radiolucent line between the lower central incisors. In cats a 'zigzag' pattern is normal.
- Palatine fissures: paired radiolucent areas, of equal size and shape, distal to the upper incisors, should appear on views obtained of the rostral maxillary area.

Abnormal pathology on dental radiographs

- Vertical bone loss: an area of vertical bone reduction, with the surrounding bone being higher (uneven bone height around adjacent roots) (Niemiec, 2007).
- Horizontal bone loss: generalized bone loss of a similar level affecting the bone surrounding one tooth or teeth (bone is approximately the same height around adjacent roots) (Bird, 2020).
- Periapical lucency: a radiolucent area in the bone around the root or the root apex (Peralta, 2017b). Do not mistake the radiolucent mental foramina (mandibular first and second premolars) or infraorbital canal (maxillary third and sometimes fourth premolars) for periapical lucencies (Neimiec, 2007). If in doubt, expose another film using a slightly different horizontal angle. If the lucency is still centred over the root apex, it likely indicates true pathology (Woodward, 2012).
- Widened periodontal ligament: can indicate inflammation due to periodontal disease, malignant or locally aggressive lesions, orthodontic trauma resulting in excessive pressure or force upon a tooth, osteomyelitis, osteosarcoma or pulpitis (DuPont and DeBowes, 2009).

- Differing root canal diameters in contralateral teeth: since dentin deposition in teeth of the same type occurs at similar rates as a pet ages, a wider canal indicates a non-vital tooth due to the cessation of dentin deposition (Niemiec, 2007; Peralta, 2017b).
- Tooth resorption (AVDC, 2021b): teeth with Type I resorption will have normal root density in some areas, a well-defined periodontal ligament space, and a visible root canal. Teeth with Type II resorption will have different radiographic density as opposed to the surrounding teeth, areas with no discernible periodontal ligament space or root canal, and in later stages will have little discernible root structure. In multi-rooted teeth, each root may be undergoing a different type of tooth resorption, termed Type III resorption.
- Caries: radiolucent areas in the enamel, usually on the occlusal surface of the upper first and second molars in dogs (Niemiec, 2007; Lewis, 2015).
- Bone fractures: oral traumatic injuries appear radiographically similar to fractures of long bones. Mandibular symphyseal separation appears as a widened radiolucent space between the lower central incisors (Peralta, 2017b).
- Oral masses: some can invade bone, initially causing a 'moth-eaten' appearance (Peralta, 2017b), later appearing radiographically as an irregular, ragged area of bone destruction with teeth 'floating' in soft tissue (Niemiec, 2012). Oral masses may also cause bone expansion, resulting in tooth movement with distinct bony margins (Niemiec, 2007, 2012). Note: histological testing is necessary for diagnosis of oral masses because malignant, benign and infectious processes can appear similar radiographically (Niemiec, 2007).

3.3　Pain Management for Dental Procedures

Pain recognition and management is challenging in pets, because they often avoid showing signs of pain (Muir, 2002; Holzman, 2006). Animals showing signs of pain in the wild become easy targets for predators, so they have evolved to hide their pain (Stellfox and Richardson, 2019). This doesn't mean they don't feel it! Dental pain, aside from the severe pain associated with stomatitis, jaw fractures, oral cancers and a few other very painful conditions, is usually hidden by the animal, who will continue to eat (often chewing on the non-painful side of the mouth) (Lewis, 2017) until either the pain is alleviated, i.e. the compromised tooth falls out and the tissues heal; the resorbing tooth resorbs completely and the gingiva grows over it (Bellows, 2016); or until the pain becomes so severe that the animal eventually stops eating and becomes debilitated. Neglecting to recognize and treat this dental pain is inhumane (Shivni, 2015).

Pain can also cause physiological stress, prolonging recovery from anaesthesia and delaying healing (Niemiec, 2004; Berg, 2010). This is especially concerning in patients who are already suffering from conditions such as heart, renal or liver disease; diabetes; or thyroid issues (Mills, 2020). Since many animals who suffer from periodontal disease are older, the chance that they have a concurrent health condition is high, making proper pain management critical for a successful outcome (Snyder, 2010; Mills, 2020).

3.3.1 Physiology of pain

Pain response is a complex series of physiochemical interactions. The brain's processing of a noxious stimulus is called nociception (Beckman, 2006). This processing results in the perception of pain (Holzman, 2006). Nociception consists of three parts, and pain perception can be blocked or controlled at each of these (Muir, 2002; Holzman, 2006).

1. Transduction: the conversion of unpleasant sensations into electrical impulses by free afferent nerve endings (Holzman, 2006). In dental patients, this occurs within the oral cavity (Beckman, 2004).
2. Transmission: the afferent nerve fibres transmit these electrical impulses to the brain (Holzman, 2006). There are two categories of afferent nerves, each responsible for a different type of pain perception: A-delta (fast) fibres, responsible for sharp, stabbing pain (e.g. tooth fracture); and C (slow) fibres, responsible for dull, throbbing pain (e.g. tooth abscess) (Beckman, 2006; Mills, 2012).
3. Modulation: synapses of neurons in the medulla lead to the brain's perception of pain (Holzman, 2006; Berg, 2010).

Tooth-related pain can originate in the pulp, the dentin or the periodontal ligament (Lyon, 2001). Pain can also result from inflammation or trauma to the gingiva, mucosa or other oral tissues such as the hard and soft palate. Surgical extractions result in pain secondary to inflammation and nerve stimulation (Mills, 2016). Gingival incisions, gingival elevation and mucogingival flaps produce more postoperative pain than simple extractions not involving soft tissues (Beckman, 2007). The intensity of acute pain, such as a tooth fracture or oral surgery, is greatest within 24–72 hours after injury (Perrone, 2011; Stellfox and Richardson, 2019).

Factors influencing pain include the patient's health status (debilitated patients are less capable of tolerating pain), age (young patients generally have a lower tolerance to acute pain, but are less sensitive to emotional stress and anxiety associated with painful procedures), breed (some breeds, such as Huskies, seem to have a lower pain tolerance), and other factors such as body temperature, the need to urinate or defaecate, hunger, unfamiliar vs home environment, and lack of attention (National Research Council (US) Committee on Pain and Distress in Laboratory Animals (NRC), 1992; Sakman, 1994; Gruen *et al.*, 2020).

3.3.2 Multimodal pain management

The goal of managing dental pain is to decrease the pain associated with the underlying dental disease while also decreasing or eliminating the acute pain caused by the dental procedure itself (Stellfox and Richardson, 2019). A multimodal approach best achieves this goal (Kimberlin, 2010). Multimodal pain management combines drugs and methods of their administration (Stellfox and Richardson, 2019) to act on different portions of the pain pathway, providing pain relief before, during and after a dental procedure (Holzman, 2006).

Once a patient's perception of pain begins, the central nervous system (CNS) becomes more sensitized to noxious stimuli (Mills, 2012). This is known as wind-up pain (Kressler, 2012a). Dental patients commonly experience wind-up pain, since they are often in pain from chronic periodontal disease or other dental conditions long before pain management is implemented (Beckman, 2007). Patients experiencing wind-up pain require higher doses of drugs to achieve pain relief (Holzman, 2006), and may not achieve the same level of pain relief as patients not experiencing wind-up pain (Stellfox and Richardson, 2019). Providing pain relief before a painful procedure begins will decrease the total dose of analgesic drugs required (Beckman, 2006), increasing patient safety (Kressler, 2012a). It also decreases the need for high concentrations of inhalant anaesthetics during the procedure (Holzman, 2006; Snyder, 2010), and decreases the intensity and duration of postoperative pain (Mills, 2020).

3.3.3 Preoperative pain management

Systemic analgesics given prior to anaesthesia as part of a patient's premedication provide preoperative pain management (Holzman, 2006). The choice of analgesic(s) given is determined by many factors, including: the patient's age, body condition and pre-existing medical conditions such as heart or liver disease; the pain expected to be caused by the procedure (e.g. full-mouth extractions would be expected to cause more pain than a single extraction); the cost of the drug; its side effects (such as profound sedation, which may be undesirable if the patient is expected to be discharged soon after the procedure); and the veterinarian's familiarity with the drug (Berg, 2010).

Opioids such as morphine, hydromorphone, buprenorphine and butorphanol modulate pain perception both centrally (in the brain) and locally (at the site of pain transduction) (Holzman, 2006), and are often part of a patient's premedication cocktail (Pablo, 2008). Alpha-2 agonists such as dexmedetomidine block the transmission of pain (Holzman, 2006), and can also be included in premedication protocols (Mills, 2020). Non-steroidal anti-inflammatory drugs (NSAIDs) such as meloxicam can be given preoperatively to most patients (Stellfox and Richardson, 2019), though they are contraindicated in animals with gastrointestinal (GI) disease, coagulopathies or reduced liver or kidney function, or who are receiving corticosteroids (Pablo, 2008). These drugs work at the sites of transduction and modulation (Holzman, 2006).

Preoperative pain management can also consist of intravenous continuous rate infusions (CRIs) of opioids, N-methyl-D-aspartate (NMDA)-receptor antagonists such as ketamine (Beckman, 2004), and other drugs prior to and during the procedure. These are employed preoperatively if the procedure is expected to be particularly painful, such as in the case of full-mouth extractions, mandibulectomies or maxillofacial reconstruction (Mills, 2020).

3.3.4   Intraoperative pain management

In veterinary dentistry, the most common modality of intraoperative pain management is regional nerve blocks, administered at least several minutes prior to a painful procedure (Holzman, 2006; Mills, 2020). Regional nerve blocks control pain by inhibiting nerve transduction at the site of the procedure and transmission of pain signals to the brain (Snyder, 2010; Mills, 2020). If given at too high a dose or administered intravenously instead of locally, these drugs can cause cardiac depression, seizures, respiratory distress, and nerve and soft tissue damage (Holzman, 2006; Snyder, 2010). When administered appropriately, however, they are safe for almost every patient, with a low risk of toxicity, no sedation and a predictable duration of pain control. Pet owners are familiar with how nerve blocks reduce pain perception because they have experienced them first-hand in their own dentist's chair.

Nerve blocks are performed by injecting local anaesthetic in the immediate vicinity of a peripheral nerve or nerve plexus. They provide excellent analgesia (Snyder, 2010), diminish the wind-up response of the CNS to pain stimuli if administered before oral surgery begins (Holzman, 2006), can reduce the amount of inhalation anaesthetic needed to perform a procedure (Kressler, 2012b), and provide pain control during recovery.

CRIs of opioids, NMDA-receptor antagonists and other drugs can also be employed at any time during the procedure if the patient's pain does not appear to be controlled by the methods discussed above (Niemiec, 2004; Beckman, 2006).

Top-ups of opioids can be given intravenously during a procedure, especially during long procedures when the duration of action of the initial dose of the opioid is suspected to have been exceeded.

3.3.5   Postoperative pain management

The most common postoperative pain medications used in veterinary dentistry are NSAIDs such as meloxicam; opioids such as buprenorphine, fentanyl and tramadol; and other medications such as gabapentin (Pablo, 2008; Mathews *et al.*, 2014). These may be given postoperatively in hospital by injection, and/or sent home for the owner to administer orally for several days or weeks after the procedure (Mills, 2020). The owner must be made aware of any expected side effects such as drowsiness, and should also monitor the pet carefully for any undesirable side effects, such as GI upset, etc.

Liquid medications or small tablets that can be hidden in soft food are usually easier for owners to administer (Mills, 2020), since pets are often reluctant to have their sore mouths manipulated in order to administer large pills and capsules. Pet owners may also be reluctant or squeamish about handling their pet's mouth postoperatively.

3.3.6 Pain assessment and monitoring

Pain can be difficult to recognize or tease out from other conditions such as anxiety in our hospitalized small animal patients (Tabor, 2016). Regardless, every dental patient should receive pain assessments while in hospital, particularly when recovering from a procedure, to properly recognize and address any postoperative discomfort (Berg, 2010). Colorado State University has developed downloadable pain scale charts for both canines and felines (CSU, 2006a, b).

3.3.7 Dental regional nerve blocks

Materials and local anaesthetics

The following is as described by Kressler (2012b).

- Syringe (1–3-ml syringe, or aspirating syringe that accepts carpules of local anaesthetic).
- 25–27 gauge, 19–38-mm needle.
- Bupivacaine 0.5% (with or without epinephrine).
- Lidocaine 2% (with or without epinephrine).

Local anaesthetic drugs

Commonly used local anaesthetic drugs in veterinary dentistry include bupivacaine and lidocaine (Kressler, 2012b). These agents are generally safe, non-allergenic, metabolized by the liver, and excreted by the kidneys (Gracis, 2015). They cause vasodilation at the site of administration, which increases systemic absorption and decreases the duration of action (Hale, 2007). To counter this, a vasoconstrictor such as epinephrine is often added. Epinephrine decreases the rate of systemic absorption, reducing the risk of systemic toxicity, increases the duration of action by approximately 50% (Niemiec, 2004; Theuns, 2008), and decreases local haemorrhage (Mills, 2020).

When using bupivacaine, do not exceed a maximum cumulative dose of 2.0 mg/kg in dogs, and 1.5 mg/kg in cats (Kressler, 2012b). When using lidocaine, do not exceed a maximum cumulative dose of 5 mg/kg in dogs, and 1 mg/kg in cats (Kressler, 2012b). If blocking the whole mouth, calculate the maximum cumulative dose volume, then divide by four (one block per quadrant), and ensure that this amount is the maximum volume administered per quadrant. In general, 1.0 mg/kg should be enough to provide adequate analgesia.

Bupivacaine (+/- epinephrine) is available in bulk bottles or in carpules as 0.5% or 5 mg/ml. A 1.8-ml carpule that fits into an aspirating syringe contains a total of 9 mg (Hale, 2007). As a rule of thumb, 0.1–0.3 ml per site is sufficient for cats and dogs weighing 6 kg or less; 0.3–0.6 ml per site is sufficient for dogs weighing 6–25 kg; and 0.7–1.0 ml per site is sufficient for dogs weighing over 25 kg (Beckman, 2014). Bupivacaine has an onset time of 15–30 minutes (Theuns, 2008). This means that it must be administered 15 to 30 minutes prior to oral surgery in order to be effective, so administration of the block(s) should be done as soon as it is known where oral surgery is to occur. Bupivacaine's duration of action is 4–6 hours (Niemiec, 2004; Theuns, 2008) which makes it ideal for most veterinary dental procedures, as the patient will remain comfortable during surgery and for a few hours after recovery, at which point oral postoperative pain medications can be given.

Adding buprenorphine (0.003 mg/kg) to the bupivacaine may increase the duration of effect for regional nerve blocks by up to 96 hours (Pablo, 2008; Mulherin and Riha, 2019).

Lidocaine (+/- epinephrine) is available in bulk bottles or carpules at 2.0% or 20 mg/ml. A 1.8-ml carpule contains a total of 36 mg (Hale, 2007). Lidocaine can be diluted with saline to achieve the small volumes required in very small patients. Lidocaine's onset time is 5–15 minutes, which is quicker than bupivacaine, but its duration of action is only 1–2 hours (Niemiec, 2004; Theuns, 2008).

3.3.8 Complications and adverse effects of dental regional nerve blocks

Complications of dental regional nerve blocks include inoculation of infection into deeper tissues (Krug, 2010). This can be avoided by cleaning the teeth and rinsing the oral tissue at the site of injection with chlorhexidine prior to block administration. Regional nerve blocks can also result in physical trauma to nerves and vessels. Minimize this by using the smallest gauge needle available, and introducing, advancing and withdrawing the needle as slowly and gently as possible (Beckman, 2004). Intravascular injection of drugs containing epinephrine can cause tachycardia, seizures and arrhythmias. Lidocaine toxicity produces neurological signs such as sedation, twitching, coma and respiratory arrest, while bupivacaine toxicity results in cardiologic signs including arrhythmias, bradycardia and cardiac arrest (Mulherin and Riha, 2019). Treat local anaesthetic toxicity with intravenous lipid emulsion (ILE) administration and supportive therapies such as intravenous fluids, oxygen administration, mechanical ventilation and cardiovascular drugs (Keating, 2016).

Cats are more sensitive to local anaesthetics than dogs, so the amount of lidocaine used to desensitize the larynx should be factored in when calculating their safe maximum dose of local anaesthetic (Keating, 2016).

Properly blocked patients should not respond to surgical stimuli such as cutting soft tissue, sectioning and extracting teeth, or performing endodontic treatment while under general anaesthesia (Beckman, 2014). If a patient's heart, respiration rate or blood pressure increase (Forsyth, 2003), the block may have been improperly placed or inadequately dosed, or has not yet taken effect. Wait for the block to take effect, try performing the block again (as long as the patient has not received their maximum safe dose of local anaesthetic) (Beckman, 2014), or add additional intraoperative pain-control measures such as CRIs (Beckman, 2006).

3.3.9 Common veterinary dental regional nerve blocks

Inferior alveolar (mandibular) nerve block (see Fig. 3.15)

Provides analgesia to the bone, all teeth, soft tissue and palatal tissue of the mandible on the infiltrated side (Berg, 2010).

1. Palpate the notch on the caudal ventral mandible just cranial to the angular process (Berg, 2010). If you cannot palpate the notch, select the point on the ventral mandible located on a vertical plane with the lateral canthus of the eye (Beckman, 2004).
2. Insert the needle intra-orally distal to the last molar at the lingual aspect of the ventral mandible at a 30-degree angle from the long axis of the mandible, or extra-orally vertically through the skin of the ventral mandible (Kressler, 2012b; Mills, 2020). In either case, keep the needle close to the surface of the mandible to prevent blocking the lingual nerve, which can result in self-trauma to the tongue during recovery (Krug, 2010; Kressler, 2012b).
3. Advance the needle to the midpoint between the ventral and dorsal borders of the mandible (approximately 0.5–1.5 cm in dogs; 0.5 cm in cats) (Kressler, 2012b), aiming toward the notch on the caudal mandible.
4. Aspirate back, and if no blood appears in the needle hub, slowly inject (Berg, 2010).
5. Hold digital pressure over the injection site for 30–60 seconds (Berg, 2010; Mills, 2020).

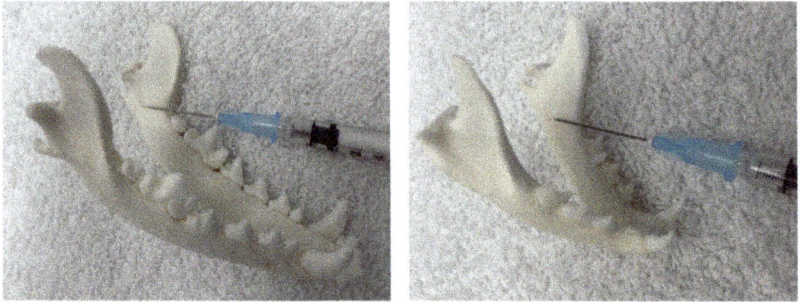

Fig. 3.15. Inferior alveolar nerve block: dog (left) and cat (right).

Maxillary nerve block (see Fig. 3.16)

Provides analgesia to the bone, all teeth, soft tissue and palatal tissue of the maxilla on the infiltrated side (Pablo, 2008).

1. With the patient's mouth open, insert the needle directly caudal to the bone surrounding the last maxillary molar (Beckman, 2004).
2. Hold the needle perpendicular to the hard palate and advance the needle until the depth of the needle extends just to the level of the root tips of the last molar (Beckman, 2004): approximately 1 cm in dogs and 0.5 cm in cats (Kressler, 2012b).
3. Aspirate back, and if no blood appears in the needle hub, slowly inject (Berg, 2010).
4. Withdraw the needle and apply digital pressure over the injection site for 30–60 seconds (Berg, 2010; Mills, 2020).

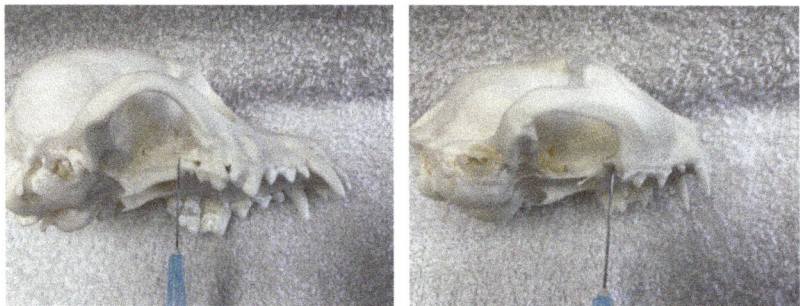

Fig. 3.16. Maxillary nerve block: dog (left) and cat (right).

Infraorbital nerve block (see Fig. 3.17)

Anaesthetizes the bone, soft tissue, and dentition rostral to and including the upper third premolar (Pablo, 2008). Caution is recommended in cats and brachycephalic breeds, as the infraorbital canal is very short, and advancing the needle may place it below or within the eyeball (Niemiec *et al.*, 2020). In these patients, advance the needle approximately 2 mm (Niemiec *et al.*, 2020) or use the maxillary nerve block instead.

1. Palpate the infraorbital foramen in the maxilla dorsal to the distal root of the maxillary third premolar (Beckman, 2004).
2. Insert the needle through the mucosa to the entrance of the foramen in a caudal direction (Beckman, 2004), holding the syringe parallel to the palate (Mills, 2020).
3. Aspirate back, and if no blood appears in the needle hub, slowly inject while holding digital pressure over the foramen (Berg, 2010).
4. Withdraw the needle and apply digital pressure over the canal for 30–60 seconds (Berg, 2010; Mills, 2020).

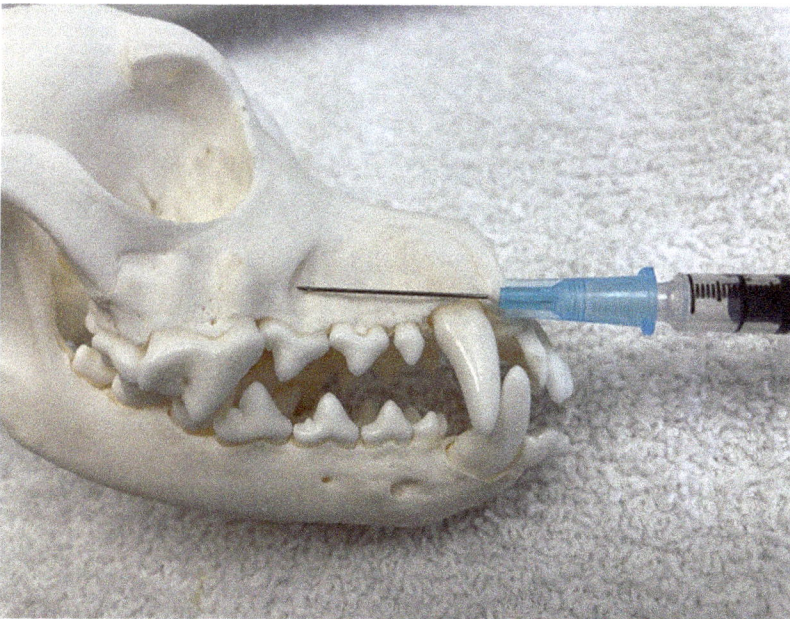

Fig. 3.17. Infraorbital nerve block: dog.

Mental nerve block (see Fig. 3.18)

Anaesthetizes all oral tissues rostral to the lower second premolar on the infiltrated side (Theuns, 2008; Berg, 2010). However, a 2010 study of this block found that it resulted in anaesthesia of only a small amount of soft tissue surrounding the lower premolars, with the canine teeth and incisors remaining unanaesthetized (Krug, 2010).

1. Palpate the middle mental foramen (the largest of the three mental foramina) just ventral to the mesial root of the second premolar (Beckman, 2004).
2. Advance the needle into the opening of the foramen in a rostral-to-caudal direction (Beckman, 2004).
3. Aspirate back, and if no blood appears in needle hub, slowly inject (Berg, 2010).
4. Withdraw the needle and apply digital pressure over the injection site for 30–60 seconds (Berg, 2010; Mills, 2020).

In cats and small dogs, the opening to the foramen cannot usually be palpated. The inferior alveolar block should be used in these patients instead (Berg, 2010; Niemiec *et al.*, 2020).

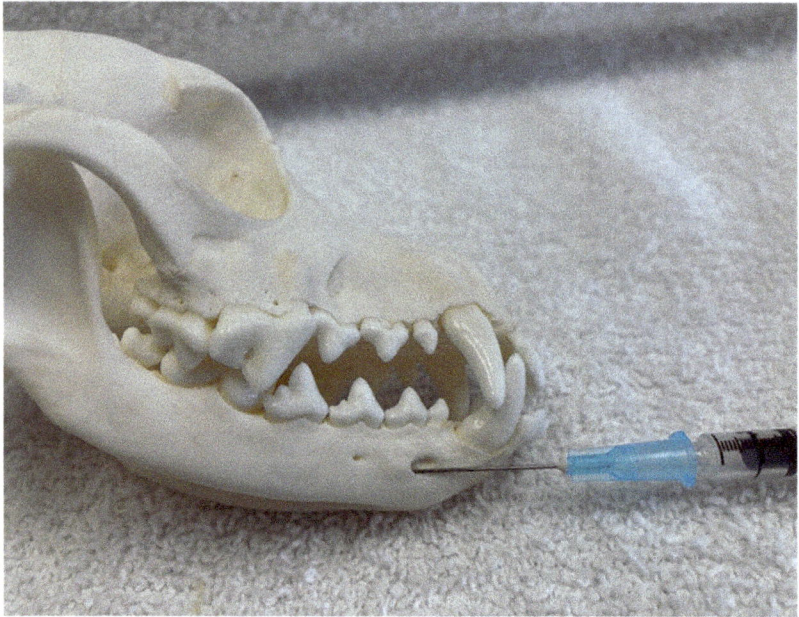

Fig. 3.18. Mental nerve block: dog.

References

AVDC (2021a) AVDC abbreviations. American Veterinary Dental College. Available at: https://avdc.org/technician-services/ (accessed 12 February 2021).

AVDC (2021b) AVDC nomenclature. American Veterinary Dental College. Available at: https://avdc.org/avdc-nomenclature/ (accessed 12 February 2021).

Beckman, B. (2004) Regional anesthesia and pain management for oral surgery part 1. In: *Proceedings of the 18th Annual Veterinary Dental Forum.* Omnipress, Madison, Wisconsin, pp. 33–37.

Beckman, B. (2006) Pathophysiology and management of surgical and chronic oral pain in dogs and cats. *Journal of Veterinary Dentistry* 23(1), 50–61. DOI: 10.1177/089875640602300110.

Beckman, B. (2007) Analgesic considerations for oral surgery. Veterinary Practice News. Available at: https://www.veterinarypracticenews.com/analgesic-considerations-for-oral-surgery/ (accessed 15 February 2021).

Beckman, B. (2012) Guide to common sense radiographic positioning. In: *Proceedings of the 26ᵗʰ Annual Veterinary Dental Forum*. Omnipress, Madison, Wisconsin (CD Rom).

Beckman, B. (2014) Nerve blocks for oral surgery in dogs. Clinician's Brief. Available at: https://www.cliniciansbrief.com/article/nerve-blocks-oral-surgery-dogs (accessed 15 February 2021).

Bellows, J. (2016) External tooth resorption in cats. Today's Veterinary Practice. Available at: https://todaysveterinarypractice.com/external-tooth-resorption-cats/ (accessed 15 February 2021).

Berg, M. (2010) Block that pain. In: *Proceedings of the 24th Annual Veterinary Dental Forum*. Omnipress, Madison, Wisconsin (CD Rom).

Berry, C.R. (2010) Basic physics and principles of making a great image: Part 2. Dvm360. Available at: https://www.dvm360.com/view/basic-physics-and-principles-making-great-image-part-2-proceedings (accessed 12 February 2021).

Bird, L. (2020) Dental radiology. In: Perrone, J. (ed.) *Small Animal Dental Procedures for Veterinary Technicians and Nurses*. Wiley Blackwell, Hoboken, New Jersey, pp. 93–130.

BVDA (2021) BVDA articles/dental charts. British Veterinary Dental Association. Available at: https://www.bvda.co.uk/bvda-articles/808-dental-charts (accessed 12 February 2021).

CADH (2014) Digital vs. conventional radiography in the dental office. The Canadian Academy of Dental Health & Community Sciences. Available at: https://www.canadianacademyofdentalhygiene.ca/blog/digital-vs-conventional-radiography-dental-office.html (accessed 12 February 2021).

CDA (2005) CDA position on control of x-radiation in dentistry. Canadian Dental Association. Available at: https://www.cda-adc.ca/en/about/position_statements/xray/ (accessed 13 February 2021).

CDA (2014) Radiation safety in dental practice. California Dental Association. Available at: https://www.cda.org/Portals/0/pdfs/practice_support/radiation_safety_in_dental_practice.pdf (accessed 12 February 2021).

CSU (2006a) Canine acute pain scale. Colorado State University. Available at: http://csu-cvmbs.colostate.edu/Documents/anesthesia-pain-management-pain-score-canine.pdf (accessed 9 September, 2020).

CSU (2006b) Feline acute pain scale. Colorado State University. Available at: http://csu-cvmbs.colostate.edu/Documents/anesthesia-pain-management-pain-score-feline.pdf (accessed 9 September, 2020).

Dalgarno, J. (2014) The use of radiographs in clinical dentistry. BDJ Team. Available at: https://www.nature.com/articles/bdjteam201426 (accessed 13 February 2021).

Devulapalli, R.V. (2015) Ideal radiography. Available at: https://www.slideshare.net/revathvyas/ideal-radiography (accessed 13 February 2021).

DIS (2021) Poor quality films – causes and corrections. Diagnostic Imaging Systems. Available at: https://vetxray.com/resource-center/continuing-education/poor-quality-films/ (accessed 13 February 2021).

Domnick, E.D. (2012) Dental charting – your best friend in medical records. In: *Proceedings of the 26th Annual Veterinary Dental Forum.* Omnipress, Madison, Wisconsin (CD Rom).

DuPont, G. and DeBowes, L. (2009) An introduction to dental radiography. In: DuPont, G. and DeBowes, L. (eds) *Atlas of Dental Radiography in Dogs and Cats.* Saunders Elsevier, Philadelphia, Pennsylvania, pp. 1–4.

Forsyth, S. (2003) Monitoring the anesthetized patient. World Small Animal Veterinary Association. Available at: https://www.vin.com/apputil/content/defaultadv1.aspx?pId=8768&catId=18831&id=3850246 (accessed 15 February 2021).

Gawor, J. (2018) Dental radiographic interpretation. In: Niemec, B.A., Gawor, J. and Jekl, V. (eds) *Practical Veterinary Dental Radiography.* CRC Press, Boca Raton, Florida, pp. 99–118.

Geha, H. (2019) The radiographic image. Dentalcare.com. Available at: https://www.dentalcare.com/en-us/professional-education/ce-courses/ce571/radiographic-contrast (accessed 13 February 2021).

Gracis, M. (2015) Techniques of locoregional anesthesia of the oral cavity. *World Small Animal Veterinary Association World Congress Proceedings, 2015.* Available at: https://www.vin.com/apputil/content/defaultadv1.aspx?id=7259186&pid=14365&print=1 (accessed 15 February 2021).

Gruen, M.E., White, P. and Hare, B. (2020) Do dog breeds differ in pain sensitivity? Veterinarians and the public believe they do. *PLOS ONE* 15(3), e0230315. Available at: https://journals.plos.org/plosone/article?id=10.1371/journal.pone.0230315 (accessed 15 February 2021).

Hale, F. (2007) Local anesthesia in veterinary dentistry. Hale Veterinary Clinic. Available at: http://www.toothvet.ca/PDFfiles/LocalAnesthesia.pdf (accessed 15 February 2021).

Heflin, M. (2018) Equipment focus: dental imaging. Veterinary Practice News. Available at: https://www.veterinarypracticenews.com/equipment-focus-dental-imaging/ (accessed 12 February 2021).

Holmstrom, S., Holmstrom, L.A., McGrath, C.J., Richey, M.T. and Wiggs, R.B. (2000a) The oral examination and disease recognition. In: Holmstrom, S. (ed.) *Veterinary Dentistry for the Technician & Office Staff.* Saunders, Philadelphia, Pennsylvania, pp. 23–64.

Holmstrom, S., Holmstrom, L.A., McGrath, C.J., Richey, M.T. and Wiggs, R.B. (2000b) Introduction. In: Holmstrom, S. (ed.) *Veterinary Dentistry for the Technician & Office Staff.* Saunders, Philadelphia, Pennsylvania, pp. 1–22.

Holmstrom, S., Holmstrom, L.A., McGrath, C.J., Richey, M.T. and Wiggs, R.B. (2000c) Dental radiology. In: Holmstrom, S. (ed.) *Veterinary Dentistry for the Technician & Office Staff.* Saunders, Philadelphia, Pennsylvania, pp. 223–246.

Holmstrom, S.E., Bellows, J., Juriga, S., Knutson, K., Niemiec, B.A. *et al.* (2013) AAHA dental care guidelines for dogs and cats. *Journal of the American Animal Hospital Association* 49(2), 75–82. DOI: 10.5326/JAAHA-MS-4013.

Holzman, G. (2006) Dental analgesic techniques. In: *Proceedings of the 20th Annual Veterinary Dental Forum.* Omnipress, Madison, Wisconsin, pp. 403–409.

Holzman, G. (2020) The basics. In: Perrone, J. (ed.) *Small Animal Dental Procedures for Veterinary Technicians and Nurses.* Wiley Blackwell, Hoboken, New Jersey, pp. 1–20.

Johnston, N. (2001) TMJs, extra oral radiographs and film interpretation. In: *World Small Animal Veterinary Association World Congress Proceedings, 2001.* Available at:

https://www.vin.com/apputil/content/defaultadv1.aspx?pId=8708&catI d=18044&id=3843695 (accessed 13 February 2021).

Keating, S. (2016) Small animal local and regional anesthesia. University of Illinois at Urbana-Champaign – Veterinary Medicine. Available at: https://vetmed. illinois.edu/wp-content/uploads/2016/09/75.-Keating-Local-and-Regional-Anesthesia-in-Small-Animals.pdf (accessed 15 February 2021).

Kimberlin, L. (2010) The pathophysiology of pain and its management in equine dental procedures. In: *Proceedings of the 24th Annual Veterinary Dental Forum.* Omnipress, Madison, Wisconsin (CD Rom).

Koenig, T. (2004) Veterinary dental terminology. In: *Proceedings of the 18th Annual Veterinary Dental Forum.* Omnipress, Madison, Wisconsin, pp. 301–305.

Kressler, A. (2012a) Prevent the pain, see what you gain. In: *Proceedings of the 26th Annual Veterinary Dental Forum.* Omnipress, Madison, Wisconsin (CD Rom).

Kressler, A. (2012b) Block that pain away. In: *Proceedings of the 26th Annual Veterinary Dental Forum.* Omnipress, Madison, Wisonsin (CD Rom).

Krug, W. (2010) Resultant area of anesthesia from mental nerve blocks in dogs. In: *Proceedings of the 24th Annual Veterinary Dental Forum.* Omnipress, Madison, Wisconsin (CD Rom).

Leary, R. (2017) Why vets we meet choose DR over CR for their dental radiographs. Veterinary Practice. Available at: https://veterinary-practice.com/article/ why-vets-we-meet-choose-dr-over-cr-for-their-dental-radiographs (accessed 13 February 2021).

Lewis, J. (2015) Do dogs and cats get cavities? Veterinary Practice News. Available at: https://www.veterinarypracticenews.com/do-dogs-and-cats-get-cavities/ (accessed 13 February 2021).

Lewis, J. (2017) How to spot signs of oral pain in your pet patients. Veterinary Practice News. Available at: https://www.veterinarypracticenews.com/how-to-spot-signs-of-oral-pain-in-your-pet-patients/ (accessed 27 January 2021).

Luechtefeld, L. (2012) Digital dental difference. Veterinary Practice News. Available at: https://www.veterinarypracticenews.com/digital-dental-difference/ (accessed 12 February 2021).

Lyon, K. (2001) Endodontic anatomy and diagnosis in the veterinary patient. *World Small Animal Veterinary Association World Congress Proceedings, 2001.* Available at: https://www.vin.com/apputil/content/defaultadv1.aspx?pId=8708&catI d=18045&id=3843706 (accessed 15 February 2021).

Mathews, K., Kronen, P.W., Lascelles, D., Nolan, A., Robertson, S. *et al.* (2014) WSAVA guidelines for recognition, assessment and treatment of pain. *Journal of Small Animal Practice* 55(6), E10–E68. Available at: https://onlinelibrary.wiley. com/doi/full/10.1111/jsap.12200 DOI: 10.1111/jsap.12200.

McMahon, J. (2020) The dental cleaning. In: Perrone, J. (ed.) *Small Animal Dental Procedures for Veterinary Technicians and Nurses.* Wiley Blackwell, Hoboken, New Jersey, pp. 65–91.

Mills, A. (2012) The general practitioner's approach to pain management – a multimodal approach. In: *Proceedings of the 26th Annual Veterinary Dental Forum.* Omnipress, Madison, Wisconsin (CD Rom).

Mills, A. (2016) Pain management for veterinary dental patients. Today's Veterinary Nurse. Available at: https://todaysveterinarynurse.com/articles/pain-man-agement-for-dental-patients/ (accessed 15 February 2021).

Mills, A. (2020) Anesthesia and the dental patient. In: Perrone, J. (ed.) *Small Animal Dental Procedures for Veterinary Technicians and Nurses.* Wiley Blackwell, Hoboken, New Jersey, pp. 51–63.

Muir, W.W. (2002) Physiology and pathophysiology of pain. In: Gaynor, J.S. and Muir, W.W. (eds) *Handbook of Veterinary Pain Management.* Mosby, St. Louis, Missouri, pp. 13–45.

Mulherin, B.L. and Riha, J.M. (2019) Regional anesthesia for the dentistry and oral surgery patient. Today's Veterinary Practice. Available at: https://todaysveterinarypractice.com/regional-anesthesia-for-the-dentistry-and-oral-surgery-patient/ (accessed 15 February 2021).

Niemiec, B.A. (2004) Pain management in veterinary dentistry. In: *Proceedings of the 18th Annual Veterinary Dental Forum.* Omnipress, Madison, Wisconsin, pp. 114–117.

Niemiec, B.A. (2007) Interpreting dental radiographs: the clues to clinical disease. Dvm360. Available at: https://www.dvm360.com/view/interpreting-dental-radiographs-clues-clinical-disease (accessed 13 February 2021).

Niemiec, B.A. (2010) Dental radiology. In: *Proceedings of the 24th Annual Veterinary Dental Forum.* Omnipress, Madison, Wisconsin (CD Rom).

Niemiec, B.A. (2011) The importance of dental radiology. Today's Veterinary Practice. Available at: https://todaysveterinarypractice.com/the-importance-of-dental-radiology/ (accessed 12 February 2021).

Niemiec, B.A. (2012) Introduction to oral neoplasia in the dog and cat. Today's Veterinary Practice. Available at: https://todaysveterinarypractice.com/practical-dentistry-introduction-to-oral-neoplasia-in-the-dog-cat/ (accessed 13 February 2021).

Niemiec, B.A., Gawor, J., Nemec, A., Clarke, D. and Tutt, C. (2020) World small animal veterinary association global dental guidelines. World Small Animal Veterinary Association. Available at: https://wsava.org/wp-content/uploads/2020/01/Dental-Guidleines-for-endorsement_0.pdf (accessed 6 February 2021).

NRC (1992) Recognition and alleviation of pain and distress in laboratory animals. National Research Council (US) Committee on Pain and Distress in Laboratory Animals. National Academies Press (US),Washington, DC. Available at: https://www.ncbi.nlm.nih.gov/books/NBK235435/#ddd00047 (accessed 15 February 2021).

Pablo, L.S. (2008) Managing perioperative pain. In: *Proceedings of the 22nd Annual Veterinary Dental Forum.* Omnipress, Madison, Wisconsin, pp. 455–460.

Peralta, S. (2017a) Interpretation of dental radiographs in dogs and cats, part 1: principles and normal findings. Today's Veterinary Practice. Available at: https://todaysveterinarypractice.com/imaging-essentialsinterpretation-dental-radiographs-dogs-catspart-1-principles-normal-findings/ (accessed 13 February 2021).

Peralta, S. (2017b) Interpretation of dental radiographs in dogs and cats, part 2: normal variations and abnormal findings. Available at: https://todaysveterinarypractice.com/imaging-essentials-interpretation-dental-radiographs-dogs-catspart-2-normal-variations-abnormal-findings/ (accessed 13 February 2021).

Perrone, J. (2008) Tighten your dentistry knowledge. Dvm360. Available at: https://www.dvm360.com/view/tighten-your-dentistry-knowledge-proceedings-0 (accessed 12 February 2021).

Perrone, J. (2011) Dental extractions: from anesthesia to send home. Dvm360. Available at: https://www.dvm360.com/view/dental-extractions-anesthesia-send-home-proceedings (accessed 15 February 2021).

RVC (2002a) Veterinary dentistry basics. Royal Veterinary College. Available at: https://www.rvc.ac.uk/review/Dentistry/Shared_Media/pdfs/Basics_print.pdf (accessed 12 February 2021).

RVC (2002b) Veterinary dentistry radiography. Royal Veterinary College. Available at: https://www.rvc.ac.uk/review/Dentistry/Radiography/radioTechniques/EOP.html (accessed 13 February 2021).

Sakman, J.E. (1994) Pain management. In: McCurnin, D. (ed.) *Clinical Textbook for Veterinary Technicians.* Saunders, Philadelphia, Pennsylvania, pp. 572–588.

Shaw, L. and Voglewede, C. (2018) Take a bite out of dental radiology: positioning for picture-perfect views. Today's Veterinary Nurse. Available at: https://todaysveterinarynurse.com/articles/take-a-bite-out-of-dental-radiology-positioning-for-picture-perfect-views/ (accessed 12 February 2021).

Shivni, R. (2015) It doesn't have to hurt. American Veterinary Medical Association. Available at: https://www.avma.org/javma-news/2015-11-01/it-doesnt-have-hurt (accessed 15 February 2021).

Snyder, C. (2010) Local blocks: proofs they work and what's new? In: *Proceedings of the 24th Annual Veterinary Dental Forum.* Omnipress, Madison, Wisconsin (CD Rom).

Stellfox, M. and Richardson, J. (2019) Pain management in surgical patients. Vet Folio. Available at: https://www.vetfolio.com/learn/article/pain-management-in-surgical-patients (accessed 15 February 2021).

Tabor, B. (2016) Pain recognition and management in critical care patients. Today's Veterinary Nurse. Available at: https://todaysveterinarynurse.com/articles/pain-recognition-and-management-in-critical-care-patients/ (accessed 15 February 2021).

Theuns, P. (2008) Local anesthesia – anatomy equipment procedures. In: *Proceedings of the 22nd Annual Veterinary Dental Forum.* Omnipress, Madison, Wisconsin, pp. 185–187.

Tompe, A. and Sargar, K. (2020) X-ray image quality assurance. StatPearls Publishing. Available at: https://www.ncbi.nlm.nih.gov/books/NBK564362/ (accessed 13 February 2021).

Williamson, G.F. (2006) Intraoral radiography: positioning and radiation protection. Available at: https://www.researchgate.net/publication/237822140_Intraoral_Radiography_Positioning_and_Radiation_Protection (accessed 12 February 2021).

Williamson, G.F. (2020) Intraoral imaging: basic principles, techniques and error correction. Dentalcare.com. Available at: https://www.dentalcare.com/en-us/professional-education/ce-courses/ce559/technique-errors (accessed 13 February 2021).

Woodward, T.M. (2012) Dental radiology – it's not so tough. Vet Folio. Available at: https://www.vetfolio.com/learn/article/dental-radiology-its-not-so-tough (accessed 13 February 2021).

Woodward, T.M. (2020) The rationale for veterinary dental radiology. Dentalaire. Available at: https://www.dentalaireproducts.com/veterinary-dental-radiology/ (accessed 13 February 2021).

If It's Broke, Fix It! Tooth Fractures, Discoloured Teeth, Abrasion and Attrition

4

Tooth fractures occur frequently in dogs and cats (Lemmons and Carmichael, 2008). Teeth can break due to trauma including being hit by a car, golf ball, rock or other hard object (Clarke, 2001), or from chewing inappropriate substances such as bones, hard toys or metal bars (Lemmons and Carmichael, 2008; Perrone *et al.*, 2020). Any tooth can break, but the most commonly fractured teeth of dogs are the canines, upper fourth premolars and lower first molars (Brine and Marretta, 1999; Clarke, 2001), and the most commonly fractured teeth of cats are the canines (Lemmons and Carmichael, 2008).

4.1 Why Treat Fractured Teeth?

Fractured teeth are painful (Perrone *et al.*, 2020). Pets will often hide this pain and continue to eat, though they may chew on the opposite side of the mouth, drop food or toys, or become reluctant to have their mouths handled (Holmstrom *et al.*, 2000; Hale, 2008). Once a tooth is fractured, the pulp is exposed, allowing bacteria from the mouth to infect the tooth. Infection can happen even in fractured teeth with no pulp exposure, with bacteria entering the exposed dentinal tubules (Hale, 2008; Klima, 2008a). This infection causes the tooth to die, and bacteria can spread from the tooth into the surrounding bone through the blood supply of the tooth root (Holmstrom *et al.*, 2000; Perrone *et al.*, 2020). Infection can destroy the bone around the tooth root (Hale, 2008), and may also enter the pet's circulating blood supply, damaging organs such as the liver, kidney and heart valves (Clarke, 2001). In some cases, this infection can cause a large abscess around the tooth root that breaks through the skin (Niemiec, 2012a). Antibiotics can reduce infection and inflammation in the short term, but the abscess will recur until the fractured tooth is treated (Hale, 2008).

DOI: 10.1079/9781789248869.0004

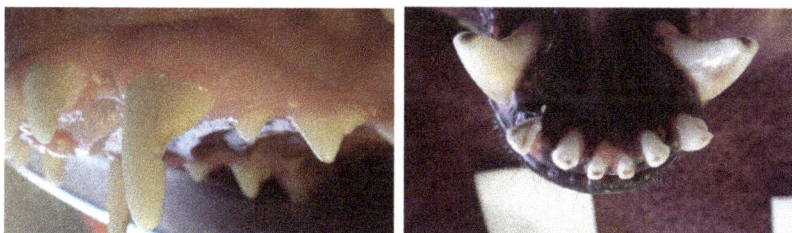

Fig. 4.1. Abrasion from chewing kennel bars (left); abrasion with reparative dentin (right).

4.2 Non-Vital Teeth

A tooth may experience trauma and not fracture, but its blood supply becomes compromised, causing the pulp to die (Hale, 2008). These dying or dead ('non-vital') teeth become discoloured, taking on a pink, purple or greyish cast due to the presence of blood within the dentinal tubules. Nearly all (>90%) of discoloured teeth are dead and require treatment (Hale, 2001). Dead pulp no longer contains immune cells, allowing bacteria to accumulate within the necrotic pulp (Hale, 2001).

4.3 Abrasion and Attrition

If a tooth regularly comes into contact with a hard or rough surface, such as kennel bars, tennis balls or even a pet's own fur, the enamel and dentin can wear away over time due to friction in a process called abrasion (see Fig. 4.1) (Hale, 2008; Lemmons and Carmichael, 2008). Wearing of a tooth from contact with another tooth due to malocclusion is called attrition. Both abrasion and attrition can lead to pulp exposure (Hale, 2008; Lemmons and Carmichael, 2008). In cases where the wearing is very gradual, the tooth may be able to repair this damage by producing reparative dentin before the pulp can become exposed. These teeth have a reddish-brown stain on the worn area, which is the reparative dentin, and the worn area feels smooth upon palpation with a dental explorer. All teeth showing wear should be radiographed to assess for signs of infection or necrosis (Hale, 2008).

4.4 Treatment Options

Treatment options for non-vital teeth or teeth with pulp exposure are currently limited to extraction or endodontic therapy (Hale, 2008; Niemiec, 2012a). While many animals can function well with the loss of a tooth, the canine teeth and carnassials are considered strategic teeth (important with regard to size and function) (Hernandez, 2008) and many pet owners prefer their pets to keep these teeth (Brine and Marretta, 1999). Keeping a functional dentition is particularly important for service dogs (Perrone *et al.*, 2020). Although endodontic treatment is most often performed on strategic teeth, almost any permanent tooth may be a candidate for endodontic treatment (Niemiec, 2012a). Endodontic treatment is not performed on teeth with severe periodontal disease (Hale, 2012), or on fractured deciduous teeth, because they will be replaced by permanent teeth (Holmstrom *et al.*, 2004).

Radiography is the most important diagnostic, prognostic and therapeutic evaluation tool in endodontics (Lemmons and Carmichael, 2008). If radiographs obtained of the injured tooth reveal little or no periodontal disease or internal root resorption, then the prognosis for endodontic treatment is generally good to excellent (Hale, 2012).

Worn or fractured teeth with no pulp exposure will benefit from a dental restoration to decrease tooth sensitivity and provide a barrier against bacteria entering the dentinal tubules (Klima, 2008a). The trauma that caused the wear or fracture must also be addressed, such as no longer allowing the pet to chew tennis balls, or preventing tooth-on-tooth contact by extraction or orthodontic movement of the opposing tooth (Lemmons and Carmichael, 2008).

4.5 Extraction

Apart from COHATs, extractions are one of the most commonly performed dental procedures in veterinary practices (Honzelka, 2012). Extraction is a treatment option any time a tooth is compromised, whether from lack of attachment due to periodontal disease, tooth fracture, non-vital teeth, fractured or persistent deciduous teeth, crowded teeth, traumatic contact with other teeth or oral tissues, or tooth resorption with an intact periodontal ligament (Juriga, 2008a; Honzelka, 2012). Extraction is often the treatment of choice for painful, difficult-to-resolve conditions like stomatitis. Extraction is considered a surgical procedure, and must be performed by a veterinarian (American Veterinary Dental College (AVDC), 2006). Nurses must still understand how extractions are performed, in order to be able to properly assist the veterinarian, prepare the required dental instruments, provide adequate patient care during and after the procedure, and educate pet owners (Mills, 2012; Sharp, 2019).

Preserving the function of fractured teeth by endodontic treatment remains the preferred treatment option for most fractured teeth (Clarke, 2001). However, if a fractured or non-vital tooth has poor periodontal health, extraction may be the best course of treatment, since the time under anaesthesia and the expense of attempting to preserve a tooth that will soon require extraction due to lack of periodontal attachment is not in our patients' or clients' best interests (Hale, 2012). If a non-vital tooth or tooth with pulp exposure has good periodontal health, but the owner declines endodontic treatment, extraction is the only remaining treatment option (Clarke, 2001). Allowing a dead or dying tooth to remain untreated or taking a 'wait and see' approach should never be presented to a pet owner as an acceptable option, as the pain and infection can be severe (Klima, 2008a).

The advantages of extracting a broken tooth are that extractions can be performed by the vast majority of veterinarians in general practice, while endodontic treatment is most commonly done by veterinary dental specialists or by veterinarians who have undergone extensive additional dental training and have made an investment in endodontic equipment (Clarke, 2001; Hale, 2012). The disadvantages of extractions include the loss of a functional tooth, postoperative pain, and aftercare including a soft diet and no chew toys for at least a week after surgery (Holmstrom *et al.*, 2004; Hale, 2012).

Possible complications of extraction include facial swelling, fractured and retained root tips, iatrogenic jaw fracture, draining tracts, perforation of eyes or sinuses by dental instruments, the creation of oronasal fistulas, iatrogenic defects in erupting permanent teeth, and potential dehiscence of the extraction site (Smith *et al.*, 2003; Juriga, 2008a; Honzelka, 2012). Postoperative radiographs should always be taken, to ensure the entire tooth was removed without iatrogenic damage to surrounding structures (Perrone *et al.*, 2020).

4.5.1   Nonsurgical extractions

Sometimes called closed extractions, nonsurgical extractions are usually performed on single-rooted teeth such as incisors and first premolars, or on significantly mobile teeth (Carmichael, 2006). Nonsurgical extractions do not require mucoperiosteal flaps or removing bone (Juriga, 2008a; Perrone *et al.*, 2020). After dental radiography and an appropriate dental regional nerve block have been performed, an intrasulcular incision is made around the tooth with a #15 or #11 scalpel blade, creating a simple envelope flap (Carmichael, 2006). Next, a dental luxator is introduced into the gingival sulcus between the tooth and the alveolar crest (Carmichael, 2006). The operator's index finger should be placed on the luxator's shank close to the tip to prevent the instrument from slipping and perforating adjacent or deeper tissues, such as the eye (DeBowes, 2012). The luxator is angled towards the tooth, and steady apical pressure is applied for a sufficient length of time to allow the periodontal ligament fibres to stretch to the point of rupture, usually 30–60 seconds (DeBowes, 2012). This is repeated at several points around the tooth until the tooth loosens, at which point extraction forceps can be used to gently rotate and pull the tooth from the alveolus (Carmichael, 2006).

If there are sharp edges of bone at the alveolar crest, these are smoothed using a round carbide bur (#2–4), or a round or cone-shaped diamond bur (Juriga, 2008a). The alveolus is then curetted to remove any bone fragments, inflammatory or necrotic tissue and debris, then flushed with water from an air-water syringe, saline or chlorhexidine solution, and the gingiva is closed without tension with an absorbable suture material, size 3-0 to 5-0, on a reverse cutting needle (Perrone *et al.*, 2020).

4.5.2 Surgical extractions

Surgical extractions, also called open extractions, are performed on canine teeth, multi-rooted teeth, non-mobile teeth, fractured deciduous teeth and teeth with Type I and III resorption, and involve creating a surgical flap and removing bone (Juriga, 2008a; Perrone *et al.*, 2020). After dental radiography and an appropriate dental regional nerve block have been performed, a mucoperiosteal flap is created by cutting either one or two vertical releasing incision(s) on the caudal and/or rostral line angles of the tooth with a #15 or #11 scalpel blade (Carmichael, 2006; Juriga, 2008a). The base of the flap should be wider than the top, to preserve the flap's blood supply. A periosteal elevator (e.g. EX9 or EX7) is used to lift the tissue flap away from the bone. This will expose the buccal cortical bone and the root or root furcations of multi-rooted teeth. A round bur (#1 or #2) or pear-shaped bur (#330) on a high-speed handpiece can be used to remove bone in the furcation area to improve visualization of the roots if needed (Juriga, 2008a; Honzelka, 2012). The tooth is sectioned using a cross-cut tapered-fissure bur (Perrone *et al.*, 2020) (ie. #699 or #701, or the longer #699L and #701L for wider teeth), cutting from the furcation toward the crown, then a luxator is used to elevate each root as described above in Section 4.5.1 (Carmichael, 2006; Honzelka, 2012). In some cases, a round bur is used to remove buccal cortical bone from the coronal area of each root before luxation is performed, to allow easier placement of the luxator (Juriga, 2008a).

An alveoplasty is performed to smooth rough or sharp bone using a round carbide bur (#2–4), or a round or cone-shaped diamond bur (Juriga, 2008a). The alveolus is curetted to remove any bone or tooth fragments, inflammatory or necrotic tissue, or debris (Honzelka, 2012), then flushed with water from an air-water syringe, saline or chlorhexidine solution (Carmichael, 2006; Juriga, 2008a). The gingival flaps must close without tension, which usually requires undermining the connective tissue with a periosteal elevator or iris scissors (Juriga, 2008a). The gingiva is then sutured with an absorbable suture material, size 3-0 to 5-0, on a reverse cutting needle (Perrone *et al.*, 2020).

4.5.3 Homecare following extraction

Patients receiving extractions should receive pain medication for at least 7 days (Niemiec, 2012b). If the extractions were extensive or the pre-extraction pathology was particularly painful, such as stomatitis (see Chapter 8), postoperative pain medication(s) should be continued for longer (Watanabe *et al.*, 2019). In most cases, antibiotics following extraction are not required; however, they may be sent home when a patient is immunocompromised, or has severe systemic disease or osteomyelitis (AVDC, 2019; Animal Dentistry & Oral Surgery (ADOS), 2021).

Patients should be fed only soft food for 7–10 days following extraction, to reduce pain during chewing and to help prevent dehiscence of the extraction site(s) (Juriga, 2008a). This can consist of canned food, or the owner can soak the pet's usual dry food in warm water or broth for several minutes to soften the kibble. They should also restrict their pet's access to toys and hard treats during this time (Juriga, 2008a; Honzelka, 2012).

If there is postoperative facial swelling, the owner can place an ice pack or bag of frozen vegetables wrapped in a thin towel on the area for up to 15 minutes, two to three times daily, if the pet will tolerate it (Zeltzman, 2021). Make sure the owner is aware that the pet's saliva may contain traces of blood for 1–2 days postoperatively, until the sutured tissues begin to heal (Taylor, 2004). Instruct the client to return for recheck as soon as possible if profuse bleeding occurs (Perrone, 2020).

Tooth brushing is usually discontinued temporarily following extraction (Khuly, 2020). This prevents trauma to the healing gingival tissues, and prevents the pet from associating tooth brushing with oral pain (Perrone, 2020). During this time, the owner should use oral rinses and/or water additives to discourage plaque formation (Perrone *et al.*, 2020).

Schedule a recheck 10–14 days postoperatively (Sacramento Veterinary Dental Services (SACVDS), 2021) to ensure the extraction sites have healed and the pet is eating well and maintaining their weight, and to discuss establishing or re-starting a tooth-brushing routine (Hale, 2008).

4.6 Endodontic Treatments

The branch of dentistry called endodontics involves the prevention, diagnosis and treatment of conditions and injuries of the dental pulp (Perrone *et al.*, 2020). The most commonly performed endodontic treatment is standard root canal therapy (Davis, 2021). Other endodontic treatments include vital pulp therapy, surgical root canal therapy, indirect pulp capping and apexification (Perrone *et al.*, 2020).

Endodontic treatments are usually faster and less traumatic than extracting periodontally healthy teeth, particularly large teeth such as canines and carnassials (Holmstrom *et al.*, 2000). This reduces anaesthetic time, causes less postoperative pain, requires minimal postoperative care, allows the pet to continue eating their current diet, and maintains a healthy, functional dentition (Hale, 2012; Perrone *et al.*, 2020). Disadvantages of endodontic treatment include expense, the need for access to a veterinary dental specialist or veterinarian with advanced training, structural or pathological problems with the root(s) that may complicate or hinder treatment, and the possibility of treatment failure (Girard *et al.*, 2006; Hernandez, 2008; Hale, 2012).

4.6.1   Standard root canal therapy

Standard root canal therapy is recommended for the treatment of endodontic disease in dogs and cats who are at least 18 months of age (Niemiec, 2008a). (Younger patients should be treated with vital pulp therapy – see Section 4.6.2, this volume). Indications for standard root canal therapy are tooth fractures with pulp exposure (Holmstrom *et al.*, 2000; Perrone *et al.*, 2020); fractures without pulp exposure that have become infected through exposure of the dentinal tubules to oral bacteria; deep caries which have exposed the pulp (see Chapter 5, this volume); non-vital teeth without fracture (due to blunt trauma, avulsion or luxation, or whose blood supply has been disrupted by jaw fracture); and worn teeth which have become infected or non-vital (Holmstrom *et al.*, 2000; Hale, 2008). To be candidates for root canal therapy, all cases must involve mature teeth with a closed root apex and have no significant periodontal disease or root fractures (Queck and Runyon, 1987; Hernandez, 2008; Kling, 2018).

A standard root canal treatment involves removing dead or infected pulp tissue, shaping and sterilizing the root canal, filling the canal and pulp chamber with an inert material, then sealing the tooth to prevent bacterial contamination (Perrone *et al.*, 2020). This leaves a tooth that is dead, but sterile and functional. Root canal therapy has a very high success rate when performed properly (Clarke, 2001). In some cases, a metal crown to protect the tooth from further trauma may be recommended (Perrone *et al.*, 2020).

An initial radiograph is performed of the tooth to assess the depth of the fracture (if any) and the size and shape of the pulp chamber, to confirm that the root apex is closed, and to ensure there is no root fracture, pulp stone (calcified area within the pulp), periodontal disease or other pathology which would complicate or contraindicate endodontic treatment (Hale, 2012). Regional nerve blocks should be placed to minimize pain intra- and postoperatively (Perrone *et al.*, 2020).

There are four basic steps involved in standard root canal therapy: access, debridement and sterilization, obturation and restoration.

Access

An access hole into the tooth's pulp chamber is made by burring through the enamel and dentin, usually with a round or pear-shaped carbide bur (Holmstrom *et al.*, 2004). In some cases, access into the pulp chamber can be made through the fracture site, providing that the site allows straight-line access to the middle third of the canal (Boyd and Ross, 2008). Football-shaped Gates Glidden drills can also be used to flare the access hole if necessary, to allow for easier passage of files into the canal, and to shape the coronal third of the canal (Holmstrom *et al.*, 2004).

Debridement and sterilization

Once the access hole is made, debridement (removal of the pulp and any diseased dentin) is performed by the use of long, thin metal files; or, in some cases, the entire pulp can be pulled out using an instrument called a barbed broach (Holmstrom *et al.*, 2000). There are many types of files that can be used for debridement. Hand files, such as Hedstrom files (H-files), Kerr files (K-files) and K-reamers are most commonly used (Holmstrom *et al.*, 2000). Hedstrom files have a spiral groove and must be used only in a push-and-pull motion within the canal, as they are fragile and can snap off in the tooth if rotated within the canal (Colmery, 2021). K-files have a twisted triangular shape and can be rotated in the canal as well as being used in a push-and-pull motion (Stein *et al.*, 2004). K-reamers are shaped like K-files and are used in the same way, but have fewer twists (Peak, 2012). Rotary files operated on an electric handpiece can also be used; these consist of a thin, straight, nickel-titanium shaft with a cutting tip (Boyd and Ross, 2008). Rotary files have better flexibility than hand files for cleaning long, curving canals such as large canine teeth, are quick and efficient at debriding and shaping canals, and place less strain on the wrist and fingers of the operator (Stein *et al.*, 2004; Boyd and Ross, 2008). The disadvantage of electric rotary systems is that the handpiece, rotary files and special obturating points that must be used with them are expensive to purchase.

Both hand and rotary files are available in various widths and lengths for debriding and shaping different-sized canals (Stein *et al.*, 2004). File widths are denoted by a colour-coded band, which indicates the file's diameter in increments of 0.05–0.1 mm (Holmstrom *et al.*, 2000). A #40 file is 0.4 mm in diameter at the tip, while a #45 file is 0.45mm. Common file lengths used in veterinary dentistry are 25 mm, 31 mm, 45 mm and 60 mm (Holmstrom *et al.*, 2000).

A chelating agent such as ethylenediaminetetraacetic acid (EDTA) is placed on the files to lubricate them as they move inside the canal, and to soften dentin to facilitate its removal (Holmstrom *et al.*, 2004). Once a file reaches the bottom of the canal, a radiograph is taken to verify the length of file necessary to reach the root apex. This is called the working length (Boyd and Ross, 2008). This length is measured with an endodontic ruler (Peak, 2012) and a rubber stopper (endodontic stop) is placed on each subsequent file at this length to ensure that the root apex isn't perforated during debridement (Holmstrom *et al.*, 2000). As the canal is debrided, the interior is cleaned and shaped by gradually increasing the diameter of the files (Boyd and Ross, 2008). Once healthy, white dentinal filings rather than darker, diseased dentinal material are seen on two or three files of increasing diameter, debridement is usually complete (Holmstrom *et al.*, 2004). Another radiograph is then taken to determine the largest-diameter file able to reach the root apex (Holmstrom *et al.*, 2004). This is called the master file or final apical size (Boyd and Ross, 2008), and confirms that the entire length of the root canal has been properly cleaned and shaped.

Smaller-diameter files are used after the master file has been determined, in a process called recapitulation (Brine and Marretta, 1999), which removes any debris packed deep within the canal.

During and after debridement, the canal is irrigated to flush out debris and to disinfect the canal (Brine and Marretta, 1999). Several solutions are used, such as EDTA to soften the dentin, sodium hypochlorite (bleach) to sterilize the canal, and sterile saline to remove the bleach and flush the canal (Brine and Marretta, 1999). Make sure to prevent bleach from coming into contact with the patient's soft tissues, and rinse copiously to prevent tissue damage if inadvertent contact occurs (Peak, 2012). After the final irrigation, absorbent paper points are placed in the canal to dry it (Holmstrom *et al.*, 2000).

Obturation

The root canal is filled with an inert material to prevent the tooth from becoming re-infected (Hale, 2012). There are several acceptable materials and techniques used to obturate root canals. First, a sealer cement is applied to the inside of the pulp chamber to fill any canal irregularities and to seal off the dentinal tubules and canals of the apical delta (Holmstrom *et al.*, 2000). Sealer cements can be placed using a file called a spiral (Lentulo) filler on a reduction slow-speed handpiece gear, or may be placed directly onto a gutta percha point (see below), which is then inserted into the canal (Boyd and Ross, 2008). Types of sealers include calcium hydroxide, epoxy resins, glass ionomers, and zinc oxide powder with eugenol (ZOE) (Niemiec, 2008b).

To complete the obturation, a radio-opaque, rubber-based material called gutta percha is used to fill the canal (Holmstrom *et al.*, 2000). Gutta percha points are tapered cones that are placed into the canal and then compacted with thin, pointed metal instruments called pluggers (downward compaction) and spreaders (lateral compaction) (Holmstrom *et al.*, 2000). Gutta percha points can also be heated, either in a small oven or

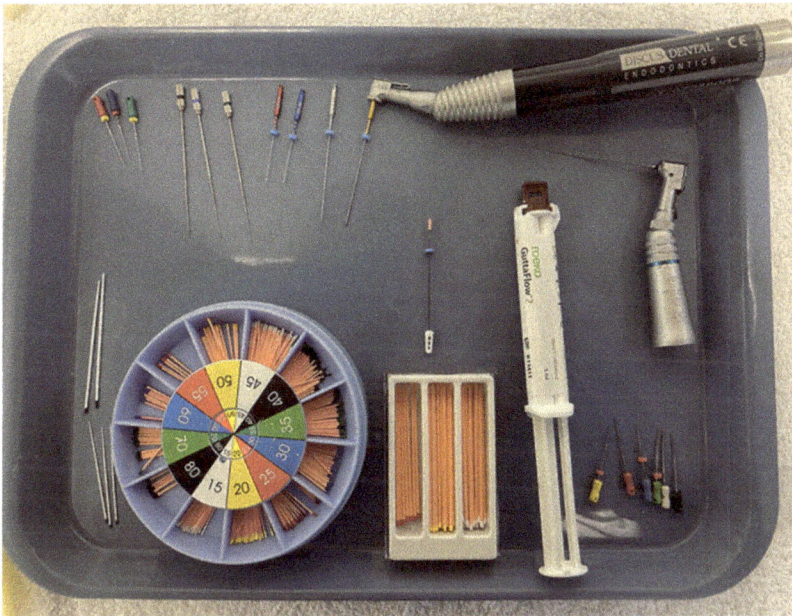

Fig. 4.2. Endodontic materials. Clockwise from top left: K-files; H-files; rotary files; rotary file on handpiece; spiral (Lentulo) filler on reduction slow-speed handpiece; pluggers; flowable gutta percha; gutta percha points; paper points.

with a hot metal instrument, which softens the gutta percha, enabling it to be carried into the canal by K-reamers, or more easily condensed within the canal (Niemiec, 2008b). Flowable gutta percha can be injected directly into the canal. Special gutta percha obturating tips are used in canals debrided with rotary files to deliver the gutta percha to the root apex, after which the remainder of the canal can be obturated with the methods discussed above (Boyd and Ross, 2008). In all cases, the gutta percha is packed into the canal, leaving several millimetres free at the coronal end of the access hole (Holmstrom *et al.*, 2004). A radiograph is taken to ensure there are no voids in the fill, which could be colonized by bacteria and lead to treatment failure (Holmstrom *et al.*, 2004; Peak, 2012).

Restoration

This is the final step in root canal therapy (Holmstrom *et al.*, 2004). A restoration fills the access hole and fracture site (if any), preventing leakage of bacteria into the tooth (Hale, 2012). Restorations are covered in greater detail in Section 4.7, this volume.

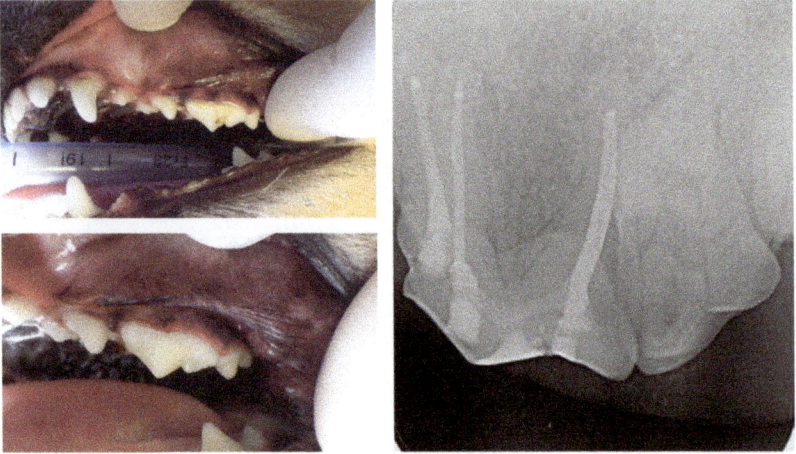

Fig. 4.3. Root canal therapy. Top left: fractured tooth 208. Right: post-treatment radiograph showing filled canals and restorations. Bottom left: tooth 208 after root canal treatment.

The access hole is conditioned with an acid-etching agent to remove any debris from the dentinal tubules (Storli, 2012). This improves the mechanical adhesion of the restorative agent. The etchant is rinsed off and bonding agent(s) are applied with a small, brush-tipped applicator (Legendre, 2001).

Next, a restorative compound is placed upon the tooth to fill the access hole. Several types of restoratives can be used: see Section 4.7.1 (this volume) for more details. Glass ionomers made of silica, quartz or similar substances form a chemical bond with dentin (Girard *et al.*, 2006), so do not require the use of bonding agents; however, they are not very strong. Composite resins are organic polymers which provide greater strength than glass ionomers, and come in both flowable and packable options. These are available in many colours to mimic the colour of the enamel. Restoratives may be chemically cured or light-cured, which requires the use of a light-curing gun (Holmstrom *et al.*, 2000).

A polishing disk or diamond bur is used to smooth the restoration, and an unfilled resin is painted on as a final sealant to protect against microleakage (Klima, 2008a).

4.6.2   Vital pulp therapy (direct pulp capping)

Vital pulp therapy is performed only in cases of either very fresh tooth fracture (fracture occurred less than 48 hours prior to treatment) (Clarke, 2001), fracture with pulp exposure of a still vital immature permanent tooth with thin dentinal walls and open root apices (patient is less than 18 months of age) (Klima, 2008a; Perrone *et al.*, 2020), or when a tooth's height needs to be reduced because of a malocclusion such as base narrow canine teeth causing trauma to the palate (see Fig. 4.4) (Holmstrom *et al.*, 2000; Hernandez, 2008). Vital pulp therapy is not the preferred treatment for fractured mature teeth, because it is not as successful as standard root canal therapy due to potential bacterial contamination (Clarke, 2001; Klima, 2008a).

Vital pulp therapy involves removing a small portion of the tooth's pulp, applying calcium hydroxide to stimulate the formation of reparative dentin, then covering the opening with a filling material (Holmstrom *et al.*, 2000). This keeps the tooth alive, allowing it to mature, forming thicker dentinal walls for better strength and a closed root apex (apexogenesis), so that if vital pulp treatment ultimately fails, the tooth may be a candidate for root canal therapy (Klima, 2008a; Niemiec, 2008a).

The procedure should be done as soon as possible after the fracture occurs because as time passes, bacteria from the oral cavity migrate further down into the pulp (Klima, 2008a). After 48 hours, the probability of being able to remove the infected portion of the pulp while still keeping the tooth alive diminishes (Holmstrom *et al.*, 2000; Clarke, 2001; Perrone *et al.*, 2020).

There are five basic steps involved in vital pulp therapy: disinfection, smoothing of the fracture site or crown reduction (if necessary), pulp removal and haemorrhage control, pulp dressing, and restoration.

Disinfection

An initial radiograph is obtained to make sure that the tooth is still vital and to ensure there are no other problems such as root fracture, etc. A regional nerve block should be placed to minimize intra- and postoperative pain. The teeth are then cleaned and the mouth is disinfected with chlorhexidine (Perrone *et al.*, 2020). This is important so as not to introduce more bacteria into the fracture site and to prevent iatrogenic infection if the crown height is being reduced deliberately (Niemiec, 2008a).

Smoothing of the fracture site or crown reduction

The fracture site is smoothed of any jagged edges with a sterile diamond bur and copious amounts of water to cool it, and/or the coronal tip of the tooth's crown is lowered to the desired height (Moore, 2012). Care must be taken not to cause thermal damage to the tooth (Niemiec, 2008a), which could lead to tooth death.

Pulp removal and haemorrhage control

All diseased pulp should be removed down to healthy, bleeding tissue. In most cases, about 5–7 mm of pulp should be removed (Clarke, 2001;

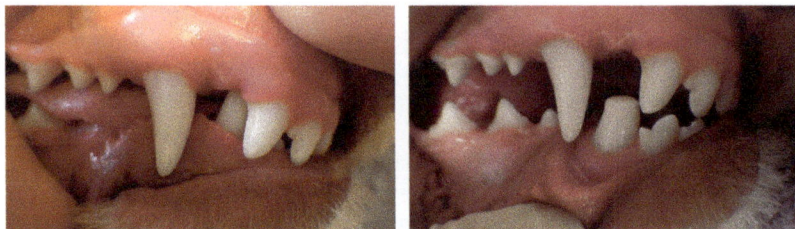

Fig. 4.4. Left: base narrow canine tooth contacting palate. Right: base narrow canine tooth after crown reduction and vital pulp therapy.

Niemiec, 2008a). Pulp removal is done with a sterile round carbide bur (#2, #3 or #4) or a coarse diamond bur (Niemiec, 2008a). Bleeding is controlled using sterile paper points. The paper points can be soaked with cold sterile saline and left inside the canal for a few minutes to allow a clot to form (Niemiec, 2008a). If the pulp continues to haemorrhage, another 1–2 mm of pulp is removed and the process repeated.

Pulp dressing

A 1-mm layer of calcium hydroxide or mineral trioxide aggregate (MTA) is applied (Niemiec, 2008a). These can consist of pastes injected or placed onto the pulp, or powders packed onto the pulp using an amalgam carrier or a sterile, moistened paper point. These materials irritate the pulp, causing it to form a reparative dentinal bridge that will protect the pulp; they have a basic pH, which helps inhibit infection (Niemiec, 2008a).

Restoration

A glass ionomer restorative material is placed over the calcium hydroxide or MTA (Perrone *et al.*, 2020). The glass ionomer forms a chemical bond with the dentin, preventing leakage of bacteria into the pulp (Girard *et al.*, 2006). A final restoration of composite resin and unfilled resin (like the final restoration in standard root canal therapy) is placed on top of the glass ionomer (Perrone *et al.*, 2020). A postoperative radiograph must be taken to ensure there are no gaps between the layers of pulp dressing and restoratives, which could lead to treatment failure (Perrone *et al.*, 2020). If there are gaps, the restoration must be removed and repeated until radiographs show a void-free restoration (Niemiec, 2008a).

4.6.3   Surgical root canal therapy (apicoectomy)

This is performed when standard root canal therapy has failed (though often, the failed root canal therapy can be redone in the standard manner) (Hennet and Girard, 2005), when there is a problem accessing the apical portion of the root due to a pulp stone or oddly shaped root, or when there is disease at the root apex (Holmstrom *et al.*, 2000). Surgical root canal therapy is performed rarely in veterinary dentistry (Holmstrom *et al.*, 2000), and is used in conjunction with or after standard root canal therapy (Hennet and Girard, 2005).

Surgical access to the root is obtained by making an incision into the alveolar mucosa over the root apex, and burring away the overlying bone to the level of the root (Hennet and Girard, 2005; Niemiec, 2008c). Any diseased tissue is curetted, and the area is flushed with sterile saline and dried. Two to four millimetres of the root tip are removed using a long-fissure or tapered-fissure bur (#699; #701) at an angle which allows access for debridement and retrograde filling of the root apex with MTA or ZOE (Niemiec, 2008c), after which the flap is sutured closed (Hennet and Girard, 2005).

4.6.4   Indirect pulp capping

This procedure is performed when there is near-exposure of the pulp (where the enamel and dentin have been damaged, causing the pulp to be close to the tooth surface but not exposed), such as the case of some caries lesions (Holmstrom *et al.*, 2000) and some fractured teeth (Klima, 2008a). Calcium hydroxide is placed over the area of damage to stimulate reparative dentin formation, then a restoration is placed (Holmstrom *et al.*, 2000).

4.6.5   Apexification

Apexification is performed to salvage a fractured, non-vital, immature tooth which does not have a closed root apex (Juriga, 2008b). The goal of apexification is to stimulate closure of the root apex with a calcified barrier so that standard root canal therapy can be performed, preserving tooth function.

The pulp is removed and the root canal is sterilized with bleach, then calcium hydroxide or MTA is packed within the canal to stimulate closure of the root apex. The tooth is sealed with a restoration (Juriga, 2008b).

Regular recheck radiographs are necessary every 3–6 months to monitor apex formation, after which time the calcium hydroxide or MTA is removed and standard root canal obturation is completed. Repeat-fills of the tooth with calcium hydroxide may be necessary to cause apexification, and it may not be successful at all, requiring extraction (Juriga, 2008b).

Teeth that have undergone apexification will always remain thin-walled and weak due to their immaturity at the time of pulp death.

4.6.6 Homecare following endodontic treatment

Once a tooth has had root canal therapy, the pet can eat and chew normally (hard kibble, treats and toys are acceptable) (Hale, 2012). If the patient is considered to be at a high risk of re-fracturing the tooth (such as a kennel-chewer or service dog), if there is little tooth crown remaining, or if the tooth is fairly young and its dentinal walls are not strong, a prosthodontic metal crown may be recommended (Brine and Marretta, 1999; Perrone *et al.*, 2020) (see Section 4.7, this volume).

Additional postoperative pain relief is usually not required for patients who have received a standard root canal treatment (Hale, 2012), but patients who have undergone vital pulp therapy or surgical root canal therapy should receive non-steroidal anti-inflammatory drugs (NSAIDs) for several days postoperatively to reduce inflammation and pain (Niemiec, 2008c; Perrone *et al.*, 2020).

Antibiotics are usually not needed following standard root canal therapy, though they may be used if periapical disease is present (Hale, 2012). A course of antibiotics is recommended following surgical root canal therapy (Perrone *et al.*, 2020) or vital pulp therapy (Niemiec, 2008a). Instruct the owner to feed only soft food for 14 days following surgical root canal therapy (Niemiec, 2008c).

Follow-up radiographs are recommended 6 months after standard (Perrone *et al.*, 2020) or surgical root canal therapy (Niemiec, 2008c), and yearly thereafter to monitor the success of treatment (Brine and Marretta, 1999) and to check the state of the restoration (Perrone *et al.*, 2020). Follow-up radiographs are imperative to ensure the success of vital pulp therapy (Clarke, 2001). Depending upon the length of time that the tooth was fractured prior to treatment, radiographs may be performed as early as 3 months postoperatively; however, it is most common to radiograph the tooth 6 months after treatment and at least yearly thereafter to monitor for continued tooth vitality (Clarke, 2001; Niemiec, 2008a). If the tooth becomes non-vital, it must undergo root canal therapy or extraction (Niemiec, 2008a).

4.7 Dental Restorations and Prosthodontics

Restorations fill tooth fracture sites (Klima, 2008a), access holes for endodontic treatments (Holmstrom *et al.*, 2000), and repair defects such as enamel hypoplasia (see Fig. 4.5) (Klima, 2008b) and caries (Holmstrom *et al.*, 2000). Prosthodontics provide structure and restore function, as in the case of a metal crown (Brine and Marretta, 1999; Perrone *et al.*, 2020).

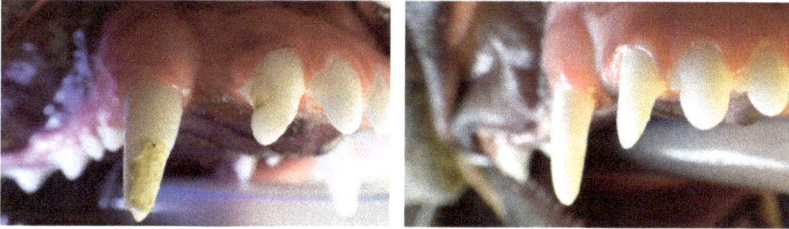

Fig. 4.5. Enamel hypoplasia before (left) and after (right) composite restoration.

There are two main types of dental restorations (Azeem and Sureshbabu, 2018):

1. Direct restorations: filling material is inserted directly into the tooth.
2. Indirect restorations (prosthodontics): restorations are placed onto the tooth instead of within the tooth structure, as in the case of crowns and bridges (Coffman, 2012). These require two anaesthetic procedures to complete: the first to shape the affected tooth or teeth to allow for placement of the prosthodontic with normal occlusion, and to take impressions (see Chapter 6, this volume) of the prepared tooth or teeth to send to a dental lab for manufacturing of the prosthodontic (Klima, 2008b; Lemmons and Carmichael, 2008). At the second procedure, a week or two later, the prosthodontic is cemented into place (Lemmons and Carmichael, 2008). The most common prosthodontics used in veterinary dentistry are metal crowns (Coffman, 2012).

4.7.1   Direct restoration materials

- Amalgam: a mixture of mercury and a powdered alloy consisting of silver, tin, zinc and copper (U.S. Food & Drug Administration (FDA), 2021). It requires a machine called an amalgamator to triturate the mercury and powder alloy together (Sakaguchi, 2019a). Amalgam does not adhere on its own to the tooth structure but requires cements or techniques to physically lock it to the tooth. It is inexpensive, self-hardening at body temperature and resistant to wear, but is prone to chipping (Sakaguchi, 2019a). Amalgam can expand with age, causing the tooth to crack. It is metallic in colour, and mercury is a known toxin (FDA, 2021).
- Composite resin (filled resin): a plastic resin filled with powdered glass, quartz or silica particles (Klima, 2008c). It mimics natural tooth colours, and can be polished for a smooth, aesthetically pleasing result, though it may discolour over time (Sakaguchi, 2019b). It is light-cured, which requires the use of a light-curing gun (Holmstrom *et al.*, 2000). Composite resin tends to shrink slightly upon curing, making the restoration vulnerable to microleakage (Legendre, 2001). Moisture adversely affects

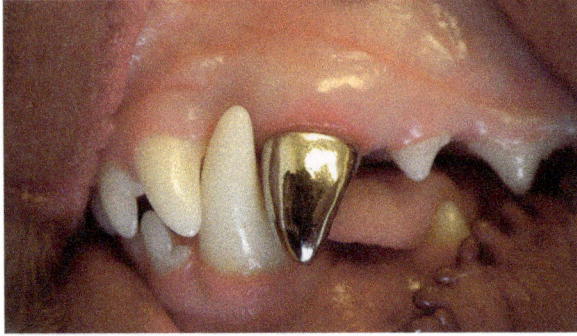

Fig. 4.6. Gold alloy crown.

bonding of composite resin to the tooth, and composite resins are more expensive and less resistant to wear than amalgam (Sakaguchi, 2019b). Composite resins can be macrofilled (small particles within the resin), which may be difficult to polish; microfilled (fine particles within the resin), which polishes well and retains shine (Hiscox, 2012); or hybrid (a combination of small and fine particles), which is easy to polish and highly resistant to fracture and wear (Legendre, 2001).

- Unfilled resin (sealant): a plastic resin that does not contain particles. Unfilled resins are less viscous and less resistant to wear than filled resins. They are often used as adhesives and sealants as an alternative to replacing large portions of tooth structure. Unfilled resins are applied over restorations to prevent microleakage, or directly onto the exposed dentin of a worn tooth, or onto a tooth with an uncomplicated enamel fracture to seal it against bacterial invasion and prevent sensitivity (Klima, 2008c).
- Glass ionomer: a mixture of glass and organic acid that bonds chemically to dentin (Girard *et al.*, 2006; Menezes-Silva *et al.*, 2019). Glass ionomers are tooth-coloured, but vary in translucency (Cho and Cheng, 1999). They are chemically cured, so do not require the use of a light-curing gun, but take time to fully set and harden. They are not subject to shrinkage and microleakage, but are not as durable as composite resins (Holmstrom *et al.*, 2000).
- Compomer: a combination of composite resin and glass ionomer (Sakaguchi, 2019b). They have better aesthetics than glass ionomers, but require a bonding system to adhere to the tooth. Compomers have a low tendency for leakage, but are not as durable as composite resins (Sakaguchi, 2019b).

4.7.2   Indirect restoration (prosthodontic) materials

- Porcelain: made of ceramic or glass (Lemmons and Carmichael, 2008). These are very brittle with a high tendency to fracture, and therefore are not suitable for most veterinary applications (Cherry, 2012). Their colour and texture can match natural tooth appearance (American Dental Association (ADA), 2002).

- Porcelain fused to metal: porcelain fused over a metal base to provide more strength while resembling a natural tooth (Lemmons and Carmichael, 2008). However, the porcelain can crack off, revealing the metal base beneath (Cherry, 2012). Some patients may have allergies to the base metals (ADA, 2002).
- Gold alloys (high noble): alloys of gold and other noble metals such as palladium or platinum (see Fig. 4.6) (ADA, 2002). They are resistant to corrosion, very strong, and durable. The appearance is metallic (silver- or gold-coloured). They are more expensive than base metal alloys, but have a low incidence of allergic reactions (ADA, 2002).
- Base metal alloys (non-noble): alloys of non-noble metals such as silver, nickel and tin (ADA, 2002). These are very strong and durable, less expensive than gold alloys, and are silver in colour. Some patients may have allergies to base metals (ADA, 2002).

4.7.3 Bonding agents

These allow restorations and prosthodontics to adhere to teeth by creating micromechanical bonds to enamel and/or dentin, and chemical bonds to restorative materials, which are placed over the bonding agents. Bonding-agent systems contain three components (Storli, 2012):

- Etchant: 30–40% phosphoric acid used to dissolve hydroxyapatite crystals in the enamel or dentin. The etching agent must be rinsed away and enamel dried completely, though dentin should be only partially dried, to keep moisture within its collagen fibres. If dentin is completely dried, its collagen fibres can collapse, impeding penetration of the primer. If etchant comes into contact with soft tissues, immediately rinse with copious amounts of water to prevent tissue damage (Gracis, 2015).
- Primer: a hydrophilic monomer applied after etching, which infiltrates the spaces of the demineralized enamel or dentin. After application, the primer is thinned and dried with air from an air-water syringe (Moore, 2012).
- Adhesive: a liquid adhesive material applied after priming and cured, usually by a light-curing gun (Moore, 2012). When a prosthodontic such as a crown is placed, a self-curing bonding agent called luting cement is used to anchor the crown to the tooth (Coffman, 2012).

4.7.4 Homecare following dental restoration

After receiving a composite restoration, the pet can resume normal eating and chewing postoperatively, though restricting access to hard food or

treats for 24 hours is recommended following amalgam restoration placement, to allow for complete curing of the material (Hecht, 2020).

Indirect restorations such as crowns require two procedures to complete, and the patient's shaped tooth may be more fragile and prone to
fracture until after the second procedure, when the prosthodontic is
placed (Brine and Marretta, 1999). Access to hard toys, treats and anything
else the patient may chew or bite inappropriately must be restricted during
this time. Once the prosthodontic has been placed, the tooth is stronger,
but not indestructible (Perrone *et al.*, 2020). Owners should be advised that
the bonding materials can fail if the pet is a determined chewer, resulting
in the loss of the prosthodontic (Perrone *et al.*, 2020). In some cases, a
crowned tooth can shear off at the gumline, with the crown still adhered
to the tooth!

References

ADA (2002) Comparison of indirect restorative dental materials. American Dental
    Association. Available at: https://www.ada.org/~/media/ADA/Member%20
    Center/FIles/materials.pdf?la=en (accessed 9 March 2021).
ADOS (2021) Antimicrobial therapy for veterinary dental and oral surgical pro-
    cedures. Animal Dentistry and Oral Surgery. Available at: https://animalde
    ntalspecialist.com/antimicrobial-therapy-vet-dentistry/ (accessed 16 February
    2021).
AVDC (2006) Veterinary dental healthcare providers. American Veterinary Dental
    College. Available at: https://avdc.org/about/#pos-stmts (accessed 16
    February 2021).
AVDC (2019) The use of antibiotics in veterinary dentistry. American Veterinary
    Dental College. Available at: https://avdc.org/about/ (accessed 16 February
    2021).
Azeem, R.A. and Sureshbabu, N.M. (2018) Clinical performance of direct versus in-
    direct composite restorations in posterior teeth: A systematic review. *Journal of
    Conservative Dentistry* 21(1), 2–9. Available at: https://www.ncbi.nlm.nih.gov/
    pmc/articles/PMC5852929/ (accessed 16 February 2021).
Boyd, R.C. and Ross, D.L. (2008) How to improve the quality and speed of your
    endodontic procedures with lightspeed instruments, endo vac irrigation and
    simplifill obturation. In: *Proceedings of the 22nd Annual Veterinary Dental Forum.*
    Omnipress, Madison, Wisconsin, pp. 21–23.
Brine, E.J. and Marretta, S. (1999) Endodontic treatment and metal crown restor-
    ation of a fractured maxillary right fourth premolar tooth: A case report. *Journal
    of Veterinary Dentistry* 16(4), 159–163. DOI: 10.1177/089875649901600401.
Carmichael, D. (2006) Dental extraction. In: *Proceedings of the 20th Annual Veterinary
    Dental Forum.* Omnipress, Madison, Wisconsin, pp. 185–190.
Cherry, B. (2012) The crown is in place. In: *Proceedings of the 26th Annual Veterinary
    Dental Forum.* Omnipress, Madison, Wisconsin (CD Rom).
Cho, S.-Y. and Cheng, A.C. (1999) A review of glass ionomer restorations on
    the primary dentition. *Journal of the Canadian Dental Association* 65(9),

491–495. Available at: http://cda-adc.ca/jcda/0/issue-9/491.html (accessed 16 February 2021).

Clarke, D. (2001) Vital pulp therapy for complicated crown fracture of permanent canine teeth in dogs: A three-year retrospective study. *Journal of Veterinary Dentistry* 18(3), 117–121. DOI: 10.1177/089875640101800301.

Coffman, C.R. (2012) Crown therapy: Introduction to veterinary prosthodontics. In: *Proceedings of the 26th Annual Veterinary Dental Forum*. Omnipress, Madison, Wisconsin (CD Rom).

Colmery, B.H. (2021) Endodontics. Vet Dentistry. Available at: http://www.vet dentistry.com/endodontics.html (accessed 16 February 2021).

Davis, E.M. (2021) Sound bites: Any time you discover a broken tooth, remember the 3 R's. Animal Dental Specialists of Upstate New York. Available at: https://www.adsuny.com/remember-the-3-rs.pml (accessed 17 February 2021).

DeBowes, L. (2012) Surgical extraction in dogs and cats. In: *Proceedings of the 26th Annual Veterinary Dental Forum*. Omnipress, Madison, Wisconsin (CD Rom).

FDA (2021) Dental amalgam fillings. U.S. Food & Drug Administration. Available at: https://www.fda.gov/medical-devices/dental-devices/dental-amalgam-fillings (accessed 10 March 2021).

Girard, N., Southerden, P. and Hennet, P. (2006) Root canal treatment in dogs and cats. *Journal of Veterinary Dentistry* 23(3), 148–160. DOI: 10.1177/089875640602300304.

Gracis, M. (2015) Treatment of alveolo-dental trauma (dental luxation and avulsion) and other dental emergencies. *World Small Animal Veterinary Association World Congress Proceedings, 2015*. Available at: https://www.vin.com/apputil/content/defaultadv1.aspx?id=7259301&pid=14365 (accessed 16 February 2021).

Hale, F.A. (2001) Localized intrinsic staining of teeth due to pulpitis and pulp necrosis in dogs. *Journal of Veterinary Dentistry* 18(1), 4–20. DOI: 10.1177/089875640101800102.

Hale, F.A. (2008) Endodontic anatomy and physiology. In: *Proceedings of the 22nd Annual Veterinary Dental Forum*. Omnipress, Madison, Wisconsin, pp. 189–193.

Hale, F.A. (2012) What is root canal treatment? Hale Veterinary Clinic. Available at: http://www.toothvet.ca/PDFfiles/root_canal_treatment.pdf (accessed 16 February 2021).

Hecht, M. (2020) How long does it take to get a filling? Healthline. Available at: https://www.healthline.com/health/how-long-does-it-take-to-get-a-filling (accessed 16 February 2021).

Hennet, P. and Girard, N. (2005) Surgical endodontics in dogs: A review. *Journal of Veterinary Dentistry* 22(3), 50–61. DOI: 10.1177/089875640502200301.

Hernandez, M. (2008) Alternatives to extractions. In: *Proceedings of the 22nd Annual Veterinary Dental Forum*. Omnipress, Madison, Wisconsin, pp. 337–338.

Hiscox, L. (2012) Dental materials – a composite review. In: *Proceedings of the 26th Annual Veterinary Dental Forum*. Omnipress, Madison, Wisconsin (CD Rom).

Holmstrom, S., Holmstrom, L.A., McGrath, C.J., Richey, M.T. and Wiggs, R.B. (2000) Advanced veterinary dental procedures. In: Holmstrom, S. (ed.) *Veterinary Dentistry for the Technician & Office Staff*. Saunders, Philadelphia, Pennsylvania, pp. 247–282.

Holmstrom, S., Frost, P. and Eisner, E. (2004) Endodontics. In: Eisner, E. (ed.) *Veterinary Dental Techniques for the Small Animal Practitioner*. Saunders, Philadelphia, Pennsylvania, pp. 255–318.

Honzelka, S.R. (2012) Dental extractions: Principles and techniques. In: *Proceedings of the 26th Annual Veterinary Dental Forum.* Omnipress, Madison, Wisconsin (CD Rom).

Juriga, S. (2008a) Surgical extraction techniques. In: *Proceedings of the 22nd Annual Veterinary Dental Forum.* Omnipress, Madison, Wisconsin, pp. 257–261.

Juriga, S. (2008b) Current concepts in apexification. In: *Proceedings of the 22nd Annual Veterinary Dental Forum.* Omnipress, Madison, Wisconsin, pp. 25–28.

Khuly, P. (2020) Tooth extractions in dogs: Causes, procedures, recovery and prevention. Hill's. Available at: https://www.hillspet.com/dog-care/healthcare/dog-tooth-extractions (accessed 16 February 2021).

Klima, L. (2008a) Addressing uncomplicated (no pulp exposure) and complicated (pulp exposure) crown fractures. In: *Proceedings of the 22nd Annual Veterinary Dental Forum.* Omnipress, Madison, Wisconsin, pp. 265–267.

Klima, L. (2008b) Enamel defects and the potential for rapid development of pathology. In: *Proceedings of the 22nd Annual Veterinary Dental Forum.* Omnipress, Madison, Wisconsin, pp. 307–309.

Klima, L. (2008c) Sealants for teeth: Why, where, and how? In: *Proceedings of the 22nd Annual Veterinary Dental Forum.* Omnipress, Madison, Wisconsin, pp. 333–336.

Kling, K. (2018) Root canal therapy for function and health. College of Veterinary Medicine, University of Illinois at Urbana-Champaign. Available at: https://vetmed.illinois.edu/root-canal-therapy-for-function-and-health/ (accessed 16 February 2021).

Legendre, L. (2001) Comparative review of the new restorative compounds. *World Small Animal Veterinary Association World Congress Proceedings, 2001.* Available at: https://www.vin.com/apputil/content/defaultadv1.aspx?pId=8708&id=3843726&print=1 (accessed 16 February 2021).

Lemmons, M. and Carmichael, D.T. (2008) Dental corner: Dental fracture treatment options in dogs and cats. Dvm360. Available at: https://www.dvm360.com/view/dental-corner-dental-fracture-treatment-options-dogs-and-cats (accessed 16 February 2021).

Menezes-Silva, R., Cabral, R.N., Pascotto, R.C., Borges, A.F.S., Martins, C.C. *et al.* (2019) Mechanical and optical properties of conventional restorative glass-ionmer cements – a systematic review. *Journal of Applied Oral Science* 27, e2018357. Available at: https://www.ncbi.nlm.nih.gov/pmc/articles/PMC6382318/ (accessed 16 February 2021).

Mills, A. (2012) The technician's role in extraction. In: *Proceedings of the 26th Annual Veterinary Dental Forum.* Omnipress, Madison, Wisconsin (CD Rom).

Moore, J. (2012) Vital pulp therapy in dogs. In: *Proceedings of the 26th Annual Veterinary Dental Forum.* Omnipress, Madison, Wisconsin (CD Rom).

Niemiec, B.A. (2008a) Vital pulp therapy. In: *Proceedings of the 22nd Annual Veterinary Dental Forum.* Omnipress, Madison, Wisconsin, pp. 285–288.

Niemiec, B.A. (2008b) A critical review of endodontic filling materials and methods. In: *Proceedings of the 22nd Annual Veterinary Dental Forum.* Omnipress, Madison, Wisconsin, pp. 31–39.

Niemiec, B.A. (2008c) Surgical endodontics. In: *Proceedings of the 22nd Annual Veterinary Dental Forum.* Omnipress, Madison, Wisconsin, pp. 19–20.

Niemiec, B.A. (2012a) Proper therapy for endodontic disease. Today's Veterinary Practice. Available at: https://todaysveterinarypractice.com/practical-dentistry-proper-therapy-for-endodontic-disease/ (accessed 16 February 2021).

Niemiec, B.A. (2012b) Dental extractions: Five steps to improve client education, surgical procedures, and patient care. Today's Veterinary Practice. Available at: https://todaysveterinarypractice.com/practical-dentistry-dental-extractions/ (accessed 16 February 2021).

Peak, M.R. (2012) Principles of endodontic therapy. In: *Proceedings of the 26th Annual Veterinary Dental Forum.* Omnipress, Madison, Wisconsin (CD Rom).

Perrone, J. (2020) Appendices. In: Perrone, J. (ed.) *Small Animal Dental Procedures for Veterinary Technicians and Nurses.* Wiley Blackwell, Hoboken, New Jersey, pp. 223–243.

Perrone, J., Sharp, S. and March, P. (2020) Common dental conditions and treatments. In: Perrone, J. (ed.) *Small Animal Dental Procedures for Veterinary Technicians and Nurses.* Wiley Blackwell, Hoboken, New Jersey, pp. 131–168.

Queck, K.E. and Runyon, C.L. (1987) Root canal therapy for fracture-induced endodontic disease in the dog. Available at: https://lib.dr.iastate.edu/cgi/viewcontent.cgi?article=3211&context=iowastate_veterinarian (accessed 16 February 2021).

SACVDS (2021) Oral surgery – extractions. Sacramento Veterinary Dental Services. *Iowa State University Veterinarian* 49(1), Article 1. Available at: https://www.sacvds.com/forms/faq-oral-surgery-extractions.pdf (accessed 16 February 2021).

Sakaguchi, R. (2019a) Restorative materials: Metals. In: Sakaguchi, R., Ferracane, J. and Powers, J. (eds) *Craig's Restorative Dental Materials.* Elsevier, Philadelphia, Pennsylvania, pp. 171–208.

Sakaguchi, R. (2019b) Restorative materials: Composites and polymers. In: Sakaguchi, R., Ferracane, J. and Powers, J. (eds) *Craig's Restorative Dental Materials.* Elsevier, Philadelphia, Pennsylvania, pp. 162–170.

Sharp, S. (2019) Brushing up on dentistry – endodontics vs. exodontics. Vet Folio. Available at: https://www.vetfolio.com/learn/article/brushing-up-on-dentistry-endodontics-vs-exodontics (accessed 16 February 2021).

Smith, M.M., Smith, E.M., La Croix, N. and Mould, J. (2003) Orbital penetration associated with tooth extraction. *Journal of Veterinary Dentistry* 20(1), 8–17. DOI: 10.1177/089875640302000101.

Stein, K.E., Marretta, S.M., Siegel, A. and Vitoux, J. (2004) Comparison of hand-instrumented, heated gutta percha and engine-driven, cold gutta-percha endodontic techniques. *Journal of Veterinary Dentistry* 23(1), 136–145. DOI: 10.1177/089875640402100301.

Storli, S. (2012) Dental materials: Bonding agents. In: *Proceedings of the 26th Annual Veterinary Dental Forum.* Omnipress, Madison, Wisconsin (CD Rom).

Taylor, E.M. (2004) Dental extractions: Indications, precautions, techniques, and complications. In: *Proceedings of the 18th Annual Veterinary Dental Forum.* Omnipress, Madison, Wisconsin, pp. 94–99.

Watanabe, R., Doodnaught, G., Proulx, C., Auger, J.-P., Monteiro, B. *et al.* (2019) A multidisciplinary study of pain in cats undergoing extractions: A prospective, blinded, clinical trial. *PLoS ONE* 14(3), e0213195. Available at: https://journals.plos.org/plosone/article?id=10.1371/journal.pone.0213195 (accessed 16 February 2021).

Zeltzman, P. (2021) Using cold therapy for dogs. Pet Health Network. Available at: https://www.pethealthnetwork.com/dog-health/dog-diseases-conditions-a-z/using-cold-therapy-dogs (accessed 16 February 2021).

The Hole Problem: Tooth Resorption and Caries

5

5.1 Tooth resorption pathology, clinical signs and diagnosis

Tooth resorption, previously known as resorptive lesions, feline odontoclastic resorptive lesions, cervical line lesions or neck lesions (Bellows, 2016a; Crawford and Losey, 2020) is one of the most common oral diseases experienced by cats (Gorrel, 2004), affecting up to 75% of cats over 5 years of age (Reiter, 2004; Bellows, 2016a). Tooth resorption can also occur in dogs (see Section 5.6, this volume) (Bellows, 2016a).

Resorption is the physiological removal of tissues or body products, such as the roots of deciduous teeth by the body (Ekerdt, 2021). Unlike bone, which is continually resorbed and remodelled by osteoclasts and osteoblasts, permanent teeth do not normally undergo physiological removal (Reiter, 2004; Shope and Carle, 2017). Tooth resorption of permanent teeth occurs through the inappropriate action of odontoclastic cells, which resorb dental hard tissues (Crawford and Losey, 2020). Resorption often begins in the cementum, with subsequent resorption of the dentin extending apically, coronally or both (Gorrel, 2004; Bellows, 2016a). Resorption can also originate within the pulp cavity in a process known as internal resorption (Bellows, 2016a).

5.1.1 Causes of tooth resorption

The cause(s) of tooth resorption is unknown (Niemiec *et al.*, 2019; Crawford and Losey, 2020), though there are various theories, such as periodontal inflammation stimulating odontoclastic cells near the cementoenamel junction, minor trauma to the cementum, local pH changes due to hairball regurgitation, autoimmune conditions or viral infections (Holmstrom *et al.*, 2000a; Bellows, 2016a, b; Shope and Carle, 2017). Different causes may apply to different cases (Bellows, 2016a).

© CAB International 2022. *An Introduction to Pet Dental Care: For Veterinary Technicians and Nurses* (K. Istace)
DOI: 10.1079/9781789248869.0005

5.1.2   Clinical signs of tooth resorption

Tooth resorption is very painful, and can cause tooth chattering, drooling, lethargy, oral bleeding, dysphagia and anorexia (Crawford and Losey, 2020). However, most patients do not show any clinical signs (Niemiec *et al.*, 2019). Resorption is often seen in the exam room as an inflamed red lesion or area of granulation tissue close to the cementoenamel junction, which can be mistaken for gingival hyperplasia (Crawford and Losey, 2020). If the area is probed, the cat will usually chatter their teeth or display some other pain response (Bellows, 2016a). As tooth resorption progresses, the crown of the tooth is destroyed until little or none remains. Often, cats who have had untreated tooth resorption will present with a 'missing' tooth (Shope and Carle, 2017) and a bump covered by gingiva where the tooth should be (Bellows, 2016b).

5.1.3   Diagnosis of tooth resorption

Once the patient is anaesthetized, palpate any visible suspected tooth resorption with a dental explorer (Gorrel, 2004; Crawford and Losey, 2020). The dentin lining an area of resorption will feel sharp and hard, not smooth like root furcation exposure or soft like a caries lesion (Shope and Carle, 2017).

Dental radiography is essential to diagnose tooth resorption and determine the appropriate treatment option (Holmstrom *et al.*, 2000a). Radiographs may show that the roots of the resorbing tooth are radiolucent, with loss of the periodontal ligament space and possibly the root itself, as the radiopacity of the root decreases to match that of the surrounding bone (Shope and Carle, 2017). However, some teeth undergoing resorption will maintain the integrity of their roots and/or periodontal ligament (American Veterinary Dental College (AVDC), 2021). In multi-rooted teeth, one root may be resorbing and the other may not (Beckman, 2011). Full-mouth radiographs should be performed on patients diagnosed with one resorbing tooth, because cats with one resorbing tooth are more likely to have or to develop others (Holmstrom *et al.*, 2000a; Bellows, 2016a).

5.2   Stages of Tooth Resorption

Tooth resorption is staged based upon radiographic determination of the severity of dental hard tissue loss (AVDC, 2021):

- TR Stage 1: Mild dental hard tissue loss (cementum and possible enamel loss).
- TR Stage 2: Moderate dental hard tissue loss (cementum and possible enamel loss; dentin loss not extending to the pulp cavity).

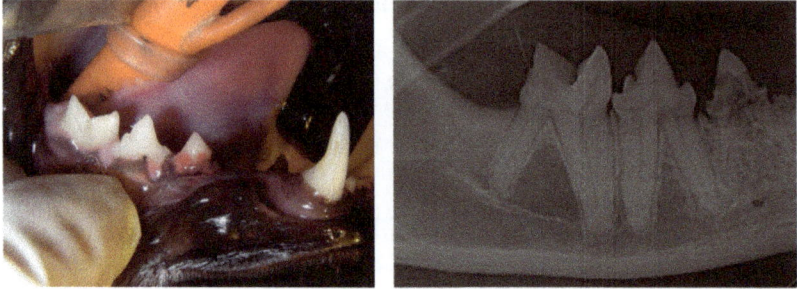

Fig. 5.1. Tooth resorption.

- TR Stage 3: Deep dental hard tissue loss (cementum and possible enamel loss; dentin loss extending to the pulp cavity); most of the tooth is intact.
- TR Stage 4: Extensive dental hard tissue loss (cementum and possible enamel loss; dentin loss extending to the pulp cavity); most of the tooth has lost its integrity. (TR4a: crown and root equally affected; TR4b: crown more severely affected than root; TR4c: root more severely affected than crown.)
- TR Stage 5: No crown remains; tooth is covered by gingiva; remnants of dental hard tissue may be visible on radiographs.

5.3   Types of Tooth Resorption

Once the stage of tooth resorption is identified, the type of tooth resorption is determined based upon its radiographic appearance (Crawford and Losey, 2020). The type of tooth resorption determines the appropriate treatment option (Klima, 2008).

- Type I: focal or multifocal areas of radiolucency of a tooth with otherwise normal radiopacity and a normal periodontal ligament space (AVDC, 2021). The dental tissues of teeth have not been replaced by bone and the root has normal density in some areas (Niemiec *et al.*, 2019). This type of resorption may be associated with inflammation, e.g. periodontal disease or stomatitis (Niemiec *et al.*, 2019).
- Type II: decreased radiopacity of part of the tooth, with narrowing or disappearing of the periodontal ligament (ankylosis) in some or all areas (AVDC, 2021). The root may appear to be disintegrating as it is being replaced by bony tissue (Klima, 2008). This type of resorption, called replacement resorption, is usually seen in an otherwise healthy mouth (Niemiec *et al.*, 2019), and may be asymptomatic if resorption is confined to the root (Gorrel, 2004).
- Type III: features of both Type I and Type II resorption are present in the same tooth (Shope and Carle, 2017; AVDC, 2021). One root may

have little discernible structure while the other is intact (Beckman, 2011; Niemiec *et al.*, 2019).

5.4 Treatment of Tooth Resorption

The prognosis for teeth undergoing resorption is grim. In the past, some veterinary dentists tried to save these teeth by filling the defects, but the vast majority of teeth continued to resorb beneath these restorations (Gorrel, 2004; Crawford and Losey, 2020). Treatment options are now limited to extraction or crown amputation (Shope and Carle, 2017; Crawford and Losey, 2020). Teeth undergoing Type II resorption with no crown involvement do not seem to be painful and may not need to be treated if the owners are willing to return for regular radiographic monitoring (Shope and Carle, 2017).

5.4.1 Extraction

Extraction (see Chapter 4, this volume) is usually limited to teeth undergoing Type I resorption, since in Type II resorption the root structure is indistinguishable from that of the surrounding bone, and attempting to extract root that is being remodelled into bone is extremely difficult and can result in jaw fracture (Lewis, 2015a). However, extraction is required for teeth with intact roots, or with resorbing roots if there are any signs of periodontal disease, endodontic disease or stomatitis (Shope and Carle, 2017; Niemiec *et al.*, 2019; Crawford and Losey, 2020). In Type III resorption, with one root undergoing resorption while the other is not, extraction of the intact root must be performed (Beckman, 2011; Lewis, 2014). Leaving an intact tooth root in place can lead to infection or osteomyelitis (Niemiec, 2012).

5.4.2 Crown amputation

Crown amputation is performed only in cases of Type II resorption and on the resorbing portion of the tooth in Type III resorption (Beckman, 2011). It must be done as aseptically as possible, and can be performed only on teeth having no signs of periodontal disease or endodontic disease, and in patients without stomatitis (Klima, 2008; Crawford and Losey, 2020). The advantage of this technique is that it causes little trauma to the patient, is relatively quick, poses no risk of fracturing the jaw, and symptomatic patients improve quickly following elimination of exposure of the resorbing tissue to the oral cavity (Klima, 2008). The disadvantage is that some root material remains in the alveolus, so there is a risk of infection (Hale, 2004).

Crown amputation is performed by creating an envelope flap, then amputating the tooth crown and the coronal portion of the root 1–2 mm beneath the alveolar margin with a round (#1, #2) or crosscut-fissure (#699, #700, #701) carbide bur (Klima, 2008; Lewis, 2014) on a high-speed handpiece, using water to cool it (Niemiec *et al.*, 2019). The bone and root(s) are smoothed with a round or pear carbide bur or a diamond bur (Lewis, 2014) and the gingiva is sutured closed with small-gauge absorbable suture material (Crawford and Losey, 2020), as is done after an extraction. Take postoperative X-rays to assess the bone smoothness of the amputation (Klima, 2008; Lewis, 2014).

5.4.3   Homecare following treatment of tooth resorption

Patients who have had extractions or crown amputations should receive pain medication for at least 7 days postoperatively (Niemiec, 2012). In most cases, antibiotics are not required (Hale, 2004). Instruct owners to feed only soft food for 7–10 days to reduce pain during chewing and to help prevent dehiscence of the extraction or crown amputation site(s) (Bellows, 2016c).

Tooth brushing should be temporarily discontinued until the tissue has healed, to prevent trauma to the healing gingiva and to prevent the pet from associating tooth brushing with oral pain (Carmichael, 2005). Oral rinses and/or water additives should be used during this time to discourage plaque formation (Bellows, 2016c).

Schedule a recheck 10–14 days postoperatively to ensure the extraction or crown amputation sites have healed and that the pet is eating well and maintaining their weight, and to discuss establishing or re-starting a dental homecare program (Carmichael, 2005).

Ideally, patients who have had crown amputations should have follow-up radiographs of the area taken 6–12 months postoperatively to ensure that the tooth roots are completing their resorption with no signs of abscess or infection (Greenfield, 2020). Pet owners should be made aware that once a cat has been diagnosed with one resorptive lesion, there is a high probability they will develop additional lesions (Hale, 2004). Yearly full-mouth radiographs are recommended to monitor for this. Since periodontal inflammation may be associated with some types of tooth resorption, dental homecare and routine COHATs are recommended, though tooth resorption can occur in the absence of periodontal disease (Hale, 2004; Carmichael, 2005).

5.5   Tooth Resorption in Dogs

Tooth resorption has been found in 17–21% of dogs, and seems to be more prevalent in older and overweight dogs (Shope and Carle, 2017).

As in cats, the exact cause of tooth resorption is unknown, but heavy mastication (chewing) forces, inflammatory conditions such as endodontic disease and periodontal disease, and traumatic injuries have all been implicated in the development of tooth resorption in dogs (Volker, 2017; Ekerdt, 2021).

Diagnosis and treatment is similar to that in cats. Root canal therapy has been successful in treating some cases of internal inflammatory resorption in dogs (Ekerdt, 2021).

5.6 Caries

Dental caries or 'cavities' are much less common in dogs than in humans, due to the animals' alkaline salivary pH; this inhibits cariogenic bacteria, which thrive in more acidic environments (Kirby, 2019). Dogs have fewer occlusal pits and wider interdental spaces than humans, which allow for less food impaction, and generally eat diets lower in carbohydrates, which also reduces the likelihood of caries formation (Reiter, 2014). However, about 5% of dogs do develop caries (Lewis, 2015b). High sugar intake, particularly from ingesting sticky human foods such as sweetened peanut butter, has been associated with the development of caries in dogs (Kirby, 2019). Dogs with poor saliva flow can also develop caries (Kirby, 2019). Caries are extremely rare in cats (Lewis, 2015b).

Caries lesions occur when certain types of bacteria ferment carbohydrates, forming acid by-products that demineralize tooth structure (McMahon, 2020). Caries typically form on the occlusal surfaces of molars, but can also form in the developmental grooves of carnassials, or on the crown close to the gingival margin (Holmstrom *et al.*, 2000b; Kirby, 2019). The lesions are brown or black in colour, and will often feel soft, sticky or

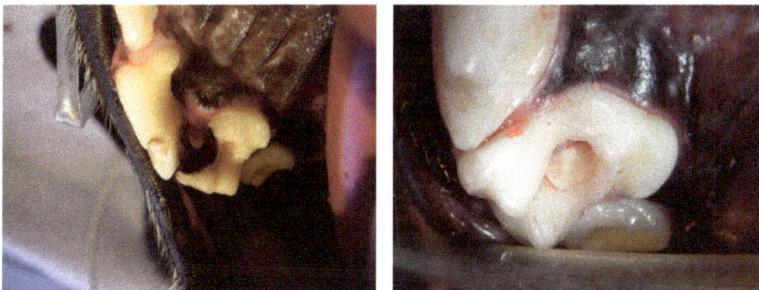

Fig. 5.2. Caries. Left: brown carious dentin close to the gingival margins of this upper carnassial and first molar. These teeth were extracted. Right: carious dentin has been removed from the occlusal surface of this first molar in preparation for a restoration.

leathery when palpated with a dental explorer (Kirby, 2019; McMahon, 2020).

Treatment options depend on how advanced the lesion is at diagnosis (Kirby, 2019). Early lesions are treated by removing the carious dentin with a bur or spoon excavator and placing a restoration (Hale, 1998). If the pulp has been exposed, root canal therapy or extraction are indicated. If there is substantial loss of tooth structure, the tooth must be extracted (Hale, 1998).

References

AVDC (2021) AVDC nomenclature. American Veterinary Dental College. Available at: https://avdc.org/avdc-nomenclature/ (accessed 12 February 2021).

Beckman, B. (2011) Tooth resorption in cats. Dvm360. Available at: https://www.dvm360.com/view/tooth-resorption-cats (accessed 17 February 2021).

Bellows, J. (2016a) External tooth resorption in cats. Today's Veterinary Practice. Available at: https://todaysveterinarypractice.com/external-tooth-resorption-cats/ (accessed 17 February 2021).

Bellows, J. (2016b) Tooth resorption in cats. Veterinary Partner. Available at: https://veterinarypartner.vin.com/default.aspx?pid=19239&id=4951295 (accessed 17 February 2021).

Bellows, J. (2016c) External tooth resorption in cats part 2: therapeutic approaches. Today's Veterinary Practice. Available at: https://todaysveterinarypractice.com/external-tooth-resorption-in-cats-part-2-therapeutic-approaches/ (accessed 17 February 2021).

Carmichael, D.T. (2005) Dental corner: how to detect and treat feline odontoclastic resorptive lesions. Dvm360. Available at: https://www.dvm360.com/view/dental-corner-how-detect-and-treat-feline-odontoclastic-resorptive-lesions (accessed 17 February 2021).

Crawford, J. and Losey, B.J. (2020) Feline dentistry. In: Perrone, J. (ed.) *Small Animal Dental Procedures for Veterinary Technicians and Nurses*. Wiley Blackwell, Hoboken, New Jersey, pp. 169–186.

Ekerdt, A. (2021) Tooth resorption in dogs. MSPCA. Available at: https://www.mspca.org/angell_services/tooth-resorption-in-dogs/ (accessed 17 February 2021).

Gorrel, C. (2004) A practical approach to managing feline odontoclastic resorptive lesions. In: *Proceedings of the 18th Annual Veterinary Dental Forum*. Omnipress, Madison, Wisconsin, pp. 103–104.

Greenfield, B. (2020) Feline Tooth Resorptions (TR)…when to extract and when to crown amputate? In: *2020 Ontario Veterinary Medical Association Conference Proceedings*. OVMA, Milton, Ontario, pp. 31–33.

Hale, F.A. (1998) Dental caries in the dog. *Journal of Veterinary Dentistry* 15(2), 79–84. DOI: 10.1177/089875649801500203.

Hale, F.A. (2004) Feline odontoclastic resorptive lesions. Hale Veterinary Clinic. Available at: http://www.toothvet.ca/VSTEP/p%20-%20forls%20and%20LPS.pdf (accessed 28 January 2021).

Holmstrom, S., Holmstrom, L.A., McGrath, C.J., Richey, M.T. and Wiggs, R.B. (2000a) Feline dentistry. In: Holmstrom, S. (ed.) *Veterinary Dentistry for the Technician & Office Staff.* Saunders, Philadelphia, Pennsylvania, pp. 283–291.

Holmstrom, S., Holmstrom, L.A., McGrath, C.J., Richey, M.T. and Wiggs, R.B. (2000b) The oral examination and disease recognition. In: Holmstrom, S. (ed.) *Veterinary Dentistry for the Technician & Office Staff.* Saunders, Philadelphia, Pennsylvania, pp. 23–61.

Kirby, S. (2019) Dental caries lesions in dogs. Veterinary Practice. Available at: https://veterinary-practice.com/article/dental-caries-lesions-in-dogs (accessed 17 February 2021).

Klima, L.J. (2008) Tooth resorption in cats: Clarifying the approach to crown amputation versus extraction. In: *Proceedings of the 22nd Annual Veterinary Dental Forum.* Omnipress, Madison, Wisconsin, pp. 245–248.

Lewis, J. (2014) How to extract teeth in cats. Veterinary Practice News. Available at: https://www.veterinarypracticenews.com/how-to-extract-teeth-in-cats/ (accessed 17 February 2021).

Lewis, J. (2015a) How to avoid the iatrogenic jaw fracture. Veterinary Practice News. Available at: https://www.veterinarypracticenews.com/how-to-avoid-the-iatrogenic-jaw-fracture/ (accessed 17 February 2021).

Lewis, J. (2015b) Do dogs and cats get cavities? Veterinary Practice News. Available at: https://www.veterinarypracticenews.com/do-dogs-and-cats-get-cavities/ (accessed 13 February 2021).

McMahon, J. (2020) The dental cleaning. In: Perrone, J. (ed.) *Small Animal Dental Procedures for Veterinary Technicians and Nurses.* Wiley Blackwell, Hoboken, New Jersey, pp. 65–91.

Niemiec, B.A. (2012) Dental extractions: five steps to improve client education, surgical procedures, and patient care. Today's Veterinary Practice. Available at: https://todaysveterinarypractice.com/practical-dentistry-dental-extractions/ (accessed 16 February 2021).

Niemiec, B.A., Morgenegg, G. and Tutt, C. (2019) Tooth resorption. Clinician's Brief. Available at: https://www.cliniciansbrief.com/article/tooth-resorption-0 (accessed 17 February 2021).

Reiter, A.M. (2004) Update on feline odontoclastic resorptive lesions. In: *Proceedings of the 18th Annual Veterinary Dental Forum.* Omnipress, Madison, Wisconsin, pp. 43–44.

Reiter, A.M. (2014) Dental caries in small animals. Available at: https://www.merckvetmanual.com/digestive-system/dentistry/dental-caries-in-small-animals (accessed 17 February 2021).

Shope, B. and Carle, D. (2017) Tooth resorption in dogs and cats. VetBloom blog. Available at: http://blog.vetbloom.com/dentistry/tooth-resorption-in-dogs-and-cats/ (accessed 17 February 2021).

Volker, M. (2017) Complications of complicated surgical extractions. Dvm360. Available at: https://www.fetchdvm360.com/wp-content/uploads/2017/11/FetchSD-2017-0130-0139-Dentistry.pdf (accessed 17 February 2021).

Out of Place: Malocclusions

6

Malocclusions are deviations in the position of individual teeth or dispari-ties in the length or width of the bones of the face (American Veterinary Dental College (AVDC), 2021). In veterinary dentistry, malocclusions are only of concern if they impair function or cause trauma or pain Hale (2018). Aesthetic concerns (including the opinions of breeders, show judges and pet owners) don't matter to our patients at all. The ethics of risking an animal's life with general anaesthesia to perform a potentially painful procedure simply for appearance are questionable (Niemiec, 2013; Bellows, 2017).

6.1 Normal Occlusion

The head and face should be symmetrical (Salter, 2004). The midline of the maxillary arches should be centred over the midline of the man-dibles where they join at the mandibular symphysis. These midlines should align with the centre of the nose and forehead. Asymmetry can be a sign of abnormal formation of the bones of the mandibles or maxilla, though some asymmetries can be attributed to infection, trauma or neoplasia (Sacramento Veterinary Dental Services (SACVDS), 2021).

There should be no missing teeth (Salter, 2004), and no teeth of the same type occupying the same space at the same time, such as in the case of retained deciduous teeth or in some instances of supernumerary teeth (Hale, 2004).

The teeth of each quadrant should line up mesial-to-distal, with none of the teeth rotated (Salter, 2004). The upper incisors should occlude labially to the lower incisors, with the lower incisors resting against or near the cingulum (enamel protrusion) on the palatal aspect of the upper incisors when the mouth is closed (AVDC, 2021). The mandibular canine teeth should occupy the diastema (space) buccally between the upper canines and the upper lateral incisors (AVDC, 2021) without excessive contact with other teeth or soft tissue. The tips of the crowns of the maxillary pre-molars should align with the interproximal spaces between the mandibular

© CAB International 2022. *An Introduction to Pet Dental Care: For Veterinary Technicians and Nurses* (K. Istace)
DOI: 10.1079/9781789248869.0006

premolars and vice versa, with the maxillary fourth premolars occluding buccally to the mandibular first molars (AVDC, 2021). In dogs, the cusps of the upper and lower molars should occlude against each other.

Brachycephalic (short-faced) breeds regularly have malocclusions due to their short maxilla, resulting in the crowding and rotation of maxillary teeth, and the disparity in the lengths between their short maxilla and normal-length mandible (Perrone *et al.*, 2020).

6.2 Abnormal Occlusion

There are four main classes of malocclusion. The class of malocclusion is recorded on the patient's dental chart and medical records, along with any specific tooth malocclusion (AVDC, 2021).

6.2.1 Class 1 malocclusion (neutroclusion / misaligned tooth)

This is a normal relationship of the maxilla and mandible, with malposition of one or more individual teeth (Holmstrom *et al.*, 2000a; AVDC, 2021). Class 1 malocclusions can include buccoversion, distoversion, labioversion, linguoversion, palatoversion and mesioversion (AVDC, 2021). Base narrow (linguoverted) canines, where the mandible is of normal length but a mandibular canine tooth or teeth contact the palate, is considered a Class 1 malocclusion (Perrone *et al.*, 2020). Rostral crossbite, in which one or more of the upper incisors occlude caudally to the lower incisors; and caudal crossbite, in which one or more maxillary premolars occlude palatally to the mandibular premolars or molars, can be types of Class 1 malocclusion if individual teeth are out of occlusion while the jaw relationship remains normal (AVDC, 2021).

6.2.2 Class 2 malocclusion (mandibular distoclusion / short mandible)

This is an abnormal rostrocaudal relationship between the maxilla and the mandible in which the mandible occludes caudal to its normal position relative to the maxilla (AVDC, 2021). A Class 2 malocclusion can sometimes cause bilateral base narrow canines (Holmstrom *et al.*, 2000a). Class 2 malocclusions have been reported more frequently in retrievers, standard poodle and poodle mixes, bull terriers and German shepherds (Thatcher, 2019).

6.2.3 Class 3 malocclusion (mandibular mesioclusion / long mandible)

This is an abnormal rostrocaudal relationship between the maxilla and mandible in which the mandible occludes rostral to its normal position

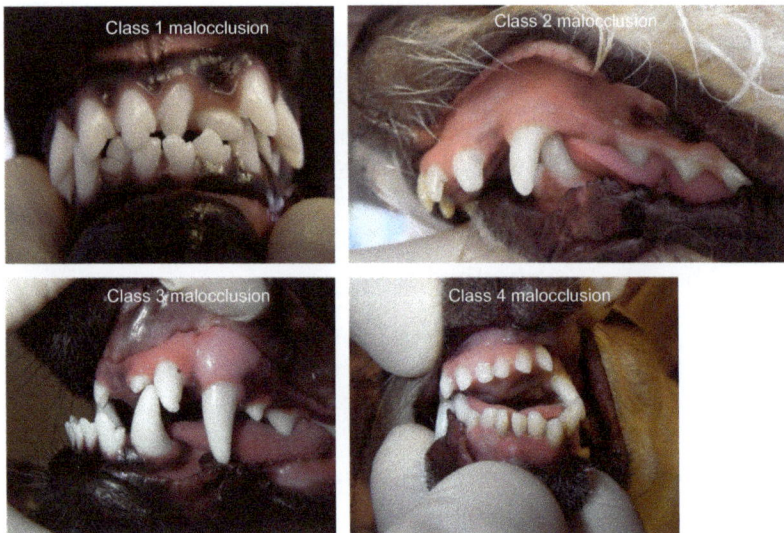

Fig. 6.1. Malocclusions.

relative to the maxilla (AVDC, 2021). Class 3 malocclusions include under-bites and level bites, in which the cusps of upper and lower incisors occlude (Holmstrom *et al.*, 2000a; Perrone *et al.*, 2020). This type of malocclusion is typical of many brachycephalic breeds, such as pugs, shih tzus, bulldogs, boxers and Persian cats (Bellows, 2017).

6.2.4   Class 4 malocclusion (maxillomandibular asymmetry)

This includes rostrocaudal asymmetry of the mandible relative to the maxilla on one side of the face only, side-to-side asymmetry of the maxilla or mandible causing loss of midline alignment between the maxilla and mandible, and dorsoventral asymmetry causing an abnormal vertical space between opposing dental arches (open bite) (AVDC, 2021).

6.3   Treatment of Malocclusions

Treatment of malocclusion is necessary only if function is impaired (the animal must be able to eat, carry toys or other objects, bite, etc.), or if pain, infection or trauma to other teeth or soft tissues is occurring due to the malocclusion (Niemiec, 2013; Hale, 2018; Perrone *et al.*, 2020).

Treatment options for malocclusion include preventive orthodontics to prevent the onset of malocclusion, interceptive orthodontics to elim-inate a developing or established malocclusion, or corrective orthodontics (AVDC, 2021). The type of malocclusion, the wishes of the owner, and the patient's general physical and periodontal health will determine the course of treatment (Hale, 2018). For example, corrective orthodontics often requires multiple procedures under general anaesthesia, and therefore would not be practical for a patient with an increased anaesthetic risk.

In all cases of malocclusion, the earlier that problems are recognized and treated, the better the outcome will be for the patient (Hale, 2018). Learning to recognize what comprises normal occlusion makes it easier to recognize abnormalities when they occur.

6.3.1 Preventive orthodontics

Preventive orthodontics aims to evaluate, predict and eliminate conditions that may predispose paediatric patients to malocclusion (AVDC, 2021). Therefore, it's essential to be able to recognize normal vs abnormal tooth eruption and occlusion in young animals (Hale, 2004).

The term deciduous (primary or baby) means a tooth that will shed. Persistent deciduous teeth are deciduous teeth that have not exfoliated once their permanent counterparts have begun to erupt (Bellows, 2019). Permanent upper canine teeth erupt mesially relative to their deciduous precursors, while permanent lower canine teeth erupt lingually to their deciduous counterparts (Hale, 2018). Permanent incisors erupt lingually or palatally to the deciduous incisors. There are no deciduous precursors for any of the molar teeth in either dogs or cats, and no deciduous precursors for the first premolars in dogs (Hale, 2004). The deciduous fourth premolar in both dogs and cats resembles and functions as a molar, but is replaced by permanent fourth premolars. If a deciduous tooth (of a tooth that normally has a deciduous precursor) fails to develop, the permanent tooth will also be absent (Hale, 2004).

All juvenile patients should be examined for malocclusions, as some malocclusions that present early in life may be correctable, giving the growing patient the best chance to achieve a normal occlusion once they have reached maturity (Hale, 2004; AVDC, 2021).

Preventive orthodontics includes client education about tooth eruption times and proper occlusion, extracting a tooth that poses a risk to the development of a malocclusion, and operculectomy, which is the surgical removal of tough, fibrous gingiva (operculum) over a permanent tooth to enable its eruption (AVDC, 2021).

Tooth eruption times

The following is as described by Holzman (2020).

Canine deciduous:

- incisors: 3–4 weeks
- canines: 3 weeks

- premolars: 4–12 weeks.
- molars: N/A

Canine permanent:

- incisors: 3–5 months
- canines: 4–6 months
- premolars: 4–6 months
- molars: 5–7 months.

Feline deciduous:

- incisors: 2–3 weeks
- canines: 3–4 weeks
- premolars: 4–6 weeks
- molars: N/A.

Feline permanent:

- incisors: 3–4 weeks
- canines: 4–5 months
- premolars: 4–6 months
- molars: 4–5 months.

6.3.2 Interceptive orthodontics

Interceptive orthodontics involves the elimination of a developing or established malocclusion (AVDC, 2021). This includes extraction of permanent or deciduous teeth in malocclusion, or crown reduction with vital pulp therapy of a permanent tooth (see Chapter 4, this volume).

The maxilla and mandible do not grow at the same rate, which can sometimes cause a condition where a deciduous tooth or teeth (usually canines and incisors) of the mandible are caught behind teeth or in the soft tissue of the maxilla or vice versa, preventing normal jaw growth (Salter, 2004; Hale, 2018). This is called a dental interlock (see Fig. 6.2) (Niemiec, 2013). Extracting the misplaced deciduous teeth should be done as soon as the condition is recognized (Hale, 2018), ideally before 12 weeks of age, to relieve this interlock, to allow the patient's jaw to grow without interference (Salter, 2004) and to alleviate any pain and/or infection caused by tooth-on-tooth or tooth-on-soft-tissue trauma every time the pet eats or closes their mouth (Hale, 2018). This does not guarantee a normal bite later in life, as some animals are genetically destined to have a dental or skeletal malocclusion (Salter, 2004). However, if the dental interlock is not corrected, the jaws are prevented from growing normally, which almost certainly guarantees a malocclusion once the animal has stopped growing (Bellows *et al.*, 2004; Hale, 2018).

Persistent deciduous teeth should be extracted if they are still present once their permanent counterpart starts to erupt (Hale, 2018). Persistent

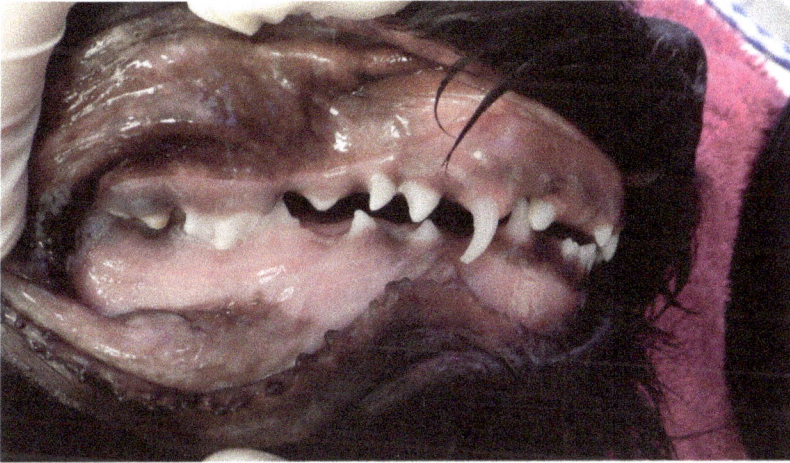

Fig. 6.2. Dental interlock.

deciduous teeth can cause Class 1 malocclusions of the permanent tooth (Perrone *et al.*, 2020), as well as periodontal disease resulting from crowding and interference with the development of a normal periodontal tissue attachment to the adult tooth (Bellows, 2019).

Deciduous teeth are thin-walled, fragile, and located very close to their adult counterparts, so extracting them can be challenging (Hale, 2018). Complications associated with extraction of deciduous teeth include the potential for root remnants to be left behind, which can cause infection progressing to osteomyelitis, and iatrogenic trauma to the developing permanent tooth bud (Bellows *et al.*, 2004). To avoid these complications, dental radiographs must be taken of the tooth to be extracted and any other teeth in the area, to determine the locations of the roots of both the deciduous and permanent teeth and to check for any abnormalities of the roots or surrounding tissues (Niemiec, 2013).

Regional dental nerve blocks are placed prior to extraction, and postoperative radiographs are taken to confirm that the entire root was removed (Charlier, 2020). Gingival flaps and bone removal may be required to remove the entire root. The extraction site is closed with absorbable suture (Bellows, 2019) (see Chapter 4, this volume).

6.3.3 Homecare following interceptive orthodontics

Pain medication should be sent home for a minimum of 7 days postoperatively (Niemiec, 2012). Instruct owners to feed soft food only and limit access to hard toys and treats until the extraction site is rechecked 7–10 days postoperatively (Juriga, 2008). Schedule a recheck of the patient's dental occlusion at 6 months of age, when all permanent teeth are expected to have erupted (Holzman, 2020). Further orthodontic treatment may be required if the malocclusion is still present (Perrone et al., 2020).

See Chapter 4, this volume, for homecare following crown reduction and vital pulp therapy.

6.3.4   Corrective orthodontics (orthodontic movement)

Corrective orthodontics corrects malocclusion by moving misaligned teeth (AVDC, 2021). Orthodontic appliances apply pressure in the direction in which a tooth needs to move (Perrone et al., 2020), relieving trauma and pain due to inappropriate tooth contact while preserving tooth structure and function and minimizing endodontic risks to the tooth. Thorough knowledge of tooth movement principles and forces are necessary to ensure success, as improperly applied orthodontic appliances can permanently damage teeth and soft tissues (Salter, 2004). The ethical implications of orthodontic movement must be considered (Holmstrom et al., 2000a). Corrective orthodontics in breeding animals is not advised, due to the potential for misleading future puppy buyers and the genetic propagation of painful dental malocclusions (Legendre, 2008; Perrone et al., 2020).

Orthodontic appliances (see Fig. 6.3) are placed and removed with the patient under general anaesthesia, and may require periodic adjustments under general anaesthesia (Bellows et al., 2004). Dental radiographs are necessary prior to movement, to ensure the tooth roots are mature and able to withstand the stresses of orthodontic movement (Salter, 2004). Radiographs are also required after orthodontic movement, to ensure the relocated tooth has remained healthy and vital (Salter, 2004; Bellows

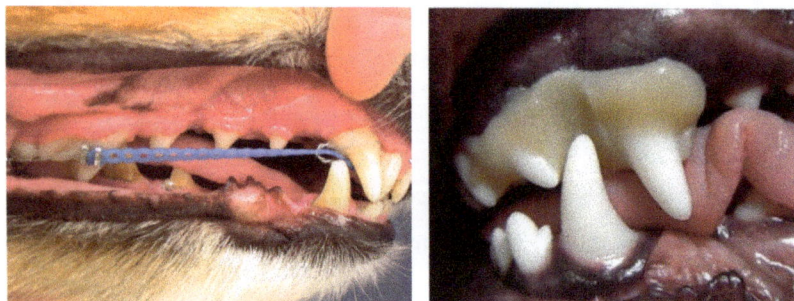

Fig. 6.3. Elastic chain (left); inclined plane (right).

et al., 2004). Orthodontic movement in veterinary patients is usually accomplished within 2–4 months (Salter, 2004). Patients between 6 and 10 months of age with completely erupted teeth are better candidates for orthodontic movement than older patients (Bellows *et al.*, 2004).

Types of orthodontic appliances

- Crown extensions: composite resin extensions bonded to the tip of an erupting permanent canine or incisor tooth (Bellows *et al.*, 2004; Hale, 2018). These cause tooth movement by directing the tooth labially and/or laterally whenever the pet closes their mouth (Bellows *et al.*, 2004; Legendre, 2008). Once the tooth has moved into the desired position, which generally takes about 4–6 weeks (Hale, 2018), the extension is removed (Bellows *et al.*, 2004).
- Inclined planes/bite plates: a composite resin or acrylic appliance fabricated within the mouth (Perrone *et al.*, 2020), or metal plate (Salter, 2004) bonded to the contralateral teeth which acts as a ramp to direct the misaligned tooth into a healthier position. These are often used to correct base narrow canines, with the appliance bonded to the upper canines and upper lateral incisors (Bellows *et al.*, 2004). When the mouth is closed, the lower canine is redirected labially and/or laterally, similar to crown extensions.
- Elastic chains: metal brackets, buttons or wires are bonded onto both the teeth to be moved and onto larger, stronger 'anchor' teeth (Salter, 2004). The canine teeth, fourth premolars and molars are commonly used as anchors (Bellows *et al.*, 2004). An elastic chain is stretched between the brackets or buttons and is shortened at regular intervals while the patient is awake, usually every 2 weeks (Legendre, 2008).
- Expansion screw devices: a metal expansion device which requires an impression taken of the patient's mouth (Bellows *et al.*, 2004). The impression is sent to a dental lab to fabricate the appliance. The appliance is then cemented into place, and the owner must use a small key to turn the screw every few days, pushing the affected teeth labially or buccally (Bellows *et al.*, 2004).
- Labial arch bar with elastics: a metal bar adhered to the dental arcade (often bonded to the canine teeth) and used with orthodontic buttons bonded onto the labial aspect of the misaligned teeth (usually incisors) (Bellows *et al.*, 2004; Legendre, 2008). Elastic chains are attached between the bar and the buttons, pulling the affected teeth into proper position.
- Palatal arch bar with spring wires: similar to an expansion screw device, but takes up less room, so is better suited to small-breed dogs (Legendre, 2008). These devices require removal at regular intervals to reactivate the spring.

6.3.5 Homecare following corrective orthodontics

The patient must not chew hard food, treats or toys (Hale, 2004), or paw at their face during the period of time that the dental appliance is in place. This may require intense owner supervision (Legendre, 2010a) and possibly an Elizabethan collar during treatment. Rechecks are scheduled weekly or at the veterinarian's discretion (Salter, 2004).

Dental homecare including tooth brushing and daily use of chlorhexidine rinse is essential while the appliance is in place (Legendre, 2010b), since dental appliances can trap food, hair and other debris, predisposing the pet to excessive plaque and calculus formation and subsequent periodontal disease (Bellows et al., 2004). General anaesthesia is required for appliance removal, after which a professional dental cleaning is performed. Occlusion is rechecked 1 month later to ensure tooth position is maintained (Bellows et al., 2004), and recheck radiographs are taken 6 months later to check for complications of tooth movement such as root resorption (Lengendre, 2010b).

Because orthodontic appliances are expensive, time consuming, easily damaged or dislodged, and require multiple veterinary visits and anaesthetic procedures as well as attentive homecare, not every patient or pet owner is a good candidate for their use (Legendre, 2008).

6.4   Impressions and Models

Veterinary nurses can assist in procedures involving orthodontic movement by taking full-mouth impressions and/or area-specific impressions, making bite registrations, and pouring diagnostic casts or stone models, which are used in the fabrication of dental appliances (Perrone et al., 2020).

6.4.1 Full-mouth impressions

Full-mouth impressions are taken using veterinary dental impression trays filled with alginate (Holmstrom et al., 2000b). Test the dental trays for proper fit first. Gently mix the alginate powder with room-temperature water (Niemiec, 2004) in a rubber mixing bowl as per the manufacturer's instructions, using a spatula in a figure-of-eight pattern to reduce the formation of bubbles, which could cause defects in the impression (Holmstrom et al., 2000b). Carefully move the patient's endotracheal tube out of the way and press the posterior of the filled tray firmly against the caudal mandible or maxilla, then press the rest of the tray into place until it covers the entire dental arcade from the molars to the incisors

(Holmstrom *et al.*, 2000b). Hold the tray still until the alginate sets. Depending upon the type of alginate used, set-up will take place within 2–5 minutes (Perrone *et al.*, 2020). Once set, pull the tray off the teeth in one brisk motion to minimize tearing of the impression (Niemiec, 2004). Inspect the impression for any voids or defects. Alginate impressions can be wrapped in damp paper towels and sealed in plastic bags (Holmstrom *et al.*, 2000b) for immediate transport to a dental laboratory, or a stone model can be poured in-clinic (see below), which is later transported to a dental laboratory.

6.4.2 Area-specific impressions

Area-specific impressions are taken with rubber-based impression materials to provide greater detail than can be obtained using alginate (Carlson, 2007). A tooth-specific or area-specific tray can be fabricated from a large syringe cap, pill vial, or other disposable container trimmed to fit over the tooth/teeth. Cutting or drilling a hole in the base of the tray allows excess impression material to escape, which helps prevent the formation of voids in the impression. Fill the tray with a low-viscosity elastic impression material, e.g. polyvinyl siloxane, and press it over the area until it has cured (the material will feel firm, not sticky) (Carlson, 2007; Coffman, 2012). Using a scalpel blade, carve a small amount of material from the hole made by the tooth crown, creating a custom mould which can then be filled with higher-viscosity polyvinyl siloxane to provide greater detail in the resulting impression (Carlson, 2007; Coffman, 2012). Place the filled tray over the area and hold the tray without moving until the material is cured. Once cured, pull the tray carefully from the mouth and inspect it to make sure there are no voids, tears or other defects. Polyvinyl siloxane impressions do not need to be kept damp when sending to dental laboratories (Carlson, 2007; Coffman, 2012). Label area-specific impressions with the Triadan number(s) and directional aids, such as buccal and palatal.

6.4.3 Bite registrations

A bite registration is taken with a flat, rectangular sheet of dental wax softened in warm water (Niemiec, 2004; Carlson, 2007). Remove the patient's endotracheal tube and place the softened wax sheet within the mouth (Niemiec, 2004; Carlson, 2007). Close the mouth over the wax, causing the tips of the teeth to create depressions within the wax, creating an impression of how the teeth occlude. Remove the wax and re-intubate the patient (Niemiec, 2004).

6.4.4 Models

Stone models can be poured in the veterinary hospital, or, if there is a dental laboratory nearby, impressions can be sent to have models poured there. Ideally, models should be poured within 30 minutes of taking impressions, though up to 6 hours is acceptable if the impression material is alginate (Perrone *et al.*, 2020). After 6 hours, the impressions may shrink or warp, resulting in inaccurate models (Carlson, 2007).

Pouring models requires powdered dental stone, a small rubber mixing bowl, a spatula and a dental vibrator: a machine which removes air bubbles from the stone mix to prevent voids and defects in the finished model (Holmstrom *et al.*, 2000b).

Measure the powdered stone by weight according to the size of the impressions, then mix it with the amount of water directed by the manufacturer. Mix gently with the spatula until it is the consistency of toothpaste, trying to minimize trapping air bubbles within the mix. Place the bowl on the vibrator for a few seconds to bring any air bubbles within the stone mix to the top (Holmstrom *et al.*, 2000b; Niemiec, 2004).

Hold the tray containing the impression on the vibrator with the rostral portion angled downward and slowly dribble the stone mix into the impression using a small spatula (Niemiec, 2004). Fill the crown impressions of each tooth first, then fill the rest of the impression. Small strips of metal (e.g. pieces of paper clips) may be placed into the impressions of the crowns of the canine teeth while pouring the stone to reinforce the stone (Niemiec, 2004). Once the teeth impressions are filled, fill the rest of the tray using the large mixing spatula (Niemiec, 2004). Set the model aside in an area where it will be left undisturbed to set for the time specified in the manufacturer's instructions, usually 30–60 minutes (Carlson, 2007).

As soon as possible after setting is complete, remove the impression tray from the alginate and carefully cut the alginate impression from the stone model with a scalpel blade, taking care not to break off the delicate stone tips of the tooth crowns (Niemiec, 2004).

Wrap stone models in bubble wrap when sending to dental laboratories, to ensure they are protected from breakage. Send along the bite registration and instructions detailing what type of appliance is to be fabricated (Carlson, 2007). Photographs of the mouth can be sent for clarification. Indicate the date you wish the appliance to arrive, which should be at least a day before the patient returns for appliance placement. The turn-around time for most dental laboratories is 7 days.

References

AVDC (2021) AVDC Nomenclature. American Veterinary Dental College. Available at: https://avdc.org/avdc-nomenclature/ (accessed 12 February 2021).

Bellows, J. (2017) The ABCs of veterinary dentistry: M is for Malposition and Malocclusion. Dvm360. Available at: https://www.dvm360.com/view/abcs-veterinary-dentistry-m-malposition-and-malocclusion (accessed 18 February 2021).

Bellows, J. (2019) The ABCs of veterinary dentistry: R is for retained, primary, deciduous teeth. Dvm360. Available at: https://www.dvm360.com/view/abcs-veterinary-dentistry-r-retained-primary-deciduous-teeth (accessed 18 February 2021).

Bellows, J., Carmichael, D., Chamberlain, T. and Eisner, E. (2004) Orthodontics panel discussion. In: *Proceedings of the 18th Annual Veterinary Dental Forum*. Omnipress, Madison, Wisconsin, pp. 23–32.

Carlson, P. (2007) Prosthodontics. In: *Proceedings of the 21st Annual Veterinary Dental Forum*. Omnipress, Madison, Wisconsin, pp. 417–421.

Charlier, C. (2020) Tooth extraction complications in dogs and cats. Today's Veterinary Practice. Available at: https://todaysveterinarypractice.com/tooth-extraction-complications-in-dogs-and-cats/ (accessed 18 February 2021).

Coffman, C.R. (2012) Crown therapy: introduction to veterinary prosthodontics. In: *Proceedings of the 26th Annual Veterinary Dental Forum*. Omnipress, Madison, Wisconsin (CD Rom).

Hale, F.A. (2004) Pediatric dentistry. Hale Veterinary Clinic. Available at: http://www.toothvet.ca/VSTEP/o%20-%20pediatric.pdf (accessed 28 January 2021).

Hale, F.A. (2018) Malocclusions. Hale Veterinary Clinic. Available at: http://www.toothvet.ca/PDFfiles/malocclusions.pdf (accessed 18 February 2021).

Holmstrom, S., Holmstrom, L.A., McGrath, C.J., Richey, M.T. and Wiggs, R.B. (2000a) The oral examination and disease recognition. In: Holmstrom, S. (ed.) *Veterinary Dentistry for the Technician & Office Staff*. Saunders, Philadelphia, Pennsylvania, pp. 23–61.

Holmstrom, S., Holmstrom, L.A., McGrath, C.J., Richey, M.T. and Wiggs, R.B. (2000b) Advanced veterinary dental procedures. In: Holmstrom, S. (ed.) *Veterinary Dentistry for the Technician & Office Staff*. Saunders, Philadelphia, Pennsylvania, pp. 247–282.

Holzman, G. (2020) The basics. In: Perrone, J. (ed.) *Small Animal Dental Procedures for Veterinary Technicians and Nurses*. Wiley Blackwell, Hoboken, New Jersey, pp. 1–20.

Juriga, S. (2008) Surgical extraction techniques. In: *Proceedings of the 22nd Annual Veterinary Dental Forum*. Omnipress, Madison, Wisconsin, pp. 257–261.

Legendre, L. (2008) Review of techniques used to correct rostral cross bite malocclusions. In: *Proceedings of the 22nd Annual Veterinary Dental Forum*. Omnipress, Madison, Wisconsin, pp. 311–313.

Legendre, L. (2010a) Corrective orthodontic techniques. *World Small Animal Veterinary Association World Congress Proceedings, 2010*. Available at: https://www.vin.com/apputil/content/defaultadv1.aspx?pId=11310&catId=33745&id=4516409 (accessed 18 February 2021).

Legendre, L. (2010b) Building of a telescopic inclined plane intraorally. *Journal of Veterinary Dentistry* 27(1), 62–65. DOI: 10.1177/089875641002700113.

Niemiec, B. (2004) Impressions and model making. In: *Proceedings of the 18th Annual Veterinary Dental Forum.* Omnipress, Madison, Wisconsin, pp. 322–324.

Niemiec, B.A. (2012) Dental extractions: five steps to improve client education, surgical procedures, and patient care. Today's Veterinary Practice. Available at: https://todaysveterinarypractice.com/practical-dentistry-dental-extractions/ (accessed 16 February 2021).

Niemiec, B.A. (2013) The basics of orthodontics. *World Small Animal Veterinary Association World Congress Proceedings, 2013.* Available at: https://www.vin.com/apputil/content/defaultadv1.aspx?id=5709808&pid=11372 (accessed 18 February 2021).

Perrone, J.R., March, P.A. and Sharp, S. (2020) Common dental conditions and treatments. In: Perrone, J. (ed.) *Small Animal Dental Procedures for Veterinary Technicians and Nurses.* Wiley Blackwell, Hoboken, New Jersey, pp. 131–168.

SACVDS (2021) Malocclusions and orthodontic treatment. Sacramento Veterinary Dental Services. Available at: https://www.sacvds.com/forms/malocclusions-orthodontic-treatment.pdf (accessed 18 February 2021).

Salter, R. (2004) Introduction to veterinary orthodontics. In: *Proceedings of the 18th Annual Veterinary Dental Forum.* Omnipress, Madison, Wisconsin, pp. 18–22.

Thatcher, G. (2019) Diagnosis and management of class II malocclusion. *Canadian Veterinary Journal* 60(7), 791–795.

7

Lumps and Bumps: Oral Masses and Cysts

Though we and our clients wish it were otherwise, benign and malignant oral masses are often similar in appearance, so must be diagnosed by biopsy and histopathology (Niemiec *et al.*, 2020). Clinical signs of oral tumours are widely variable, ranging from no signs to pain, discomfort upon opening or closing the mouth, anorexia, dysphagia, weight loss, oral bleeding, halitosis, epistaxis, nasal discharge, exophthalmos (bulging of the eye), facial deformity and dyspnoea (Kristel, 2008; Perrone *et al.*, 2020; Perrone, 2012). Exam-room findings include an abnormal mass of tissue or swelling in the mouth, tissue ulcerations or other oral lesions, and possibly enlarged lymph nodes (Perrone *et al.*, 2020). Oral cancer should also be considered whenever a loose tooth is found in a patient with an otherwise healthy mouth (Crowder, 2007).

Bloodwork including a complete blood count (CBC) and chemical profile, urinalysis, three-view chest radiographs, CT and MRI scans, and aspirates or biopsies of enlarged lymph nodes are recommended to rule out metastases, stage the tumour, and determine the patient's prognosis (Crowder, 2007; Taney, 2007; Perrone *et al.*, 2020).

Prior to biopsy or other reduction of oral masses, dental radiography and regional nerve blocks should be performed. Take photographs prior to biopsy to send along to the histopathologist (Parry, 2017). These can also be shown to the patient's owner, who often can't see the full extent of the mass while their pet is awake.

7.1 Oral Biopsies

Small oral masses may be completely excised and sent for histopathology (Taney, 2007). Larger oral masses should have incisional biopsies taken first in order to diagnose and plan treatment (Reiter, 2008). Incisional biopsies are performed with a scalpel blade or biopsy punch (Reiter, 2008). They should be obtained from within the tumour, not near the edges of the tumour, to prevent spreading potentially cancerous cells (Parry, 2017). In

© CAB International 2022. *An Introduction to Pet Dental Care: For Veterinary Technicians and Nurses* (K. Istace)
DOI: 10.1079/9781789248869.0007

large masses, multiple samples should be taken from different locations in the mass (Reiter, 2008). Biopsies should be deep, since many oral tumours are covered with a layer of gingiva (Kristel, 2008; Reiter, 2008). The margins of oral tumours removed by excisional biopsy should be marked with India ink or a commercial marking system, to allow the pathologist to accurately determine the margins once the sample is sliced for microscopic analysis (Boston, 2015). This is done by blotting the specimen dry and painting the margins using a cotton-tipped applicator (Boston, 2015).

Place the sample in 10% buffered formalin. There should be at least ten times more formalin per volume than tissue (Reiter, 2008). Large tumours should be partially sliced into 1-cm sections, leaving the base of the specimen intact, to allow for better formalin penetration (Boston, 2015). Record the oral examination findings including the location, size and gross appearance of the mass on the histopathology requisition form, and attach or email the pathologist any photographs, dental radiographs and CT or MRI scans (Parry, 2017).

7.2 Benign Lesions

Benign lesions can be locally aggressive, but do not spread to other organs (Perrone *et al.*, 2020). The following is not a comprehensive list, but describes commonly seen benign oral masses and cysts.

7.2.1 Gingival hyperplasia/enlargement

Gingival hyperplasia is an enlargement or overgrowth of the gingival tissue (Niemiec *et al.*, 2020). It can be seen in any breed of dog or cat, but is over-represented in boxers (Niemiec *et al.*, 2020) and bulldogs (Perrone *et al.*, 2020). Gingival hyperplasia can be plaque-induced, genetic, or a potential side effect of medications such as cyclosporine, anti-seizure medications and calcium-channel blockers (Hale, 2008a; Niemiec *et al.*, 2020). This gingival enlargement leads to the formation of pseudopockets. Although gingival attachment at the cementoenamel junction is maintained, pseudopockets can trap food and hair, leading to periodontal disease (Hale, 2008a). Treatment involves surgical reduction (gingivectomy) of the excessive tissue to a normal pocket depth (Niemiec *et al.*, 2020) with either a scalpel blade, electrocautery or laser (see Chapter 2, this volume) (Perrone *et al.*, 2020). If a scalpel blade is used, gingival bleeding must be controlled with pressure and/or haemostatic solution (Hale, 2008a).

7.2.2 Papilloma

Most commonly affecting puppies, these usually present as small white, grey or pink bumps or clusters of bumps on the lips, tongue, gingiva or palate (Niemiec *et al.*, 2020). They are caused by the canine oral papilloma virus (COPV1) (Crowder, 2007) and often resolve on their own in a few months (Perrone *et al.*, 2020), though in rare cases they can develop into carcinomas (Niemiec *et al.*, 2020). They do not require removal unless they are causing pain or problems with eating (Perrone *et al.*, 2020).

7.2.3 Peripheral odontogenic fibroma

Once referred to as fibromatous epulis (Niemiec *et al.*, 2020) or ossifying epulis (Crowder, 2007), this is the most common type of benign oral canine neoplasm. They are slow-growing, firm, smooth, discrete masses in the gingiva near or surrounding a tooth, but originate from the periodontal ligament (Niemiec *et al.*, 2020; Perrone *et al.*, 2020). Though they rarely grow more than 2 cm in diameter, they can displace teeth (Kristel, 2008). Treatment requires extraction of the tooth and thorough curettage of the periodontal ligament from the alveolus.

7.2.4 Acanthomatous ameloblastoma

Acanthomatous ameloblastoma, previously referred to as acanthomatous epulis, often has a cauliflower-like or fleshy appearance (Kristel, 2008; Niemiec *et al.*, 2020) and is locally aggressive, with the potential for bone infiltration (Eroshin *et al.*, 2007). These masses originate from odontogenic epithelium (Eroshin *et al.*, 2007). Treatment involves complete resection of the mass, adjacent tissue, teeth and bone, with 1–2-cm margins (Niemiec *et al.*, 2020; Perrone *et al.*, 2020). Radiation therapy may be indicated when complete removal is unachievable (Niemiec *et al.*, 2020).

7.2.5 Eosinophilic granuloma

These lesions can be raised, pink or yellow in colour, or have an ulcer-like appearance, and are found most commonly on the upper lip, tongue, soft palate and pharynx (Niemiec *et al.*, 2020; Perrone *et al.*, 2020). While they are usually painless, if the ulcers are severe they can affect eating. They can be seen in both cats and dogs, though are more common in cats (Perrone *et al.*, 2020). They may have various causes, including an immune response from various stimuli such as food allergies or fleas, genetic predisposition, or trauma (Niemiec *et al.*, 2020). Secondary infections may occur (Niemiec, 2012). They are usually treated with steroids, antibiotics, flea prevention or allergy testing (Niemiec *et al.*, 2020; Perrone *et al.*, 2020). Surgical debulking may be required if the lesion is so large that it prevents the patient from eating (Crawford, 2010).

7.2.6 Dentigerous cysts

Unerupted teeth that remain within the bone of the jaw may lead to the formation of a fluid-filled cyst around the unerupted tooth (see Fig. 7.1)

(Hale, 2008b; Niemiec *et al.*, 2020). These dentigerous cysts can cause destruction of the adjacent teeth, periodontal tissues and bone, leading to loss of adjacent teeth and potential jaw fracture (Hale, 2008b). Tumours such as ameloblastomas or odontogenic tumours can also arise from dentigerous cysts (D'Astous, 2011). Studies have shown that over 30% of 'missing' teeth are actually unerupted (Bellows, 2004), so any areas of unexplained missing teeth in patients with permanent dentition should be radiographed (Niemiec *et al.*, 2020), and all unerupted teeth should be extracted (Hale, 2008b). This can easily be done when the pet is under general anaesthesia for spay or neuter. In older patients, where an unerupted tooth has been in place for years and there is no radiographic evidence of a cyst, regular radiographic monitoring may also be an option (Hale, 2008b).

Once a patient has developed a dentigerous cyst, it must be treated surgically as soon as possible to prevent further damage to the jaw and adjacent teeth (Hale, 2008b). In addition to extracting the unerupted tooth, the entire cyst lining must be removed by thorough curettage to prevent the cyst from recurring (Niemiec *et al.*, 2020). If the cyst is large, teeth and bone on either side may need to be removed to ensure complete excision (Hale, 2008b). Osteoconductive materials or bone grafts (Marretta, 2004) should be placed if there has been extensive bone destruction. Histologic examination of the removed cyst can rule out any tumour formation and confirm the diagnosis of a dentigerous cyst (D'Astous, 2011).

7.2.7 Odontoma

Odontomas occur in dogs, most commonly at less than 1 year of age, and are rare in cats. They originate from the dental follicle of developing teeth (Milella, 2012). There are two types of odontoma: compound and complex. Compound odontomas contain numerous denticles, which are tooth-like structures (Niemiec *et al.*, 2020), though they may be tiny and misshapen. Complex odontomas also contain dentinal or calcified tissue, but it is not differentiated into tooth-like structures (Niemiec *et al.*, 2020). Like dentigerous cysts, these tumours can cause bone destruction. Treatment for either type of odontoma is complete surgical removal (Milella, 2012).

7.2.8 Salivary mucocele

Also known as sialoceles or ranulas, salivary mucoceles present as painless, fluctuant swellings in the neck, beneath the jaw, or sublingually, caused by accumulated saliva from a damaged salivary gland or duct (Lobprise and Wiggs, 2000; American College of Veterinary Surgeons (ACVS), 2021), or duct blockage due to inflammation, sialoliths (calcified debris) or mucin (Niemiec, 2007). They are most often seen in dogs, possibly due to trauma from collars or bites, or chewing on foreign objects (ACVS, 2021).

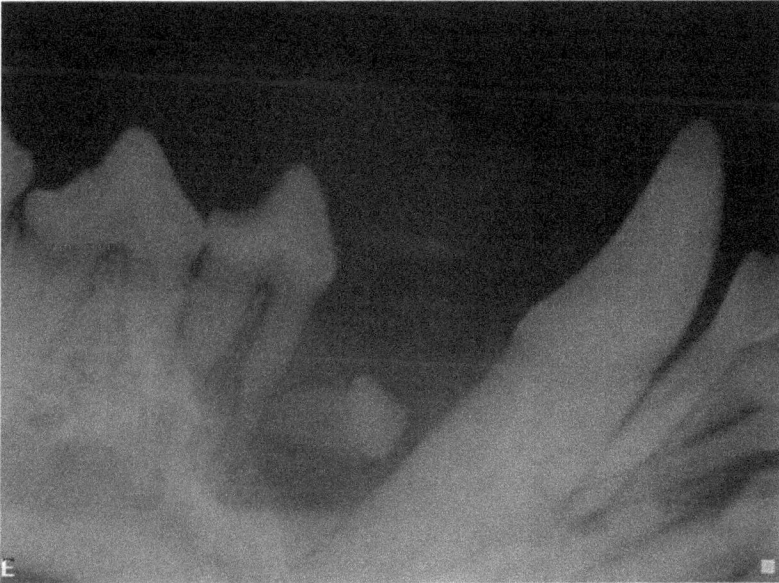

Fig. 7.1. Dentigerous cyst.

Sublingual mucoceles can cause difficulty with eating or bleeding due to chewing on the mucocele, while mucoceles in the pharyngeal area can cause difficulty with breathing and swallowing (ACVS, 2021). Diagnostics include physical examination, skull and dental radiographs, fluid cytology and histopathology (Niemiec, 2007). Treatment for all types of salivary mucoceles is complete surgical removal of the salivary gland(s) associated with the mucocele (Niemiec, 2007) and possible drain placement (ACVS, 2021). Marsupialization of the mucosa overlying sublingual mucoceles may also be performed (Niemiec, 2007; ACVS, 2021).

7.3 Malignant Lesions

These lesions are locally destructive and may metastasize to other organs (Perrone *et al.*, 2020), making them potentially fatal. The following is not a comprehensive list, but describes commonly seen oral malignancies.

7.3.1 Malignant melanoma

The most common oral malignancy in dogs (Niemiec *et al.*, 2020), though rare in cats, these lesions are fast-growing and highly metastatic (Perrone *et al.*, 2020). They are often (but not always) pigmented, may have an ulcerated or necrotic appearance, and can be found in the gingiva, mucosa, palate and tongue (Kristel, 2008). Prognosis is usually poor, because metastasis often occurs prior to diagnosis (Kristel, 2008). Treatment requires complete surgical excision (Niemiec *et al.*, 2020). Removal of regional lymph nodes is recommended (Kristel, 2008).

A canine melanoma vaccine is available through veterinary oncologists that may help prevent metastasis and prolong survival time, though it does not prevent growth of the primary tumour (Perrone *et al.*, 2020).

7.3.2 Squamous cell carcinoma

Squamous cell carcinoma (SCC) is the most common oral cancer of cats and the second most common of dogs (Niemiec *et al.*, 2020). It originates from squamous epithelial cells and is often found on the palate or under the tongue, though can occur almost anywhere in the mouth (Lobprise and Wiggs, 2000; Perrone *et al.*, 2020). The lesions are often ulcerated, nodular, and pink or grey in colour (Perrone *et al.*, 2020). SCC is locally invasive and can metastasize to the lungs in dogs, but does not metastasize quickly in cats unless it is on the tonsils (Lobprise and Wiggs, 2000; Perrone *et al.*, 2020). Bone involvement is common (Niemiec *et al.*, 2020). Treatment requires complete surgical excision with wide margins, with or without radiation therapy (Niemiec *et al.*, 2020). Regional lymph node removal is recommended (Kristel, 2008).

The prognosis for cats with SCC is poor, with a 1-year survival rate of less than 10% even with treatment (University of Florida Small Animal Hospital (UFL), 2021), because it is not usually diagnosed until the cancer is advanced (Perrone *et al.*, 2020).

7.3.3 Fibrosarcoma

Fibrosarcoma is the second most common malignant oral tumour in cats (Kristel, 2008) and the third most common in dogs (Lobprise and Wiggs, 2000; Taney, 2007). It is often found in the maxilla, including the gingiva, palate and mucosa, and usually appears as proliferative and ulcerated tissue (Kristel, 2008). It does not metastasize quickly, but it is very aggressive locally, with invasion into the bone (Kristel, 2008), and recurrence is common (Taney, 2007; Niemiec *et al.*, 2020). Complete surgical excision with minimum 2-cm margins is recommended (Kristel, 2008).

7.3.4 Osteosarcoma

Osteosarcoma is the fourth most common malignant oral tumour in dogs (Farcas *et al.*, 2012), and can also occur in cats. It can be found in either the mandible or maxilla, occurs more frequently in large breeds, and is usually diagnosed in pets aged 9–10 years (Farcas *et al.*, 2012). Wide surgical resection (>1-cm margins) is recommended, with or without radiation and

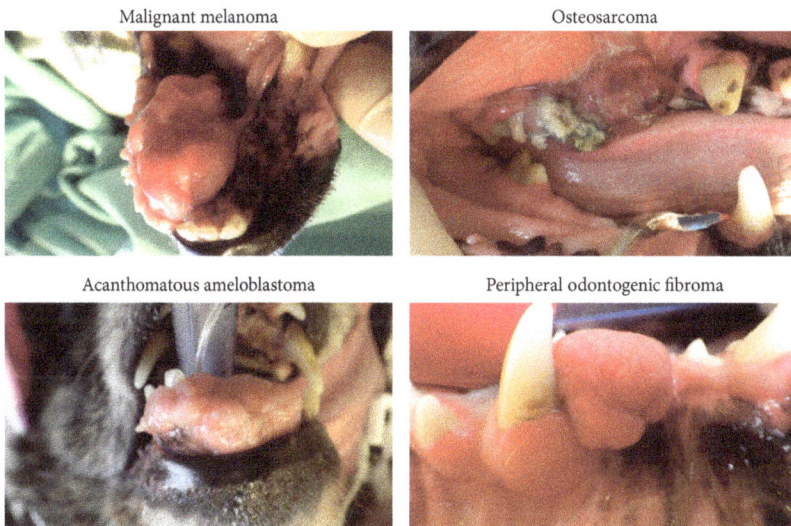

Fig. 7.2. Oral masses.

chemotherapy (Niemiec *et al.*, 2020). Local recurrence is common (Farcas *et al.*, 2012).

7.3.5 Oral malignancy treatment considerations

Owners should always be made aware of the long-term prognosis and potential complications of oral cancer surgeries (Kristel, 2008). For large malignant masses, total or partial mandibulectomy, partial maxillectomy, or partial resection of the palate may be required to obtain adequate margins (Perrone *et al.*, 2020). A major risk of these surgeries is potentially fatal blood loss intraoperatively, so preoperative blood typing should be done and blood products should be on hand in case transfusion is required (Reiter, 2012). Potential postoperative complications include incision dehiscence (Crowder, 2007), mesial drifting of the remaining mandible following mandibulectomy causing trauma to the palate from the remaining lower canine tooth, increased drooling, difficulty with eating, changes to the pet's appearance including tongue protuberance, and tumour recurrence (Taney, 2007). For patients who must undergo large oral cancer surgeries, particularly cats, placement of a temporary feeding tube should be considered to ensure adequate nutrition postoperatively (Taney, 2007; Perrone *et al.*, 2020).

Radiation therapy and/or chemotherapy may be considered as adjuncts to surgical resection when complete resection cannot be accomplished, or when metastasis has already occurred (Perrone *et al.*, 2020).

Side effects from radiation therapy include inflammation of the skin and mucous membranes, anorexia, hair loss, excessive salivation, halitosis and secondary mucosal infections (Perrone *et al.*, 2020; Animal Cancer & Imaging Center (ACI), 2021; Stoewen and Pinard, 2021). Side effects of chemotherapy include lethargy, anorexia, vomiting, diarrhoea, cystitis, kidney or liver damage, and heart failure (Fullerton, 2018; Perrone *et al.*, 2020).

Debulking surgery can be used for palliative care to lessen pain and to remove tissue that is interfering with chewing, allowing patients to continue to eat in cases where the prognosis is poor; however, tumour regrowth is often rapid (Perrone *et al.*, 2020).

7.4   Homecare following oral mass biopsy or removal

Provide patients with postoperative pain medications until the area has completely healed (Lantz, 2010). If the tumour was not completely removed, pain medications may be required indefinitely (Reiter, 2012). An Elizabethan collar may be needed for patients who paw at their mouths postoperatively (Reiter, 2012).

If a feeding tube has been placed, instruct the pet owner in its use and maintenance, including appropriate feeding volume and frequency, cleaning and rechecks (Reiter, 2012). All patients should be fed a soft diet until the surgical site has completely healed, with hard treats and toys restricted (Reiter, 2012). Patients who have had large areas of resection, such as mandibulectomy or maxillectomy, may have difficulty picking up or masticating their food (Taney, 2007), and may be able to eat better if they are hand-fed canned-food 'meatballs'. Make owners aware that their pets' feeding and drinking may be significantly messier after mandibulectomy or maxillectomy (Lantz, 2010). Any skin incisions must be kept clean during healing. If the pet's tongue hangs from the mouth, they may drool more (Lantz, 2010), and the tongue can dry out over the course of the day (Wag!, 2020). Owners should moisten the tongue when they notice that it is becoming dry. Ongoing rechecks may be required to monitor for tumour regrowth and/or metastasis (Lantz, 2010).

Following mandibulectomy, crown reduction with vital pulp therapy may be required on the remaining lower canine tooth if mandibular drift occurs and begins to cause trauma to other oral tissues (Taney, 2007).

References

ACI (2021) Veterinary radiation therapy. Animal Cancer & Imaging Center. Available at: http://www.veterinarycancer.com/radiation-therapy (accessed 22 February 2021).

ACVS (2021) Salivary mucocele. American College of Veterinary Surgeons. Available at: https://www.acvs.org/small-animal/salivary-mucocele (accessed 22 February 2021).

Bellows, J. (2004) Where did the premolars go? In: *Proceedings of the 18th Annual Veterinary Dental Forum.* Omnipress, Madison, Wisconsin, p. 263.

Boston, S. (2015) Advanced surgical oncology. *World Small Animal Veterinary Association World Congress Proceedings, 2015.* Available at: https://www.vin.com/apputil/content/defaultadv1.aspx?id=7259386&pid=14365 (accessed 22 February 2021).

Crawford, J. (2010) Feline oral diseases. In: *Proceedings of the 26th Annual Veterinary Dental Forum.* Omnipress, Madison, Wisconsin (CD Rom).

Crowder, S.E. (2007) 'Benign' oral tumors in the dog and cat. In: *Proceedings of the 21st Annual Veterinary Dental Forum.* Omnipress, Madison, Wisconsin, pp. 211–214.

D'Astous, J. (2011) An overview of dentigerous cysts in dogs and cats. *Canadian Veterinary Journal* 52(8), 905–907.

Eroshin, V., Lewis, J.R. and Reiter, A. (2007) Treatment of acanthomatous ameloblastoma by rostral mandibulectomy. In: *Proceedings of the 21st Annual Veterinary Dental Forum.* Omnipress, Madison, Wisconsin, pp. 63–64.

Farcas, N., Arzi, B. and Verstraete, F.J.M. (2012) Oral and maxillofacial osteosarcoma in dogs: a review. *Veterinary and Comparative Oncology* 12(3), 169–180. Available at: https://onlinelibrary.wiley.com/doi/pdf/10.1111/j.1476-5829.2012.00352.x (accessed 22 February 2021).

Fullerton, E. (2018) Chemotherapy-induced side effects: prevention and treatment. Today's Veterinary Nurse. Available at: https://todaysveterinarynurse.com/articles/chemotherapy-induced-side-effects-prevention-and-treatment/ (accessed 22 February 2021).

Hale, F.A. (2008a) Surgical treatment of gingival enlargements. In: *Proceedings of the 22nd Annual Veterinary Dental Forum.* Omnipress, Madison, Wisconsin, pp. 329–332.

Hale, F.A. (2008b) Dentigerous cysts. In: *Proceedings of the 22nd Annual Veterinary Dental Forum.* Omnipress, Madison, Wisconsin, pp. 235–237.

Kristel, J.A. (2008) It's not a tumor – or is it? recognizing oral tumors in dogs and cats. In: *Proceedings of the 22nd Annual Veterinary Dental Forum.* Omnipress, Madison, Wisconsin, pp. 491–493.

Lantz, G.C. (2010) Management of oral tumors: partial maxillectomy and mandibulectomy. In: *Proceedings of the 26th Annual Veterinary Dental Forum.* Omnipress, Madison, Wisconsin (CD Rom).

Lobprise, H.B. and Wiggs, R.B. (2000) Oral examination and recognition of pathology. In: Lobprise, H.B. and Wiggs, R.B. (eds) *The Veterinarian's Companion for Common Dental Procedures.* AAHA Press, Lakewood, Colorado, pp. 11–37.

Marretta, S.M. (2004) Diagnosis and treatment of unerupted teeth in the dog. In: *Proceedings of the 18th Annual Veterinary Dental Forum.* Omnipress, Madison, Wisconsin, pp. 70–71.

Milella, L. (2012) Compound odontoma in a kitten. In: *Proceedings of the 26th Annual Veterinary Dental Forum.* Omnipress, Madison, Wisconsin (CD Rom).

Niemiec, B. (2007) Update on salivary disorders. In: *Proceedings of the 21st Annual Veterinary Dental Forum.* Omnipress, Madison, Wisconsin, pp. 25–28.

Niemiec, B. (2012) Unusual feline oral pathology. In: *Proceedings of the 26ᵗʰ Annual Veterinary Dental Forum.* Omnipress, Madison, Wisconsin (CD Rom).

Niemiec, B.A., Gawor, J., Nemec, A., Clarke, D. and Tutt, C. (2020) World Small Animal Veterinary Association global dental guidelines. World Small Animal Veterinary Association. Available at: https://wsava.org/wp-content/uploads/2020/01/Dental-Guidleines-for-endorsement_0.pdf (accessed 6 February 2021).

Parry, N.M. (2017) AVMA 2017: managing oral tumors in dogs. Dvm360. Available at: https://www.dvm360.com/view/avma-2017-managing-oral-tumors-in-dogs (accessed 22 February 2021).

Perrone, J.R. (2012) Common tumors of the oral cavity: are we looking for them or snipping them off? In: *Proceedings of the 26th Annual Veterinary Dental Forum.* Omnipress, Madison, Wisconsin (CD Rom).

Perrone, J.R., March, P.A. and Sharp, S. (2020) Common dental conditions and treatments. In: Perrone, J. (ed.) *Small Animal Dental Procedures for Veterinary Technicians and Nurses.* Wiley Blackwell, Hoboken, New Jersey, pp. 131–168.

Reiter, A. (2008) Oral biospy – when and how. In: *Proceedings of the 22nd Annual Veterinary Dental Forum.* Omnipress, Madison, Wisconsin, pp. 271–272.

Reiter, A.M. (2012) Mandibulectomy procedures in the dog and cat. In: *Proceedings of the 26th Annual Veterinary Dental Forum.* Omnipress, Madison, Wisconsin (CD Rom).

Stoewen, D. and Pinard, C. (2021) Radiation therapy. VCA. Available at: https://vcahospitals.com/know-your-pet/radiation-therapy (accessed 22 February 2022).

Taney, K. (2007) Fundamental principles of oncologic surgery. In: *Proceedings of the 21st Annual Veterinary Dental Forum.* Omnipress, Madison, Wisconsin, pp. 157–158.

UFL (2021) Oral squamous cell carcinoma in cats. University of Florida Small Animal Hospital. Available at: https://smallanimal.vethospital.ufl.edu/clinical-services/oncology/types-of-cancer-and-treatment/oral-squamous-cell-carcinoma-in-cats/ (accessed 22 February 2021).

Wag! (2020) Hanging tongue syndrome in dogs. Available at: https://wagwalking.com/condition/hanging-tongue-syndrome (accessed 22 February 2021).

8

Seeing Red: Stomatitis, Feline Juvenile Gingivitis and Contact Mucositis

8.1 Stomatitis

Stomatitis (also known as gingivostomatitis, lymphocytic plasmocytic stomatitis, chronic ulcerative stomatiti and chronic gingivitis-stomatitis-faucitis) is an extremely painful disease characterized by widespread, severe inflammation of the soft tissues of the mouth including the gingiva, buccal mucosa and caudal mucosa (Holmstrom *et al.*, 2000; Crawford and Losey, 2020). Clinical signs include red and swollen gingival and mucosal tissues (Crawford and Losey, 2020), which may also be ulcerated and/or proliferative (Crawford, 2010); oral bleeding; pawing at the mouth; anorexia; weight loss; hypersalivation and halitosis (Bellows, 2010). Tooth resorption and/or periodontitis may also be present (Holmstrom *et al.*, 2000). Stomatitis occurs most frequently in cats, but has also been diagnosed in dogs (Lewis, 2017).

8.1.1 Diagnosis of stomatitis

Stomatitis can be frustrating to diagnose (Lobprise and Wiggs, 2000a) and treat, due to the wide variety of clinical presentations and the lack of knowledge about its causes (Niemiec, 2012). Suspected causes include viral infections such as feline leukaemia virus (FeLV), feline immunodeficiency virus (FIV) and feline calicivirus (FCV); and the blood parasite *Haemobartonella felis* (Crawford and Losey, 2020). However, many cats with stomatitis test negative for these, and the most widely accepted theory is that stomatitis is caused by an immune hypersensitivity reaction to plaque bacteria (Lobprise and Wiggs, 2000b; Bellows, 2010).

Stomatitis can usually be differentiated from gingivitis upon oral examination, since the inflammation is not confined to the gingiva, as in gingivitis, but extends beyond the mucogingival line, often involving the tissues of the caudal oropharynx lateral to the palatoglossal folds (Lewis, 2014a). However, early stages of stomatitis may present similarly to gingivitis (Crawford and Losey, 2020).

© CAB International 2022. *An Introduction to Pet Dental Care: For Veterinary Technicians and Nurses* (K. Istace)
DOI: 10.1079/9781789248869.0008

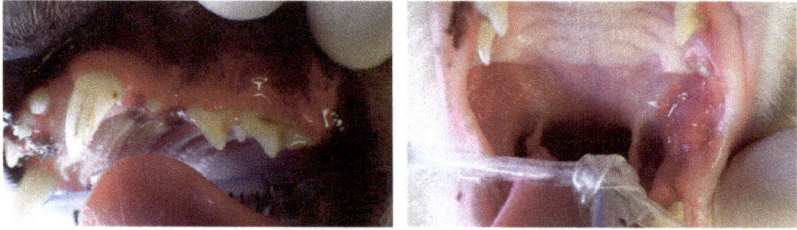

Fig. 8.1. Stomatitis.

A thorough physical examination, history from the pet owner and labwork including a complete blood count (CBC), chemistry profile and FeLV/FIV status (Crawford and Losey, 2020) should be performed to rule out any other conditions, including eosinophilic granuloma complex, periodontitis, uremic ulcers, chemical or electrical burns, food allergies and autoimmune diseases (Holmstrom *et al.*, 2000). In the case of stomatitis, these tests are unrevealing, though the serum total protein and serum globulins may be elevated (Holmstrom *et al.*, 2000). A biopsy may be recommended to rule out other conditions (Holmstrom *et al.*, 2000) such as squamous cell carcinoma.

8.1.2 Treatment of stomatitis

In all cases, pain medications (Crawford, 2010) such as buprenorphine, fentanyl, tramadol, gabapentin and non-steroidal anti-inflammatory drugs (NSAIDs) should be initiated as soon as possible to alleviate the patient's discomfort (Crawford and Losey, 2020). If necessary, appetite stimulants such as mirtazapine can be administered (Greenfield, 2017), or a feeding tube placed to provide nutrition preoperatively in debilitated patients (Rochette, 2012).

Frequent professional dental cleanings and diligent dental homecare were once recommended to keep the plaque bacteria population in the mouth under control (Greenfield, 2017). However, this conservative treatment is usually unsuccessful because plaque bacteria recolonize quickly (Greenfield, 2017), and the condition is so painful that most cats will not tolerate the thorough twice-daily tooth brushing required to sufficiently reduce plaque bacteria (Lewis, 2014a, b).

Complete tooth removal, including the roots of teeth affected by tooth resorption, is the recommended treatment for stomatitis, since any root remnants can cause continued inflammation (Bellows, 2010; Niemiec, 2012; Lewis, 2014a). If inflammation is confined to the caudal oral mucosa, extraction of the molars and premolars may be sufficient to cure the condition, but if inflammation is present near the canines and incisors, full-mouth extractions are necessary (Bellows, 2010; Niemiec, 2012;

Lewis, 2014a). Full-mouth extractions have been successful in curing this condition in 60–90% of patients (Niemiec, 2012). Before proceeding with full-mouth extractions, clients should be made aware that some patients may require adjunct therapy following extractions (see below).

Dental regional nerve blocks are performed, and preoperative dental radiographs are taken (Bellows, 2010). If full-mouth extractions are performed, an oesophagostomy feeding tube should be placed to ensure that the cat is able to receive adequate nutrition postoperatively (Bellows, 2010; Crawford and Losey, 2020). Alternatively, the teeth on one side of the mouth can be extracted first (Crawford and Losey, 2020), allowing the cat to eat on the untreated side, and 3–4 weeks later the teeth on the opposite side of the mouth can be extracted. Postoperative dental radiographs are essential to ensure no roots remain (Lyon, 2004).

Anti-inflammatory drugs, systemic antibiotics, antiviral treatments and CO_2 laser therapy (Lewis *et al.*, 2007) have met with varying degrees of success, and are usually recommended only for refractory cases where oral inflammation is still present several months following full-mouth extractions (Lewis, 2014b; Greenfield, 2017). The immunosuppressive drug cyclosporine has been shown to be successful in resolving inflammation, particularly in patients who have not previously received corticosteroids (Greenfield, 2017). Side effects of cyclosporine include reduced liver or kidney function, anaemia, and transient vomiting and diarrhoea (Lyon, 2004; Greenfield, 2017). Corticosteroids such as prednisolone may also relieve stomatitis inflammation, though usually with less success than cyclosporine (Greenfield, 2017). Therapy with antibiotics such as clindamycin, doxycycline, amoxicillin-clavulanic acid and metronidazole may reduce inflammation in some refractory cases (Hennet, 2014). CO_2 laser therapy can be used in refractory cases to char the inflamed tissue, resulting in scar tissue formation, which is less likely to become inflamed (Lewis *et al.*, 2007; Crawford and Losey, 2020). This therapy requires general anaesthesia, operator skill and proficiency in usage of the laser, and possible placement of a feeding tube for postoperative nutrition.

8.1.3 Homecare following full-mouth-extraction treatment of stomatitis

Pain medications such as buprenorphine, fentanyl, gabapentin and NSAIDs (Lewis, 2014b), usually in combination, are required for several weeks to months postoperatively. Liquid, injectable or transdermal medications are usually easier for owners to administer (Lewis, 2014b; Crawford and Losey, 2020) to these patients than tablets or capsules (Rochette, 2012).

If a feeding tube has been placed, instruct the pet owner in its use and maintenance, including appropriate feeding volume and frequency, cleaning, rechecks and removal. All patients should be fed a soft diet until the surgical sites have completely healed (Crawford and Losey, 2020), and hard treats and toys restricted during this time. Many patients who have had full-mouth extractions require a soft diet for life; however, there are some kibble-loving cats who prefer to eat hard food (swallowing it whole) after their mouths have healed, and they are pain-free (Sacramento Veterinary Dental Services (SACVDS), 2021).

Since many of these cats have suffered with chronic oral inflammation for some time before they are diagnosed and treated, the inflammation may take some time to resolve after extractions are performed (Lewis, 2014b). Schedule postoperative rechecks every 2 weeks until the inflammation subsides (Rochette, 2012) to ensure that adequate pain relief is being provided and that the cat is eating well enough to maintain their body weight. Rechecks also help in identifying refractory cases.

8.2   Feline Juvenile Gingivitis

Feline juvenile gingivitis is severe generalized inflammation and hyperplasia of the attached gingiva of kittens (Lobprise and Wiggs, 2000b). Unlike stomatitis, there is no inflammation of the caudal oral mucosa (Niemiec, 2014). Juvenile gingivitis can be seen as early as 4 months of age when permanent tooth eruption begins (Niemiec, 2012), but is most often diagnosed between 6 and 12 months of age (Ruhnau, 2017). Most kittens with juvenile gingivitis have few clinical signs beyond gingival inflammation (Force, 2010), but if left untreated this condition can progress to feline juvenile periodontitis, in which tissue destruction and loss of the periodontium occurs (Force, 2010; Byard, 2018).

The cause of juvenile gingivitis is unknown (Niemiec, 2012) but is likely multifactorial (Van de Wetering, 2011). Inflammation instigated by the exfoliation of primary teeth, viral and bacterial agents, an immune hypersensitivity reaction to plaque bacteria, and genetics may all play a role in this disease (Force, 2010; Van de Wetering, 2011).

8.2.1   Diagnosis of feline juvenile gingivitis

The patient's FeLV, FIV and FCV status should be evaluated, as these diseases may also cause oral inflammation (Beckman, 2019). Histopathology should be performed if an underlying condition is suspected or if the gingival inflammation appears atypical (Niemiec, 2012). Dental radiographs are essential to distinguish feline juvenile gingivitis from its more advanced form, feline juvenile periodontitis (Niemiec, 2012, 2014).

8.2.2   Treatment of feline juvenile gingivitis

Treatment involves keeping the bacterial load of the oral cavity low by a combination of frequent professional dental prophylaxis every 3–6 months

(Ruhnau, 2017; Byard, 2018), even when calculus and visible plaque are not present; gingivectomy of hyperplastic tissue to reduce any pseudopockets; extraction of any persistent deciduous teeth; and meticulous dental homecare including daily tooth-brushing and rinsing with antimicrobial agents such as chlorhexidine (Force, 2010; Perrone, 2016).

Low-dose daily doxycycline and feline interferon have been used successfully as adjuncts to dental homecare in some cases (Beckman, 2019). Full-mouth radiographs are necessary to monitor for attachment loss (Ruhnau, 2017). Tooth resorption associated with inflammation can also occur (Ruhnau, 2017).

NSAIDs are often used to decrease the inflammation and provide pain relief. Corticosteroids should be avoided, as they have been implicated in worsening of the disease (Ruhnau, 2017).

If diligent measures are taken to keep the teeth clean, this condition may resolve (Lobprise and Wiggs, 2000b) by the time patient is 2 years of age (Force, 2010), but in some cases, multiple or full-mouth extractions may eventually be required (Ruhnau, 2017).

8.3   Contact Mucositis

Contact mucositis, also known as chronic ulcerative paradental stomatitis (CUPS), contact stomatitis, ulcerative stomatitis and contact mucosal ulceration, is a painful condition of dogs which causes ulceration of the gums and mucosa in areas that touch tooth surfaces (Niemiec, 2014; Bellows, 2016). These lesions are often called paradental, contact or 'kissing' ulcers (Bellows, 2016). The lateral mucosa of the tongue may also become inflamed and ulcerated from contact with the mandibular teeth.

Like stomatitis and feline juvenile gingivitis, contact mucositis is an inflammatory disease likely stimulated by hypersensitivity to dental plaque (Lobprise and Wiggs, 2000b; Niemiec, 2014). This inflammation can progress to gingivitis and attachment loss (Bellows, 2016). Patients with contact mucositis usually have halitosis and may be anorexic or able to eat only soft food (Niemiec, 2014), stop playing with their toys (Bellows, 2016), paw at the mouth, chatter their teeth (Carmichael, 2004) or drool excessively (Reiter, 2014). They may also have concurrent lip fold dermatitis and/ or mandibular lymphadenopathy (Carmichael, 2004). Contact mucositis can occur in any breed, but it is overrepresented in Maltese, Cavalier King Charles spaniels and, greyhounds (Bellows, 2016).

8.3.1   Diagnosis of contact mucositis

A complete physical examination and labwork including a CBC, chemistry profile and urinalysis (Bellows, 2016) should be performed. Laboratory findings commonly associated with contact mucositis are hyperproteinaemia and mild neutrophilia (Bellows, 2016). Although contact mucositis can be presumptively diagnosed based on a patient's history and oral examination findings, a definitive diagnosis can only be made by biopsy and histology in order to rule out conditions that can cause oral ulceration, such as autoimmune diseases (Niemiec, 2014; Lewis, 2017).

8.3.2 Treatment of contact mucositis

Pain medications such as buprenorphine, tramadol, gabapentin and NSAIDs should be initiated as soon as possible after diagnosis (Beckman, 2006) to alleviate discomfort and allow the dog to eat.

Treatment requires lifelong plaque-reduction therapy (Niemiec, 2014), including frequent professional dental cleanings (every 4–6 months), full-mouth dental radiography, extraction of any teeth with advanced periodontal disease, and extraction of teeth contacting the ulcerated areas (Bellows, 2016; Lewis, 2017). In severe cases, extraction of all caudal teeth or full-mouth extractions may be necessary (Lewis, 2017). Dogs who have not been eating well prior to treatment may need pre- and/or postoperative nutritional or fluid therapy or placement of a feeding tube.

If the inflammation does not resolve with professional dental cleanings and diligent dental homecare, adjunct treatments with antibiotics such as amoxicillin-clavulanic acid, clindamycin, metronidazole and tetracyclines, and/or corticosteroids such as prednisolone to suppress inflammation, may be necessary (Carmichael, 2004). A combination of metronidazole and clindamycin has been effective in severe cases (Carmichael, 2004).

8.3.3 Homecare for dogs with contact mucositis

Pain medications such as gabapentin, tramadol and NSAIDs, often in combination, may be required for several weeks to months postoperatively (Beckman, 2006; Lewis, 2017).

If a feeding tube has been placed, instruct the pet owner in its use and maintenance, including appropriate feeding volume and frequency, cleaning, rechecks and removal. All patients should be fed a soft diet until the surgical sites have completely healed, and hard treats and toys restricted during this time.

Ongoing diligent dental homecare (including daily tooth-brushing, oral rinses such as chlorhexidine, and plaque-reducing water additives) is essential to keep the plaque bacteria population low (Niemiec, 2014). This can be complicated by the fact that most of these dogs are in such pain that their owners are often unable to brush their teeth (Reiter, 2014) or may be bitten in the attempt, so appropriate pain medications should be administered to the patient for as long as necessary (Beckman, 2006).

In addition to dental homecare, frequent rechecks and COHATs are required to keep this condition under control (Carmichael, 2004; Bellows,

2016). Pet owners should also be warned that full-mouth extractions may become necessary if more conservative treatment is insufficient to keep their pet's oral inflammation and pain at bay (Carmichael, 2004; Lewis, 2017).

References

Beckman, B.W. (2006) Pathophysiology and management of surgical and chronic oral pain in dogs and cats. *Journal of Veterinary Dentistry* 23(1), 50–59. DOI: 10.1177/089875640602300110.

Beckman, B. (2019) Hyperplastic feline juvenile gingivitis. International Veterinary Dentistry Institute. Available at: https://veterinarydentistry.net/hyperplastic-feline-juvenile-gingivitis/ (accessed 26 October 2020).

Bellows, J. (2010) Feline oropharyngeal inflammation – not just stomatitis. In: *Proceedings of the 26th Annual Veterinary Dental Forum*. Omnipress, Madison, Wisconsin (CD Rom).

Bellows, J. (2016) Chronic ulcerative paradental stomatitis of dogs. Clinician's Brief. Available at: https://www.cliniciansbrief.com/article/chronic-ulcerative-paradental-stomatitis-dogs (accessed 26 October 2020).

Byard, V. (2018) A special focus on feline dentistry. Pennsylvania Veterinary Medical Association. Available at: https://cdn.ymaws.com/www.pavma.org/resource/resmgr/docs/kvc/2018/byard,_vicki/5._feline_dentistry.pdf (accessed 1 March 2021).

Carmichael, D.T. (2004) Dental corner: diagnosing and treating chronic ulcerative paradental stomatitis. Dvm360. Available at: https://www.dvm360.com/view/dental-corner-diagnosing-and-treating-chronic-ulcerative-paradental-stomatitis (accessed 27 October 2020).

Crawford, J. (2010) Feline oral diseases. In: *Proceedings of the 26th Annual Veterinary Dental Forum*. Omnipress, Madison, Wisconsin (CD Rom).

Crawford, J. and Losey, B.J. (2020) Feline dentistry. In: Perrone, J. (ed.) *Small Animal Dental Procedures for Veterinary Technicians and Nurses*. Wiley Blackwell, Hoboken, New Jersey, pp. 169–186.

Force, J. (2010) Feline dentistry. In: *Proceedings of the 26th Annual Veterinary Dental Forum*. Omnipress, Madison, Wisconsin (CD Rom).

Greenfield, B. (2017) Chronic feline gingivostomatitis: proven therapeutic approaches and new treatment options. Today's Veterinary Practice. Available at: https://todaysveterinarypractice.com/chronic-feline-gingivostamatitis-proven-therapeutic-approaches-new-treatment-optionsce-article/ (accessed 26 October 2020).

Hennet, P. (2014) Feline chronic gingivostomatitis. In: *World Small Animal Veterinary Association World Congress Proceedings, 2014*. Available at: https://www.vin.com/apputil/content/defaultadv1.aspx?pId=12886&catId=57092&id=7054896&ind=55&objTypeID=17 (accessed March 1, 2021).

Holmstrom, S., Holmstrom, L.A., McGrath, C.J., Richey, M.T. and Wiggs, R.B. (2000) Feline dentistry. In: Holmstrom, S. (ed.) *Veterinary Dentistry for the Technician & Office Staff*. Saunders, Philadelphia, Pennsylvania, pp. 283–291.

Lewis, J. (2014a) Why teeth removal is best when your patient has feline stomatitis. Veterinary Practice News. Available at: https://www.veterinarypracticenews.

com/why-teeth-removal-is-best-when-your-patient-has-feline-stomatitis/ (accessed 1 March 2021).

Lewis, J. (2014b) Feline stomatitis: medical therapy for refractory cases. Veterinary Practice News. Available at: https://www.veterinarypracticenews.com/Feline-Stomatitis-Medical-Therapy-for-Refractory-Cases/ (accessed 26 October 2020).

Lewis, J. (2017) Causes of canine stomatitis and how to treat it. Veterinary Practice News. Available at: https://www.veterinarypracticenews.com/causes-of-canine-stomatitis/ (accessed 27 October 2020).

Lewis, J.R., Tsugawa, A.J. and Reiter, A.M. (2007) Use of CO2 laser as an adjunctive treatment for caudal stomatitis in a cat. *Journal of Veterinary Dentistry* 24(4), 240–249. DOI: 10.1177/089875640702400406.

Lobprise, H.B. and Wiggs, R.B. (2000a) Feline oral and dental disease. In: Lobprise, H.B. and Wiggs, R.B. (eds) *The Veterinarian's Companion for Common Dental Procedures.* AAHA Press, Lakewood, Colorado, pp. 137–148.

Lobprise, H.B. and Wiggs, R.B. (2000b) Periodontal disease. In: Lobprise, H.B. and Wiggs, R.B. (eds) *The Veterinarian's Companion for Common Dental Procedures.* AAHA Press, Lakewood, Colorado, pp. 39–70.

Lyon, K.F. (2004) Gingivostomatitis – what do we call it – how do we treat it? In: *Proceedings of the 18th Annual Veterinary Dental Forum.* Omnipress, Madison, Wisconsin, pp. 285–291.

Niemiec, B.A. (2012) Unusual feline oral pathology. In: *Proceedings of the 26th Annual Veterinary Dental Forum.* Omnipress, Madison, Wisconsin (CD Rom).

Niemiec, B.A. (2014) Feline and canine oral ulcerative disease. Today's Veterinary Practice. Available at: https://todaysveterinarypractice.com/practical-dentistry-feline-canine-oral-ulcerative-disease/ (accessed 1 March 2021).

Perrone, J.R. (2016) Top 5 feline oral health concerns. Clinician's Brief. Available at: https://www.cliniciansbrief.com/article/top-5-feline-oral-health-concerns (accessed 1 March 2021).

Reiter, A.M. (2014) Oral inflammatory and ulcerative disease in small animals. MSD Veterinary Manual. Available at: https://www.merckvetmanual.com/digestive-system/diseases-of-the-mouth-in-small-animals/oral-inflammatory-and-ulcerative-disease-in-small-animals (accessed 1 March 2021).

Rochette, J. (2012) Feline stomatitis. Clinician's Brief. Available at: https://www.cliniciansbrief.com/article/feline-stomatitis (accessed 1 March 2021).

Ruhnau, J. (2017) Treatment of feline juvenile gingivitis in cats. In: *World Small Animal Veterinary Association Congress Proceedings, 2017.* Available at: https://www.vin.com/apputil/content/defaultadv1.aspx?pId=20539&catId=113438&id=8506389&ind=52&objTypeID=17 (accessed 22 October, 2020).

SACVDS (2021) Feline chronic gingivostomatitis. Sacramento Veterinary Dental Services. Available at: https://www.sacvds.com/forms/feline-chronic-gingivostomatitis.pdf (accessed 1 March 2021).

Van de Wetering, A. (2011) Dental and oral cavity. In: Peterson, M.E. and Kutzler, M.A. (eds) *Small Animal Pediatrics.* Elsevier, St. Louis, Missouri, pp. 340–350.

Bad to the Bone: Jaw Fractures, Temporomandibular Joint (TMJ) Luxation, and Avulsed and Luxated Teeth

9

Mandibular and maxillary fractures can occur due to trauma to the face and head, such as being hit by a vehicle, falls or animal bites; and pathologic weakening of the bones of the jaw by disease processes including periodontal disease and oral tumours (Lopes *et al.*, 2005; Perrone *et al.*, 2020) Fractures can also be iatrogenic, due to veterinary error when performing tooth extractions (Lopes *et al.*, 2005). Types of jaw fractures include:

- fractures of the body of the mandible (the most common type of jaw fracture in dogs) (Lewis, 2015a)
- fractures of the rostral mandible and maxilla
- symphyseal separation (the most common type of jaw fracture in cats) (Lewis, 2015a)
- maxillary fractures, including palatal fractures
- fractures of the ramus (vertical portion) of the mandible.

Trauma to the face and head can also cause luxation of the temporomandibular joint (TMJ), tooth luxation (partial displacement of a tooth from its alveolus) or tooth avulsion (tooth is completely removed from its alveolus).

9.1 Clinical Signs of Jaw Fractures

The clinical signs of mandibular and maxillary fractures vary depending upon their location. Common signs of maxillary fracture include pain, epistaxis, nasal obstruction, dental malocclusion and facial asymmetry (Legendre, 1998; Barbudo *et al.*, 2000; Lobprise and Wiggs, 2000). Signs of mandibular fractures include pain, difficulty eating, oral bleeding, dental malocclusion, soft-tissue swelling and an inability to close the mouth (Legendre, 1998; Barbudo *et al.*, 2000; Lantz, 2010; American College of Veterinary Surgeons (ACVS), 2021). Symphyseal separation may present

© CAB International 2022. *An Introduction to Pet Dental Care: For Veterinary Technicians and Nurses* (K. Istace)
DOI: 10.1079/9781789248869.0009

with few to no clinical signs, or with pain, lateral tipping of the mandible, difficulty with eating or an inability to close the mouth (Legendre, 1998).

9.1.1   Diagnosis of jaw fractures

Since many of these fractures occur due to trauma, the patient must be evaluated for internal injuries and stabilized if necessary (Legendre, 2003). Establish an airway, control haemorrhages, and treat shock prior to jaw fracture diagnosis and treatment (Lantz, 2010). Thoracic and abdominal radiographs may be indicated (Peak, 2012) to rule out pneumothorax, diaphragmatic hernia, etc. Labwork including a complete blood count (CBC), serum chemistry profile and urinalysis should be performed (Peak, 2012). Administer pain medications as soon as possible (Peak, 2012). If the fracture is open, intravenous antibiotics should be administered (Hall and Wiggs, 2005; Lantz, 2010).

Once the patient is sufficiently stable for general anaesthesia, take full-mouth intraoral radiographs (Peak, 2012; Legendre, 2012). Dorsoventral and lateral skull radiographs are recommended for suspected maxillary fractures or TMJ luxations (Legendre, 2003), and oblique and open-mouth skull views may be useful (Peak, 2012). CT scans can provide a complete three-dimensional view of the fracture (Lantz, 2010).

9.1.2   Temporary stabilization of jaw fractures

Patients with jaw fractures may need several days of emergency or critical care prior to jaw fracture repair (Peak, 2012), or may be referred to a veterinary dental specialist. Temporary stabilization with a muzzle (Perrone et al., 2020) during this time improves comfort, prevents further trauma, and allows the patient to be fed a soft slurry food (Lantz, 2010). Muzzles may be used as the sole treatment for minimally displaced (Marretta, 2009) or pathologic fractures (Perrone, 2009), or can be used to provide additional support when other treatment methods are used (Lobprise and Wiggs, 2000; Perrone et al., 2020). Muzzle stabilization is not recommended in brachycephalic breeds since the muzzle may interfere with breathing (Perrone, 2009; Lantz, 2010).

Prior to muzzle placement, the patient should receive pain medications so that closing the mouth does not cause undue discomfort. (Lobprise and Wiggs, 2000). Sedation and/or an Elizabethan collar may be required to prevent the patient from removing the muzzle (Lobprise and Wiggs, 2000; Stevens, 2006).

Nylon or cloth muzzles have the advantage that they can be washed after feeding (Stevens, 2006). Ideally, two muzzles are sent home with the patient, so one can be washed while the patient is wearing the other (Stevens, 2006; Perrone et al., 2020). The muzzle should be large enough to allow the pet to lap food and water, but not so large that they can open their mouth (Perrone *et al.*, 2020). The correct size and shape of commercial muzzle may not be readily available (Perrone, 2009). In these cases, you can easily create a tape muzzle.

9.1.3 How to make and place a tape muzzle

1. Gently close the patient's mouth partway, leaving a 0.5–1.5-cm opening, depending on the size of the patient, to allow lapping of slurried food and water (Lobprise and Wiggs, 2000; Stevens, 2006). The teeth should be positioned as close to proper occlusion as is achievable. The occlusion of the canine teeth is a good guide (Perrone, 2009).
2. Place a strip of 1.25–2.5-cm-wide medical tape adhesive side up around the pet's muzzle, just behind the canine teeth (Lobprise and Wiggs, 2000). Wrap another strip of tape around this circle, adhesive side down (Perrone, 2009).
3. Measure the distance between one side of the tape muzzle to the back of the head, passing below the ears (Lobprise and Wiggs, 2000). Cut four strips of tape (DentalVets, 2021) 10–20 cm longer than this length. Remove the tape circle from the patient's muzzle. Apply one of the strips adhesive side up to the inside surface of the tape circle, then apply another strip adhesive side up on the opposite side of the tape circle (DentalVets, 2021). Apply the two remaining tape strips adhesive side down on top of the first two. Now you should have a tape circle with two straps.

   Replace the tape circle on the patient's muzzle and tie the straps around the back of the patient's head. Make sure the straps do not come into contact with the patient's eyes (DentalVets, 2021). Another strip of tape can be placed over the muzzle circle to ensure the straps do not come off.

This type of tape muzzle can be easily removed to clean both it and the patient's face after eating, then retied, making it suitable when the muzzle is expected to be in place for long periods. Alternatively, a single sling can be placed from one side of the muzzle to the other around the back of the head, by measuring two longer strips of tape rather than four shorter ones (Perrone, 2009). The first sling is centred at the back of the head and placed adhesive side up with the ends wrapped under the muzzle tape circle, with the second sling placed adhesive side down over the first (Perrone, 2009). If desired, a third tape strap can be placed from the tape circle over the bridge of the nose to the sling at the back of the head, to prevent slippage (Stevens, 2006). The first strip should be placed adhesive side out, then another tape placed over it adhesive side down.

9.2 Jaw Fracture Repair Techniques

Treatment options are determined primarily by the location and severity of the fracture. The aim is to restore normal dental occlusion so the patient can eat without pain or trauma (Lobprise and Wiggs, 2000; Lantz, 2010). If the teeth are kept in proper occlusion during healing, the bones of the jaw will heal appropriately (Legendre, 2012). A feeding tube may be required to ensure adequate post-operative nutrition (Barbudo *et al.*, 2000; Lantz, 2010). Place dental regional blocks prior to fracture repair (Peak, 2012), and manage preoperative, intraoperative, and postoperative pain.

9.2.1 Treatment of fractures of the body of the mandible

These fractures can be repaired by intra-oral splints, usually made of acrylic or resin; interosseous or interfragmentary wiring; interdental wiring; interarcade bonding; titanium miniplates; or external skeletal fixation (Barbudo *et al.*, 2000; Hall and Wiggs, 2005).

In cases of jaw fracture due to trauma, any damaged teeth or teeth affected by periodontal disease involved in the fracture site may be extracted (Peak, 2012; Perrone *et al.*, 2020); however, they are often left in place initially to provide anchorage sites for wires and/or splints (Barbudo *et al.*, 2000; Legendre, 2012; Peak, 2012). Once the fracture has healed, any compromised teeth can be extracted or treated endodontically (Barbudo *et al.*, 2000; Legendre, 2012). For pathologic fractures due to periodontal disease, diseased teeth must be extracted and the area cleaned and debrided to remove the source of infection and allow the bone to heal (Hall and Wiggs, 2005; Lantz, 2010).

Intra-oral splints

These are non-invasive, relatively inexpensive, and can be used to reinforce wire repair techniques (Hall and Wiggs, 2005). Cold-curing acrylic or chemical-curing composite resins (Lantz, 2010; Peak, 2012) can be applied directly to the crowns of teeth after any open wounds have been sutured closed. Most of the splint material should be applied on the lingual aspect of the teeth, in order to maintain proper dental occlusion with the maxillary teeth (Hall and Wiggs, 2005: Perrone *et al.*, 2020). The teeth must first be cleaned, polished with non-fluoridated flour pumice, acid-etched, and bonding agents applied (Hall and Wiggs, 2005). Once cured, the acrylic or composite is shaped and any sharp edges are smoothed with a dental bur (Perrone *et al.*, 2020) or polishing disks (Peak, 2012). If there are no healthy teeth in the area, as is usually the case with pathologic fractures, the soft tissue is closed and stainless-steel wire looped around the body of the mandible of each fragment, and splint material is applied onto the wires (Hall and Wiggs, 2005; Legendre, 2012).

Interosseous/interfragmentary wiring

Soft tissue is reflected away from the mandibular bone, and holes are drilled through the bone fragments with a round carbide or diamond bur. Then 18–24-gauge (Miller, 2020) stainless-steel wire is passed through the holes, the ends of the wire are twisted together and tightened, and the soft tissues are sutured closed. Care must be taken to avoid causing injury to the tooth roots, nerves, vessels and mandibular canal (Perrone *et al.*, 2020). This technique is often reinforced by acrylic splinting to help hold the teeth in proper occlusion while the bone fragments heal (Lantz, 2010). The wiring remains in place permanently, and any splint material is removed once the fracture has healed.

Interdental wiring

Here, 24–26-gauge wire (Peak, 2012) is placed around the base of the tooth crowns of at least two adjacent teeth on each side of the fracture line, using various techniques to reduce the fracture and bring the teeth into proper occlusion (Lantz, 2010). An acrylic or composite splint is placed over the wires to ensure they stay in place while the fracture heals (Lantz, 2010). The splint and wiring must be removed once healed.

Interarcade bonding

Cold-curing acrylic or chemical-curing composite is applied bilaterally between the upper and lower canine teeth, immobilizing the mouth (Lobprise and Wiggs, 2000; Legendre, 2003). Sufficient space must be left so the patient can lap food and water, and a temporary feeding tube is often placed in these patients to ensure they receive adequate nutrition (Legendre, 2003).

Titanium miniplates

These small plates are placed directly onto the mandibular bone, with the screws angled to avoid any tooth roots and the mandibular canal (Lantz, 2010). These plates are especially useful in patients who have no teeth in the fractured area, thus making other types of repair difficult (Lewis, 2016).

External skeletal fixation (ESF)

Pins are placed through the skin of the face into each bone fragment (ACVS, 2021). The pins are connected to a rod on the outside of the jaw, bringing the fragments into occlusion and immobilizing them. The patient's skin must be kept clean and dry while the ESF appliance is in place, and an Elizabethan collar may be needed to prevent pawing at the appliance. After the fracture has healed, the pins are removed.

9.2.2 Treatment of fractures of the rostral mandible and rostral maxilla, and pathologic fractures

Interdental or interosseous wiring +/- intra-oral acrylic splinting can sometimes be used to repair rostral or pathologic fractures (Wood, 2003; Faria, 2004). It is also acceptable to perform a partial mandibulectomy or maxillectomy to remove the fractured portion (Wood, 2003; Faria, 2004; Lantz, 2010): this eliminates the risks of non-vital teeth, ankylosis and osteomyelitis (Wood, 2003). However, complications such as intraoperative bleeding, wound dehiscence and disfigurement can occur (Wood, 2003; Faria, 2004).

9.2.3 Treatment of symphyseal separation

Circumferential wiring (Perrone *et al.*, 2020) is performed by threading 22-gauge wire (Lewis, 2015b) through an 18-gauge needle, entering the oral cavity from beneath the chin after the skin is shaved and surgically scrubbed (Legendre, 2012; Lewis, 2015b). The wire is passed intra-orally around the mandible behind the distal aspect of the crowns of both lower canine teeth, then back out through the chin (Legendre, 2012). The symphysis is brought together in proper alignment, the ends of the wire are twisted together beneath the chin using forceps, then cut (Lewis, 2015b). A small blob of composite resin should be placed on the cut ends of the wires to prevent any trauma to the patient from the sharp wires (Lewis, 2015b). The wire is left in place for 3–4 weeks, then removed (Perrone *et al.*, 2020).

A less invasive technique uses cerclage wire looped in a figure-of-eight between the bases of the crowns of the lower canine teeth to bring the symphysis together. (Legendre, 1998; Barbudo *et al.*, 2000). A splint of self-curing acrylic or chemical-curing composite is placed on this figure-of-eight wire to keep it in position and prevent soft-tissue trauma from the wires (Legendre, 1998; Barbudo *et al.*, 2000). This technique can cause linguoversion of the canine teeth (Lobprise and Wiggs, 2000).

9.2.4 Treatment of maxillary fractures

If the teeth or bones are not displaced, maxillary fractures may be allowed to heal on their own (Barbudo *et al.*, 2000; Legendre, 2003), after any soft-tissue injuries are debrided and closed. However, if there is any malocclusion, facial asymmetry or deformity, nasal obstruction or communication

Maxillary fracture repair using wire and acrylic splint

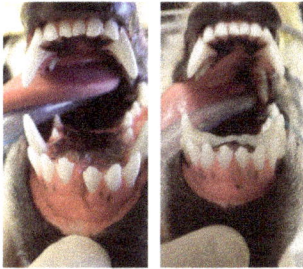

Symphyseal separation repair by circumferential wiring

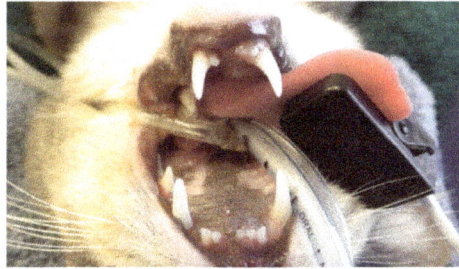

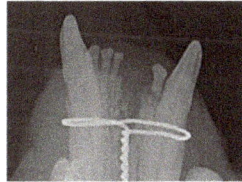

Fig. 9.1. Fracture repair techniques.

between the oral and sinus cavities, the fracture(s) will need to be repaired (Barbudo *et al.*, 2000). The techniques are similar to the treatment of mandibular fractures, though if applying an intra-oral acrylic or composite splint to the maxillary teeth, most of the material should be applied to the buccal surfaces to allow for proper occlusion with the mandibular teeth (Legendre, 2003).

9.2.5 Treatment of fractures of the ramus of the mandible

Displacement of the bones in these types of fractures is often minimal, so a muzzle may be all that is required to stabilize the jaw during healing (Lobprise and Wiggs, 2000). If there is bone displacement, then interosseous/interfragmentary wiring, titanium miniplates or interarcade bonding between the upper and lower canine teeth can be used to repair these fractures (Verstraete, 2006). A condylectomy may need to be performed if any arthritic changes develop after healing, which usually results in the patient's inability to close their mouth (Barbudo *et al.*, 2000).

9.2.6 Homecare following jaw fracture repair

Pain medications such as buprenorphine, gabapentin, tramadol and nonsteroidal anti-inflammatory drugs (NSAIDs), usually in combination, may be required for several weeks postoperatively (Legendre, 2012). Oral antibiotics may be administered for 7–10 days if the fracture was open

(Legendre, 2003; Hall and Wiggs, 2005). Liquid or injectable medications are often easier for owners to administer to these patients (Perrone *et al.*, 2020) than tablets or capsules.

All patients should be fed a soft, slurry (semi-liquid) diet until the fracture has completely healed (Legendre, 1998; Barbudo *et al.*, 2000). Pet owners can make this slurry by mixing either the pet's regular canned food or a high-calorie recovery canned diet with water in a blender. Hard treats and toys should be restricted until the fracture has completely healed and any appliance removed (Hall and Wiggs, 2005; Perrone *et al.*, 2020). If a feeding tube has been placed, instruct the pet owner in its use and maintenance, including appropriate feeding volume and frequency, cleaning, rechecks and removal (ACVS, 2021).

An Elizabethan collar is recommended to prevent the patient from pawing at or rubbing their face and damaging any appliances, wiring or splints (Stevens, 2006). If a splint, interarcade bonding or ESF is in place, the owner should be sent home with chlorhexidine oral rinse to clean both it and the mouth twice daily (Legendre, 2003; Lantz, 2010). Schedule rechecks every 1–2 weeks, with radiographs to check for bone healing between 4 and 8 weeks (Perrone *et al.*, 2020). Once the fracture has healed, splints and any interdental wire is removed from the teeth using a carbide or diamond bur on a high-speed handpiece, wire cutters, and extraction forceps to break off pieces of splint (Perrone *et al.*, 2020), and the teeth are cleaned and polished (Legendre, 2003; Lantz, 2010).

9.3 Temporomandibular Joint (TMJ) Luxation

TMJ luxation is considered a dental emergency, since if it is not reduced soon after the initial injury, blood clots and tissue fibrosis may make it impossible to reduce (Klima, 2007).

TMJ luxation occurs most often in cats (Reiter, 2007). Patients with TMJ luxation usually have a history of head trauma and present with a rostrally and laterally displaced lower jaw, causing a malocclusion and an inability to close their mouths (Reiter, 2007). Haemorrhages may be visible in the caudal mucosa and/or soft palate. If only one temporomandibular joint is luxated, the mandibles will be displaced to the opposite side (Reiter, 2007). If both temporomandibular joints are luxated (not as common), both mandibles will be displaced rostrally.

Dorsoventral and left and right lateral oblique skull radiographs (Gawor, 2017) are taken to evaluate the TMJ and rule out other conditions such as mandibular or maxillary fractures. CT or MRI scans are also helpful in evaluating this condition.

The patient is anaesthetized and a fulcrum such as a small syringe or pencil (Gawor, 2017) is placed between the upper and lower carnassial teeth on the luxated side. The mandible of the luxated side is gently pulled rostrally (Gawor, 2017), then the mouth is closed over the fulcrum while directing the mandible caudally (Reiter, 2007). Skull radiographs are repeated to confirm the procedure has been successful (Thatcher, 2017).

If TMJ reduction was difficult or there are any concurrent fractures, interarcade bonding between the upper and lower canine teeth or a tape muzzle can ensure jaw stability during healing (Lobprise and Wiggs, 2000; Klima, 2007).

The patient should receive pain medications including a NSAID for 7–10 days postoperatively, to help relieve inflammation in the joint and surrounding tissues (Thatcher, 2017). They should be fed soft food only for at least 2 weeks, to minimize chewing while the area is healing (Thatcher, 2017).

9.4   Luxated and Avulsed Teeth

A luxated or avulsed tooth is considered a dental emergency, since there is a short time frame in which a tooth that has been partially or completely displaced from its alveolus can be successfully re-implanted (Niemiec, 2012).

Luxated teeth are partially displaced from the alveolus due to a traumatic injury (Gracis, 2015). They may be pushed further into the alveolus, pulled partially out of the alveolus, or displaced laterally within the alveolus. The alveolus is usually fractured (Gracis, 2015).

An avulsed tooth is completely displaced from the alveolus (Gracis, 2015). It should be placed into milk or physiologic saline as soon as possible to preserve the vitality of the periodontal cells (Klima, 2007). Avulsed teeth should not be placed in water, as water can cause cell destruction. If the tooth has been outside the mouth for less than 20 minutes before being placed into milk or saline, there is a good chance of successful re-implantation (Klima, 2007). Stored in milk or saline, periodontal tissues will remain alive for up to 3 hours. The longer a tooth is allowed to remain outside the mouth, the higher the chances that periodontal tissues will dry out and die, leading to root resorption and re-implantation failure (Klima, 2007).

In cases of both luxation and avulsion, the blood supply to the teeth has been compromised, which will result in tooth death, and the pet owner must commit to treating the tooth endodontically once it has been re-implanted and the tissues have healed (Klima, 2007). If they are unwilling to do so, the luxated tooth should be extracted, or the alveolus of the avulsed tooth should be cleaned and debrided, and the area sutured closed.

9.4.1 Treatment of luxated and avulsed teeth

The patient is anaesthetized, a dental regional nerve block is placed, intravenous (IV) antibiotics are administered, and dental radiographs are taken of the area to assess if there are any fractures of the alveolus (Gracis, 2015). The tooth and alveolus are gently rinsed with saline to remove any debris, hair, blood clots, etc. while avoiding causing damage to the periodontal tissues (Klima, 2007; Gracis, 2015). The tooth is replaced into the alveolus and the patient's occlusion is evaluated (Klima, 2007). Any soft-tissue injuries are repaired, then the tooth is acid-etched and fixed into place with interdental wiring and a self-curing acrylic or cold-curing composite resin splint (Gracis, 2015). This splint is left in place for 7–10 days in the case of avulsed teeth with no alveolar fractures, or up to 8 weeks for luxated teeth with extensive alveolar fractures (Klima, 2007).

9.4.2 Homecare following re-implantation

The patient should receive postoperative pain management for at least 7 days, antibiotics, and be fed a soft diet with no access to hard treats or toys (Gracis, 2015). Instruct the owner to rinse the splint and mouth twice daily with a chlorhexidine solution (Gracis, 2015). Once the splint is removed, the tooth must be endodontically treated with standard root canal therapy. Schedule follow-up radiographs every 6–12 months to monitor for signs of re-implantation failure such as root resorption and loss of the periodontal ligament (ankylosis) (Gracis, 2015).

References

ACVS (2021) Mandibular fractures. American College of Veterinary Surgeons. Available at: https://www.acvs.org/small-animal/mandibular-fractures (accessed 20 January 2021).

Barbudo, G.R., Selmi, A.L. and Canola, J.C. (2000) Oral and maxillofacial reconstruction in a cat using wire and acrylic. *Journal of Veterinary Dentistry* 14(4), 168–172. DOI: 10.1177/089875640001700401.

DentalVets (2021) Trauma to jaws. Available at: https://www.dentalvets.co.uk/common-cases/trauma-to-jaws (accessed 25 January 2021).

Faria, M.L.E. (2004) Successful maxilla reimplantation after traumatic injury in a dog. Dvm360. Available at: https://www.dvm360.com/view/successful-maxilla-reimplantation-after-traumatic-injury-dog (accessed 26 January 2021).

Gawor, J. (2017) Treatment of TMJ rostral luxation in a cat. In: *World Small Animal Veterinary Association Congress Proceedings, 2017.* Available at: https://www.vin.com/apputil/content/defaultadv1.aspx?pId=20539&catId=113438&id=8506392&ind=54&objTypeID=17 (accessed 26 January 2021).

Gracis, M. (2015) Treatment of alveolo-dental trauma (dental luxation and avulsion) and other dental emergencies. In: *World Small Animal Veterinary Association World Congress Proceedings, 2015*. Available at: https://www.vin.com/apputil/content/defaultadv1.aspx?id=7259301&pid=14365 (accessed 27 January 2021).

Hall, B.P. and Wiggs, R.B. (2005) Acrylic splint and circumferential mandibular wire for mandibular fracture repair in a dog. *Journal of Veterinary Dentistry* 22(3), 170–175. DOI: 10.1177/089875640502000304.

Klima, L.J. (2007) Dental and oral emergencies. In: *Proceedings of the 21st Annual Veterinary Dental Forum*. Omnipress, Madison, Wisconsin, pp. 51–53.

Lantz, G.C. (2010) Management of facial fractures. In: *Proceedings of the 24th Annual Veterinary Dental Forum*. Omnipress, Madison, Wisconsin (CD Rom).

Legendre, L. (1998) Use of maxillary and mandibular splints for restoration of normal occlusion following jaw trauma in a cat: a case report. *Journal of Veterinary Dentistry* 15(4), 179–181. DOI: 10.1177/089875649801500406.

Legendre, L. (2003) Intraoral acrylic splints for maxillofacial fracture repair. *Journal of Veterinary Dentistry* 20(2), 70–78. DOI: 10.1177/089875640302000201.

Legendre, L. (2012) Minimally-invasive techniques for mandibular fracture repairs. In: *Proceedings of the 26th Annual Veterinary Dental Forum*. Omnipress, Madison, Wisconsin (CD Rom).

Lewis, J. (2015a) How to repair non-invasive jaw fracture. Veterinary Practice News. Available at: https://www.veterinarypracticenews.com/how-to-repair-non-invasive-jaw-fracture/ (accessed 2 March 2021).

Lewis, J. (2015b) Cerclage wire for rostral instability. Veterinary Practice News. Available at: https://www.veterinarypracticenews.com/cerclage-wire-for-rostral-mandibular-instability/ (accessed 2 March 2021).

Lewis, J. (2016) When to use miniplates for mandibular fractures. Veterinary Practice News. Available at: https://www.veterinarypracticenews.com/when-to-use-miniplates-for-mandibular-fractures/ (accessed 2 March 2021).

Lobprise, H.B. and Wiggs, R.B. (2000) Oral and dental emergencies. In: Lobprise, H.B. and Wiggs, R.B. (eds) *The Veterinarian's Companion for Common Dental Procedures*. AAHA Press, Lakewood, Colorado, pp. 115–135.

Lopes, F.M., Gioso, M.A., Ferro, D.G., Leon-Roman, M.A., Venturini, M.A.F.A. *et al.* (2005) Oral fractures in dogs of Brazil – a retrospective study. *Journal of Veterinary Dentistry* 22(2), 86–90. DOI: 10.1177/089875640502200202.

Marretta, S.M. (2009) Managing jaw fractures. Dvm360. Available at: https://www.dvm360.com/view/managing-jaw-fractures-proceedings (accessed 2 March 2021).

Miller, J. (2020) Jaw fractures. Clinician's Brief. Available at: https://www.cliniciansbrief.com/article/jaw-fractures (accessed 2 March 2021).

Niemiec, B.A. (2012) Dental emergencies. In: *Proceedings of the 26th Annual Veterinary Dental Forum*. Omnipress, Madison, Wisconsin (CD Rom).

Peak, M.R. (2012) Noninvasive jaw fracture repair techniques for the dog and cat. VetFolio. Available at: https://www.vetfolio.com/learn/article/noninvasive-jaw-fracture-repair-techniques-for-the-dog-and-cat (accessed 2 March 2021).

Perrone, J. (2009) Arts and crafts in veterinary dentistry: the tape muzzle. Dvm360. Available at: https://www.dvm360.com/view/arts-and-crafts-veterinary-dentistry-tape-muzzle-proceedings (accessed 25 January 2021).

Perrone, J.R., March, P.A. and Sharp, S. (2020) Common dental conditions and treatments. In: Perrone, J. (ed.) *Small Animal Dental Procedures for Veterinary Technicians and Nurses.* Wiley Blackwell, Hoboken, New Jersey, pp. 131–168.

Reiter, A.M. (2007) Differentiation between temperomandibular joint luxation and open-mouth jaw locking. In: *Proceedings of the 21st Annual Veterinary Dental Forum.* Omnipress, Madison, Wisconsin, p. 153.

Stevens, A.G. (2006) Acrylic for repair of mandibular fractures. Clinician's Brief. Available at: https://www.cliniciansbrief.com/article/acrylic-repair-mandibular-fractures (accessed 25 January 2021).

Thatcher, G. (2017) Temperomandibular joint luxation in the cat: diagnosis and management. *Canadian Veterinary Journal* 58(9), 989–993.

Verstraete, F.J.M. (2006) Decision-making in maxillofacial fracture repair. In: *Proceedings of the 20th Annual Veterinary Dental Forum.* Omnipress, Madison, Wisconsin, pp. 281–285.

Wood, B.C. (2003) Management of rostral mandible fracture including lateral luxation of a mandibular canine tooth in a dog. *Journal of Veterinary Dentistry* 20(2), 91–94. DOI: 10.1177/089875640302000204.

Common Dental Problems of Rabbits, Rodents and Other Small Mammals

Like dogs and cats, small caged pets can develop dental problems that must be addressed to ensure their overall health. Owners often have less close personal contact with these types of pets, and are less likely to bring them to the veterinary hospital to be examined on a regular basis (Donnelly, 2007), limiting our ability to detect oral problems until they are advanced and the pet presents with clinical signs such as dysphagia, anorexia, weight loss, drooling, facial swellings, epiphora, nasal discharge and inability to close the mouth (Hoefer, 2001; Legendre, 2003; Osofsky, 2006). Many veterinary practices see these species less often than canine and feline patients, and staff may lack familiarity with handling (Tynes, 2013), recognizing pathology, and anaesthesia.

10.1 Oral Anatomy and Dentition

10.1.1 Lagomorphs, caviomorph rodents and murine rodents

Dental formulae (Lobprise, 2009):

Lagomorphs – rabbit: 2(I2/1, C0/0, PM3/2, M2–3/3) = 26–28.
Caviomorph rodents – guinea pig / degu / chinchilla: 2(I1/1, C0/0, PM1–2/1, M3/3) = 20–22.
Murine rodents – rat / mouse / hamster / gerbil: 2(I1/1, C0/0, PM0/0, M2–3/2–3) = 12–16.

There are significant differences in the dentition between lagomorphs, caviomorph rodents and murine rodents. Lagomorphs have four maxillary incisors: two anterior and two posterior (Lobprise, 2009), while all rodents have only two maxillary incisors (Legendre, 2003). The extra posterior incisors of rabbits are commonly referred to as 'peg teeth' (Lobprise, 2009). Rabbits chew in a lateral fashion, with the lower incisors occluding between the peg teeth and the anterior upper incisors (Hoefer, 2001; Okuda *et al.*, 2007). The incisors of most rodents are sharp and chisel-like (Holmstrom *et al.*, 2000), and those of murine rodents are normally yellow-orange in colour (Osofsky, 2006).

All teeth of lagomorphs and caviomorph rodents grow continuously (Legendre, 2003), as they are worn down by the animals' abrasive diet of fibrous plant material (Okuda *et al.*, 2007). However, in murine rodents only the incisors continue to grow, allowing mice, rats, hamsters and gerbils to chew through hard obstacles to gain access to food and shelter (Michigan State University (MSU), 2001). Their diet of seeds, grains, tubers and meat is not particularly abrasive, so it is not necessary for their molars to grow continuously (Hoefer, 2001; Donnelly, 2007).

Conscious oral examination of these patients is difficult, as they have a small, long and narrow oral cavity and often only the anterior portion of the mouth can be examined (Lobprise, 2009). An otoscope can be used to increase visualization of the oral cavity in awake patients (Hoefer, 2001), but approximately 50% of dental pathology will be missed (Crossley, 2003a).

10.1.2 Ferrets

Dental formula: 2(I3/3, C1/1, PM3/3, M1/2) = 34 (Cooper, 2017).

Ferrets are obligate carnivores (Cooper, 2017), and their oral anatomy and dentition appears similar to that of the cat (Lobprise and Wiggs, 2000). They have long, narrow, flat skulls, with a short facial area (He *et al.*, 2002). Oral examination can usually be performed on conscious patients (Lobprise and Wiggs, 2000).

10.1.3 Hedgehogs

Dental formula: 2(I2–3/2, C1/1, P3–4/2–3, M3/3) = 34–40 (Crossley, 2003b).

Hedgehogs are insectivores, with a unique oral anatomy including a primitive tooth structure (Chaprazov *et al.*, 2014). Their incisors are used to prehend prey, and their canines resemble incisors or premolars (Crossley, 2003b). Hedgehogs often curl into a spiny ball when stressed, thus requiring sedation or anaesthesia to perform an oral examination (Tynes, 2013).

10.2 Anaesthesia

10.2.1 Preanaesthetic fasting

Preanaesthetic fasting should be limited to less than 1 hour in lagomorphs and rodents, as these patients have a high risk of hypoglycaemia (Legendre, 2003) and intestinal ileus (Osofsky, 2006). Fasting of ferrets and hedge-hogs should be limited to 2 hours, as they are prone to hypoglycaemia

(Cooper, 2017). Water should not be withheld from any small mammal (Bilhun *et al.*, 2020).

10.2.2 Preanaesthetic lab testing

A preanaesthetic blood panel consisting of, at minimum, a packed cell volume/total protein (PCV/TP), blood urea nitrogen (BUN), blood glucose and urine specific gravity (USG) should be performed (Bennett, 2009). Blood can be collected from the lateral saphenous or cephalic veins of some conscious rabbits, guinea pigs and ferrets; if larger blood volumes are required, blood can be collected from the jugular or cranial vena cava of sedated patients (Crowder, 2006; Cooper, 2017). Blood can also be collected from the auricular vessels in rabbits, but care must be taken not to damage the vessels (Maddamma and Lennox, 2012). The cranial vena cava is the preferred collection site for murine rodents and hedgehogs, with the patient sedated (Donnelly, 2007; Maddamma and Lennox, 2012). Butterfly catheters (25–27-gauge) or 25–27-gauge needles on a 1-ml syringe (Maddamma and Lennox, 2012), tuberculin syringes (Donnelly, 2007) or a haematocrit tube placed into the hub of a 25-gauge needle inserted into a vein can be used for blood collection.

10.2.3 Premedication

Premedication reduces the stress associated with induction and provides pain management. Some procedures, such as oral examinations, can be done using only chemical restraint. Commonly used premedication drugs in small mammals include ketamine, midazolam, medetomidine, glycopyrrolate, buprenorphine and butorphanol (Osofsky, 2006; Hawkins and Pascoe, 2012).

10.2.4 Intravenous (IV) access

It is challenging to gain intravenous access in very small patients (Maddamma and Lennox, 2012). IV catheters of 24-gauge or smaller can be placed into the cephalic or lateral saphenous veins of most guinea pigs, rabbits and ferrets (Rosenthal, 2001; Cooper, 2017). Smaller mammals such as mice and hamsters have limited venous access (Donnelly, 2007). Subcutaneous medications and fluids can be administered in these patients.

10.2.5 Anaesthetic induction and maintenance

Injectable induction can be performed on patients who have IV catheters. Commonly used induction drugs include ketamine/diazepam (Osofsky, 2006), propofol (Bennett, 2009) and alfaxan (Jurox, 2021).

Mask induction with isoflurane and O_2 can be performed (Osofsky, 2006) using a small anaesthetic mask on a non-rebreathing system (Bennett, 2009). For very small patients, chamber induction or a large anaesthetic mask placed over the patient can be used (Holmstrom *et al.*, 2000).

Intubation can be performed on larger patients, with direct visualization using a laryngoscope with a small blade and an endotracheal tube of 2 mm or greater; however, due to the small oral cavity, large tongue and the caudal location of the glottis in rabbits, this can be challenging (Johnson, 2011). A canine otoscope or an endoscope can also be used to achieve visualization of the vocal folds, then either the endotracheal tube or a French size 5 polypropylene urinary catheter guide is fed along the scope into the trachea (Johnson, 2011). If a catheter guide is used, remove the scope and thread the endotracheal tube over the catheter into the larynx, then remove the catheter (Holmstrom *et al.*, 2000; Johnson, 2011).

Blind intubation can be attempted in rabbits by hyperextending the neck while in a sternal position (Okuda *et al.*, 2007). The endotracheal tube is advanced during inhalation while listening for respiratory sounds at the end of the tube (Johnson, 2011). Condensation inside clear tubes or movement of the non-rebreathing bag can also confirm proper placement (Johnson, 2011). No more than two intubation attempts in rabbits should be made, to avoid tracheal traumatization (Holmstrom *et al.*, 2000). Reusable, species-specific endotracheal tubes for rabbits called v-gel® are available, which can be positioned quickly and safely, but they are bulkier within the mouth (Docsinnovent, 2020).

When intubation is unsuccessful, a small anaesthetic mask can be placed over the noses of lagomorphs and rodents, as they are obligate nose breathers, to allow anaesthetic delivery while still allowing access to the oral cavity (Legendre, 2003). If a sufficiently small mask is unavailable, a dental dam or the palm of an examination glove can be stretched over the end of a non-rebreathing-system anaesthetic hose (Osofsky, 2006). Cut a slit into the stretched glove with a scalpel blade, then place the patient's nose through it to maintain anaesthesia while allowing access to the mouth. Alternatively, a French size 4–8 red rubber catheter can be inserted into one nostril and advanced to the depth of the pharynx (Hawkins and Pascoe, 2012). The catheter is attached to the anaesthetic hose using a small endotracheal tube adapter (Lobprise, 2009).

Intubation is challenging in very small patients, though the use of 1.5-mm small exotic straight silicone endotracheal tubes in hedgehogs (Johnson, 2011) and 12–14-gauge IV catheters with the stylet removed used as endotracheal tubes in smaller rodents (Holmstrom *et al.*, 2000) have been described, with placement guided by a scope as outlined above.

Ferrets have tight jaw tone following anaesthetic induction, but intubation is fairly straightforward using 2–3-mm endotracheal tubes (Crowder, 2006; Cooper, 2017) and an assistant to hold the mouth open (Johnson,

2011). Topical lidocaine should be applied to the arytenoids or endotracheal tube to prevent laryngospasm (Cooper, 2017).

10.2.6 Anaesthetic monitoring

Monitoring can be performed with a multiparameter monitor, paediatric stethoscope, Doppler blood-pressure monitor, thermometer and pulse oximetry sensor placed on the foot, ear or scrotum (Osofsky, 2006; Crowder, 2006). Visualization of mucous-membrane colour and the chest movements of respirations is essential (Osofsky, 2006). Ensure the patient's body temperature is maintained during anaesthesia and recovery using forced-air blankets, resistive heating systems or circulating water blankets (Osofsky, 2006; Bennett, 2009).

10.3 Pain Management

Multimodal pain management should be used, including opioids in premedication protocols and constant-rate infusions (Lichtenberger, 2008). Non-steroidal anti-inflammatory drugs (NSAIDs) such as meloxicam can also be given pre-, intra- and postoperatively (Osofsky, 2006; Lichtenberger, 2008). Dental regional nerve blocks can be performed in rabbits and ferrets with lidocaine or bupivacaine (Lichtenberger, 2008) at a dose of 1 mg/kg using a 27-gauge needle on a 1 ml syringe (Cooper, 2017). Assessing pain in these small mammals can be difficult, so every patient who has undergone a potentially painful procedure should be given pain relief (Lichtenberger, 2008). Several 'grimace scales' are available to help recognize changes in facial expression indicating pain in rabbits and rodents (National Centre for the Replacement, Refinement & Reduction of Animals in Research (NC3Rs), 2020). Other signs of pain include anorexia, tooth grinding, aggression or abnormal behaviour, hiding and lethargy (Kolb, 2017).

10.4 Dental Radiography

10.4.1 Lagomorphs and rodents

Extra-oral skull radiographs allow assessment of crown and root length, the occlusal plane and periapical lucencies (Hoefer, 2001). Dental radiography units provide better detail than standard X-ray machines (Holmstrom *et al.*, 2000). Size 4 dental films or phosphor plates can capture the entire skull of most small patients (Lobprise, 2009). Using Size 2 digital sensors may require taking several exposures of each view. If Size 0, 1 and 2 dental films or phosphor plates are available, rabbit intra-oral radiographs can be obtained using bisecting angle technique (Regalado and Legendre, 2017) (see Chapter 3, this volume).

Computed tomography (CT) including cone-beam CT (CBCT) is used increasingly in these patients to produce high-resolution, cross-sectional images without superimposition of anatomic structures (Osofsky, 2006).

Extra-oral skull views (Kolb, 2017):

- Lateral: place the patient in lateral recumbency with the head extended and the film, plate or sensor beneath the skull. Ensure the head is parallel to the table, not tilted or rotated. Aim the X-ray beam perpendicular to the skull.
- Right and left lateral obliques: place the patient, film and X-ray beam as per the lateral view (above), then rotate the head 40 degrees dorsally, so the mandible is elevated. Use foam wedges, towels, etc. beneath the mandible as necessary. Turn the patient onto their opposite side and repeat.
- Dorsoventral: place the patient in sternal recumbency with the head extended and the film, plate or sensor beneath the skull. Ensure the head is parallel to the table, not tilted or rotated. Aim the X-ray beam perpendicular to the skull.

10.4.2 Ferrets and hedgehogs

Intra-oral radiographs can be taken with Size 0, 1 and 2 dental film or phosphor plates (Cooper, 2017) using bisecting angle technique. Size 2 digital sensors also can be used intra-orally in ferrets.

10.5 Dental Instruments

Specialized dental instruments exist for the long, narrow mouths of rabbits and small mammals (see Fig. 10.1). A set of lagomorph and rodent instruments includes the following (Holmstrom *et al.*, 2000; Crossley, 2003a; Legendre, 2003):

- rodent incisor luxator
- rodent molar/premolar luxator
- Crossley rabbit luxator
- rodent molar/premolar extraction forceps
- rodent mouth gag
- pouch dilators
- molar/premolar rasp
- rodent tongue depressor (or regular tongue depressor cut in half lengthwise)
- low-speed burs to use for odontoplasty (e.g. HP5, HP558)
- high-speed burs for use in incisor trimming and extraction (e.g. FG330, FG701)

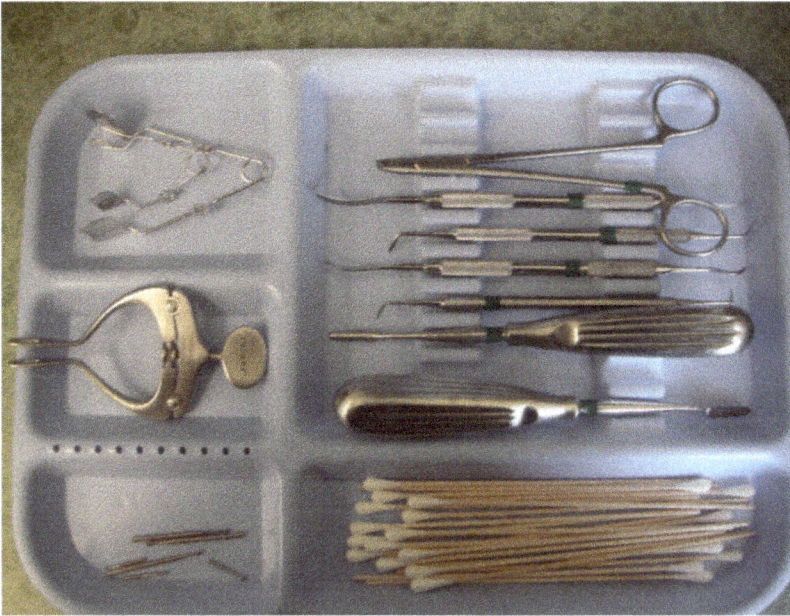

Fig. 10.1. Lagomorph and rodent dental instrument tray. Clockwise from top left: pouch dilators; extraction forceps; Crossley rabbit luxator; rodent molar luxator; rodent incisor luxator; rodent premolar luxator; molar/premolar rasps; cotton-tipped applicators; burs; rodent mouth gag.

Magnifying loupes, 18-gauge needles used as small luxators, low-volume suction (saliva ejector) with the tip cut to fit a urinary catheter, and cotton-tipped applicators to absorb blood and fluid from the mouth are also useful.

The treatment of ferrets can be accomplished with dental instruments designed for small canine or feline patients (Cooper, 2017).

10.6   Oral Pathology of Lagomorphs and Rodents

10.6.1   Malocclusion

The most common dental problem of both lagomorphs and rodents is malocclusion, causing overgrowth of incisors and/or cheek teeth (Legendre, 2003; Lobprise, 2009). Patients may present with tongue entrapment, sharp points causing soft-tissue lacerations of the tongue and buccal mucosa, excess salivation (slobbers) and tooth root elongation causing lacrimal discharge, eye prolapse or a lumpy mandible (Legendre, 2003; Lobprise, 2009).

Malocclusions can be traumatic or atraumatic (Lobprise, 2009). Traumatic malocclusion results from an injury to the tooth, causing a loss of a portion of the crown and subsequent loss of normal wear on the opposing tooth (Holmstrom *et al.*, 2000). Atraumatic malocclusions may result from a lack of roughage in the diet, which allows the teeth to overgrow (Legendre, 2003); or hereditary conditions such as jaw-length disparity between the mandible and the maxilla (Lobprise, 2009). Regardless of the cause, untreated tooth overgrowth results in altered tooth curvature, preventing the occlusal surfaces of the teeth from meeting normally, which can widen interdental spaces, causing food or bedding impaction and periodontal abscesses (Legendre, 2003; Okuda *et al.*, 2007).

Traumatic malocclusions are treated by smoothing the crown of the traumatized tooth with a dental bur to reduce soft-tissue injuries, capping any exposed pulp with calcium hydroxide, and performing crown reduction (see below) on the opposing tooth until the traumatized tooth regrows (Legendre, 2003). Atraumatic malocclusions can be treated with routine crown reduction every 6–8 weeks (Hoefer, 2001), tooth extraction (Lobprise, 2009) (see Section 10.6.2, this volume), and dietary changes such as increasing the amount of roughage vs pellets in the diet (Holmstrom *et al.*, 2000).

Crown reduction (odontoplasty) should be performed with dental burs, not tooth trimmers or clippers, due to the risk of longitudinal tooth fractures (Legendre, 2003; Lobprise, 2009). Incisors can be trimmed in some patients while conscious or with sedation; crown reduction of premolars and molars always requires general anaesthesia (Lobprise, 2009). A #330 pear bur, #701 tapered- fissure bur or a coarse diamond bur on a high-speed handpiece without water are used to reduce the crowns of incisor teeth (Legendre, 2003). The patient is held in sternal recumbency, a cotton-tipped applicator or tongue depressor is placed behind the incisors to prevent soft-tissue injury to the tongue and oral mucosa (Lobprise, 2009), and the incisors are trimmed one at a time, with care taken not to cut into the pulp chamber. To reduce the crown height of premolars and molars, the patient must be anaesthetized (Kolb, 2017) and placed either in sternal recumbency in a tabletop dental positioner (Lennox, 2008) or in dorsal recumbency. Cheek dilators and a mouth gag are necessary to visualize the oral cavity, and care must be taken to protect the oral tissues from laceration (Kolb, 2017). HP5, HP558 or conical lab burs on a low-speed handpiece are used to trim any sharp spikes and reduce crown height (Kolb, 2017). Premolar/molar rasps can be used for additional smoothing (Lobprise, 2009). Any debris, including pieces of tooth, must be removed from the mouth to prevent aspiration by the patient.

Remember: the molars of murine rodents should never be trimmed, as they don't grow continuously!

10.6.2 Tooth root abscess

Tooth root abscesses in lagomorph and caviomorph rodents are treated by extraction and curettage of infected tissue and purulent material, along with systemic or local antibiotics (Lennox and Bauck, 2012). Extra-oral abscess lancing and possible marsupialization may be required (Legendre, 2011), and infection recurrence is common (Legendre, 2003).

Extraction of these animals' long, curved roots often requires the use of specialized, long-bladed luxators (Lobprise, 2009). After the tooth has become loose, it should be pressed back into the alveolus while being rotated to remove the germinal tissue that causes the continuing growth of these teeth (Lobprise, 2009). The alveolus should also be curetted to remove any remaining germinal tissue, since if any is left behind, the tooth may regrow (Lennox, 2008). The extraction site is then closed with fine, absorbable suture (Lennox, 2008). If several teeth in the same quadrant are extracted, the opposing teeth will not be worn down, and will require monitoring and periodic crown reduction (Lobprise and Wiggs, 2000).

10.6.3 Miscellaneous conditions

Other oral conditions include oral viral papillomas in rabbits; gingival haemorrhage and loose teeth in guinea pigs secondary to scurvy (Legendre, 2003; Osofsky, 2006); and gingivitis, stomatitis and/or excessive salivation caused by rough edges on water bottles, feeders or cages (Holmstrom *et al.*, 2000; Legendre, 2003). Rodents and lagomorphs can experience cheek pouch impaction causing stomatitis (Holmstrom *et al.*, 2000; Legendre, 2003). This is treated by removing the impacted material and administering antibiotics. Cheek pouch eversion can also occur in hamsters (Miwa and Sladsky, 2016). The pouch is replaced and sutured through the cheek to prevent re-eversion. Murine rodents may present with facial swelling ventral or rostral to the eye resulting from abscessed tooth roots due to periodontal disease (Osofsky, 2006).

10.7   Oral Pathology of Ferrets

Fractured teeth, especially canine teeth (Crowder, 2006), and periodontal disease are common in ferrets (Cooper, 2017). COHATs, extractions and endodontic procedures are very similar to those performed in the cat (Crowder, 2006).

10.8   Oral Pathology of Hedgehogs

Hedgehogs can develop periodontal disease, presenting with inappetence and/or pawing at the face (Chaprazov *et al.*, 2014). Treatment includes supportive care, pain management, professional dental hygiene, extraction

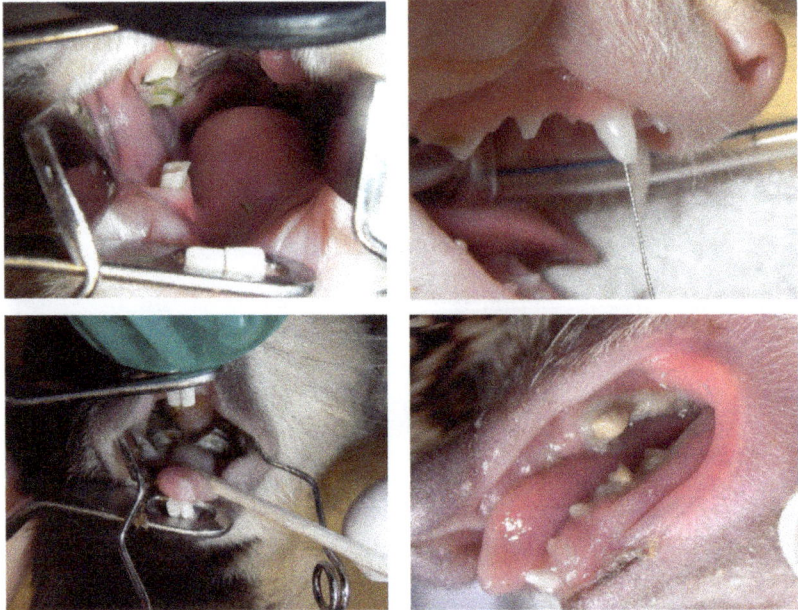

Fig. 10.2. Clockwise from top left: sharp points on rabbit premolars; root canal therapy in a ferret; periodontal disease in a hedgehog; tongue entrapment in a guinea pig.

of any diseased teeth and possible antibiotic administration (Chaprazov *et al.*, 2014).

10.9 Husbandry and Homecare

10.9.1 Postoperative care

Patients who have had oral surgery will need nutritional support until healed (Osofsky, 2006). Rodents and lagomorphs may be offered or assist-fed a variety of soft foods, such as Oxbow Critical Care® (Oxbow, 2021), yogurt, hay or soaked pellets puréed with water in a blender (Osofsky, 2006). Ferrets and hedgehogs may be fed high-protein canned (Crowder, 2006) or liquid food (Cooper, 2017). For assist-feeding, 35-ml syringes with catheter tips work for ferrets and larger rabbits; 12-ml curved-tip syringes with the tips cut down work well for smaller rabbits, chinchillas and guinea pigs; and 1–3-ml syringes can be used to feed tinier patients. Oral medications like enrofloxacin may be mixed with ice cream or yogurt, or flavoured by a compounding pharmacy to improve palatability (Donnelly, 2007). Owners can be taught to administer subcutaneous injections of antibiotics such as penicillin G, which is often used for the treatment of rabbit abscesses (Legendre, 2014).

If the patient has had extra-oral surgery such as abscess lancing, their cage bedding and debris may stick to the site. Owners can gently clean the area using a cloth and warm water several times daily (Legendre, 2014). A dilute solution of povidone-iodine and water can be used to flush marsupi-alized abscesses daily (Noonan, 2021).

10.9.2 Preventing dental problems

To help prevent tooth overgrowth, owners should be encouraged to feed rabbits, guinea pigs, degus and chinchillas the majority of their diets as roughage, such as Timothy hay, fresh greens and vegetables (Legendre, 2003). Commercial pellets, which require little chewing, are not necessary and if used should make up only a minor portion of the diet of lagomorphs and caviomorph rodents (Kolb, 2017). Chew aids, such as wooden blocks, can help wear down the incisors of lagomorphs and rodents (Donnelly, 2007). Guinea pigs must be given vitamin C supplementation to prevent scurvy (Legendre, 2003; Osofsky, 2006). Stress, which can lead to traumatic malocclusions, can often be reduced by enlarging the animal's cage, removing or adding companions, and adding stimulation such as toys and mazes (Lobprise and Wiggs, 2000).

Like cats and dogs, ferrets can be trained to have their teeth brushed daily to prevent periodontal disease, using the same products (Cooper, 2017) (see Chapter 14, this volume). Annual COHATs under general anaesthesia are recommended (Johnson-Delaney, 2008).

References

Bennett, A.R. (2009) Small mammal anesthesia – rabbits and rodents. Dvm360. Available at: https://www.dvm360.com/view/small-mammal-anesthesia-rabbits-and-rodents-proceedings (accessed 3 March 2021).

Bilhun, C.G., Boisvert, D.P.J., Carter, K.K., Cross, B.M. and Demers, G. (2020) Guide to the care and use of experimental animals. Canadian Council on Animal Care. Available at: https://www.ccac.ca/Documents/Standards/Guidelines/Experimental_Animals_Vol1.pdf (accessed 3 March 2021).

Chaprazov, T., Dimitrov, R., Stamatova-Yovcheva, K. and Uzunova, K. (2014) Oral and dental disorders in pet hedgehogs. *Turkish Journal of Veterinary and Animal Sciences* 38, 1–6. Available at: https://www.researchgate.net/publication/270121171_Oral_and_dental_disorders_in_pet_hedgehogs (accessed 28 September 2020).

Cooper, J. (2017) Ferret dentistry: no weasling about it. Today's Veterinary Nurse. Available at: https://todaysveterinarynurse.com/articles/ferret-dentistry-no-weaseling-about-it/ (accessed 29 September 2020).

Crossley, D.A. (2003a) Oral biology and disorders of lagomorphs. *Veterinary Clinics of North America: Exotic Animal Practice* 6(3), 629–659.

Crossley, D.A. (2003b) Oral biology and disorders of chiroptera, insectivores, monotremes, and marsupials. *Veterinary Clinics of North America: Exotic Animal Practice* 6(3), 523–564.

Crowder, S.E. (2006) Principles of ferret dentistry. In: *Proceedings of the 20th Annual Veterinary Dental Forum.* Omnipress, Madison, Wisconsin, pp. 165–169.

Docsinnovent (2020) v-gel. Docsinnovent. Available at: https://docsinnovent.com (accessed 3 March 2021).

Donnelly, T.M. (2007) Rodent husbandry and care. Veterinary Partner. Available at: https://veterinarypartner.vin.com/default.aspx?pid=19239&id=4952599 (accessed 3 March 2021).

Hawkins, M.G. and Pascoe, P.J. (2012) Anesthesia, analgesia, and sedation of small mammals. In: Quesenberry, K.E. and Carpenter, J.W. (eds) *Ferrets, Rabbits, and Rodents: Clinical Medicine and Surgery.* Saunders, St. Louis, Missouri, pp. 429–451.

He, T., Friede, H. and Kiliaridis, S. (2002) Macroscopic and roentgenographic anatomy of the skull of the ferret (Mustela putorius furo). *Laboratory Animals* 36(1), 86–96. Available at: https://journals.sagepub.com/doi/pdf/10.1258/0023677021911795 (accessed 3 March 2021).

Hoefer, H.L. (2001) Small mammal dentistry. *Atlantic Coast Veterinary Conference 2001.* Available at: https://www.vin.com/apputil/content/defaultadv1.aspx?id=3843937&pid=11131 (accessed 28 September 2020).

Holmstrom, S., Holmstrom, L.A., McGrath, C.J., Richey, M.T. and Wiggs, R.B. (2000) Pocket pet dentistry. In: Holmstrom, S. (ed.) *Veterinary Dentistry for the Technician & Office Staff.* Saunders, Philadelphia, Pennsylvania, pp. 293–323.

Johnson, D. (2011) Endotracheal intubation of small exotic mammals. Dvm360. Available at: https://www.dvm360.com/view/endotracheal-intubation-small-exotic-mammals-proceedings (accessed 28 September 2020).

Johnson-Delaney, C.A. (2008) Dental disease in ferrets: more serious than we thought. Small Animal and Exotics. *Proceedings of the North American Veterinary Conference, Volume 22,* Orlando, Florida, USA, 2008, 1809–1811. The North American Veterinary Conference, Gainesville, USA. Available at: https://www.cabi.org/isc/FullTextPDF/2009/20093019003.pdf (accessed 3 March 2021).

Jurox (2021) Alfaxan multidose in pet rabbits. Alfaxan Multidose. Available at: https://www.alfaxan.co.uk/alfaxan/rabbits (accessed 3 March 2021).

Kolb, S. (2017) Rabbit dentistry. Today's Veterinary Nurse. Available at: https://todaysveterinarynurse.com/articles/rabbit-dentistry/ (accessed 3 March 2021).

Legendre, L. (2003) Oral disorders of exotic rodents. *Veterinary Clinics of North America: Exotic Animal Practice* 6(3), 601–628.

Legendre, L. (2011) Treatment of oral abscesses in rodents and lagomorphs. *Journal of Veterinary Dentistry* 28(1), 30–33.

Legendre, L. (2014) Managing rabbit and rodent dental-related abscesses. *World Small Animal Veterinary Association World Congress Proceedings, 2014.* Available at: https://www.vin.com/apputil/content/defaultadv1.aspx?pId=12886&catId=57092&id=7054757 (accessed 3 March 2021).

Lennox, A. (2008) Dentistry of rabbits. Dvm360. Available at: https://www.dvm360.com/view/dentistry-rabbits-proceedings (accessed 3 March 2021).

Lennox, A.M. and Bauck, L. (2012) Basic anatomy, physiology, husbandry, and clinical techniques. In: Quesenberry, K.E. and Carpenter, J.W. (eds) *Ferrets, Rabbits, and Rodents: Clinical Medicine and Surgery.* Saunders, St. Louis, Missouri, pp. 339–353.

Lichtenberger, M. (2008) Anesthesia, analgesia and monitoring of the critical rabbit patient. *British Small Animal Veterinary Congress 2008.* Available at: https://www.

vin.com/apputil/content/defaultadv1.aspx?pId=11254&id=3862857 (accessed 3 March 2021).

Lobprise, H. (2009) Dentistry quarterly: challenges in pocket pet dentistry. Veterinary Practice News. Available at: https://www.veterinarypracticenews. com/dentistry-quarterly-challenges-in-pocket-pet-dentisty/ (accessed 28 September 2020).

Lobprise, H.B. and Wiggs, R.B. (2000) Oral and dental disease in pocket pets. In: Lobprise, H.B. and Wiggs, R.B. (eds) *The Veterinarian's Companion for Common Dental Procedures.* AAHA Press, Lakewood, Colorado, pp. 149–160.

Maddamma, M.M. and Lennox, A.M. (2012) Venipuncture in exotic companion mammals. Today's Veterinary Practice. Available at: https://todaysveterinaryprac-tice.com/todays-technician-venipuncture-in-exotic-companion-mammals/ (accessed 28 September 2020).

Miwa, Y. and Sladsky, K.K. (2016) Common surgical procedures of rodents, fer-rets, hedgehogs, and sugar gliders. Veterinary Clinics: Exotic Animal Practice. Available at: https://www.vetexotic.theclinics.com/article/S1094-9194(15)00087-0/fulltext (accessed 28 September 2020).

MSU (2001) Rodents. Michigan State University. Available at: https://www.canr. msu.edu/ipm/uploads/files/Community_and_Schools_PDFs/rodentfs.pdf (accessed 3 March 2021).

NC3Rs (2020) Grimace scales. National Centre for the Replacement, Refinement & Reduction of Animals in Research. Available at: https://www.nc3rs.org.uk/ grimacescales (accessed 28 September 2020).

Noonan, B. (2021) Dental anatomy and disease of the domestic rabbit (*Oryctolagus cuniculus*). Available at: https://www.mspca.org/angell_services/dental-anato-my-and-disease-of-the-domestic-rabbit/ (accessed 3 March 2021).

Okuda, A., Hori, Y., Ichihara, N., Asari, M. and Wiggs, R.B. (2007) Comparative observation of skeletal-dental abnormalities in wild, domestic, and laboratory rabbits. *Journal of Veterinary Dentistry* 24(4), 224–229. DOI: 10.1177/089875640702400403.

Osofsky, A. (2006) Dentistry in pet rodents. VetFolio. Available at: https://www. vetfolio.com/learn/article/dentistry-in-pet-rodents (accessed 28 September 2020).

Oxbow (2021) Critial care – herbivore. Oxbow Animal Health. Available at: https://www.oxbowanimalhealth.com/our-products/professional-line/ critical-care (accessed 3 March 2021).

Regalado, A. and Legendre, L. (2017) Full-mouth intraoral radiograph-ic survey in rabbits. *Journal of Veterinary Dentistry* 34(3), 190–200. DOI: 10.1177/0898756417723145.

Rosenthal, K.L. (2001) Pet rabbit basics and techniques. *Atlantic Coast Veterinary Conference 2001.* Available at: https://www.vin.com/apputil/content/default-adv1.aspx?id=3844042&pid=11131 (accessed 3 March 2021).

Tynes, V. (2013) Safe and humane handling of small mammal patients. Today's Veterinary Practice. Available at: https://todaysveterinarypractice.com/to-days-technician-safe-humane-handling-of-small-mammal-patients/ (accessed 3 March 2021).

Gaining Client Compliance, Dental Estimates, and the Dangers of Anaesthesia-free Dentistry

11

11.1 Gaining Client Compliance

Pet owners are often reluctant to book their pet's needed COHAT. To make matters worse, many veterinarians and veterinary nurses hesitate to present dental estimates to clients, because talking about finances is contrary to our caregiving instincts (Hauser, 2020). We want the best for our patients, and see ourselves as healthcare providers, not salespeople. Most dental procedures, when done safely and correctly, aren't cheap; nor should they be (Eisner, 2008)! But while we may be painfully aware of the total at the bottom of the estimate that we hand to a pet owner, cost often isn't their main concern (Myers, 2007a; Byard, 2008).

To gain client compliance with dental care and treatment, we must determine the reason(s) for their reluctance, show empathy (Bellows, 2007) and, above all, be prepared to address their fears. If a client is reluctant to proceed with treatment, you can initiate this dialogue by saying, 'I know this is a difficult decision. Can we talk about your concerns?' (Myers, 2007a). There are various potential reasons why the client may be feeling hesitant.

11.1.1 General anaesthesia

Anaesthesia is one of the main reasons pet owners choose not to pursue dental treatment (Woodward, 2004; Dominguez, 2016). Fear of general anaesthesia is pervasive (Berg, 2007), and many patients with periodontal disease are older and possibly living with concurrent health problems that can increase anaesthetic risk. Owners may believe that older pets are unable to undergo general anaesthesia (Dominguez, 2016).

Let your client know that their fears are common. Explain that advances including preanaesthetic health screening, safer anaesthetic drugs and better anaesthetic monitoring have minimized the risks of anaesthesia (Berg, 2007; Dowdy, 2010a; Dominguez, 2016), even in older pets (Myers, 2013a). All patients should receive preanaesthetic labwork (Woodward,

© CAB International 2022. *An Introduction to Pet Dental Care: For Veterinary Technicians and Nurses* (K. Istace)
DOI: 10.1079/9781789248869.0011

2004), and older patients or those with health concerns may need a more involved work-up prior to anaesthesia (Dominguez, 2016). This may include chest radiographs, echocardiogram, or referral to a cardiologist, internal medicine specialist, etc. to assess anaesthetic risk and devise an appropriate anaesthetic protocol. Of course, your hospital must be capable of providing all of the above. Staying abreast of the latest anaesthetic recommendations, drugs and technology by attending continuing education seminars, completing online learning, and subscribing to veterinary journals will increase your proficiency in delivering and monitoring anaesthesia.

If the pet's health is compromised in some way, e.g. with advanced heart or kidney disease, you may wish to offer referral to a veterinary dental specialist, who can accomplish any required dental work in minimal time under anaesthesia (American Animal Hospital Association (AAHA), 2021a). Referral to a veterinary anaesthesiologist may also help ease the client's anxieties. Some veterinary specialist centres offer both services.

11.1.2 Expense/necessity

Some clients may baulk at the cost of their pet's COHAT, especially as it may be more expensive than out-of-pocket costs for their own dental care (Dominguez, 2016). In this case, the onus is on us to educate them about periodontal disease treatment in pets (Hale, 2011).

Anaesthesia and associated treatments such as preanesthetic blood testing and anaesthetic monitoring are part of the increased costs involved in pet vs human dental procedures. Because human patients are able to understand what is going on and cooperate (Dowdy, 2010b), dental scaling of our teeth can be performed by a professional hygienist without anaesthesia (Camilo, 2008). However, in pets, access to the most important areas in the mouth for periodontal disease treatment (below the gumline where periodontal disease begins) is impossible while the pet is awake (Myers, 2017). This is not only because it's unlikely that a cat or dog will lie on their back under a bright light while holding perfectly still with their mouth wide open for a prolonged procedure, but also because the areas beneath a pet's gingiva are often much more sore and diseased than comparable areas in a person's mouth (Camilo, 2008), due to their lack of oral hygiene. Even a pet without painful areas in their oral cavity may be frightened by strangers poking around in their mouth, and may be inclined to bite (American Veterinary Dental College (AVDC), 2004).

Another difference pet owners may not appreciate between human and pet dentistry is that there is usually significantly more disease present in an animal's mouth, necessitating periodontal treatments, extractions, etc. beyond the scope of a simple 'teeth cleaning' (Dowdy, 2010b). Pet owners may not recognize the need to diagnose and treat their pet's dental problems, especially in the case of conditions not traditionally associated with pets or not common knowledge, such as dead or fractured teeth, retained deciduous teeth, malocclusions or tooth resorption. These problems may be deemed unimportant or not affecting the pet's quality of life, since most clients don't often (or ever!) look in their pet's mouths (Dominguez, 2016). These 'invisible' problems are easier to ignore than more obvious health issues such as limping or vomiting. Again, client education is the key (Niemiec, 2012). A nurse with thorough knowledge of and ability to explain dental diseases, treatment options and the consequences to the pet if left untreated (i.e. pain, chronic infection, dental abscesses, oronasal fistulas, pathologic jaw fractures, etc.) is often able to get these pet owners on board with the veterinarian's treatment plan (Niemiec, 2012). The vast majority of clients want to do right by their pets. Once educated, they usually agree with the necessity for treatment (Lue *et al.*, 2008).

Some clients may wish to proceed with dental treatment for their pets but are truly financially constrained (Dominguez, 2016). The best way to prevent this is to be proactive when a client first presents with their new puppy or kitten. Encouraging clients to get pet health insurance before dental diseases develop may give them the financial ability to afford dental radiographs, extractions, biopsies, etc., though routine COHATs are usually not covered. If you need to refer the pet to a dental specialist for root canal therapy, orthodontic work or oral cancer treatment, the insured client may be better able to afford that, too. Some veterinary practices offer in-house health care 'packages' for an annual fee, to cover the cost of certain types of treatment, which may include COHATs and other dental care.

Unfortunately, we are often in the position where a client does not have insurance cover, and their pet now needs dental care. The practice may offer the option of a payment plan, whereby the pet can have a necessary procedure and the client pays the bill in instalments over an agreed period of time. If the client fails to pay, the practice is obliged to turn to a debt-collection company to recoup its losses. An alternative is third-party financing, where the client applies to a financing company for a loan, with the veterinary practice receiving immediate payment from the third-party financier (Myers, 2017). The practice therefore does not have to concern itself with bill collection, and the client then makes monthly payments to the third party. Another option is to split the dental procedure into two or more sessions, to allow time for the client to budget for the required funds. For example, the first procedure may be a COHAT and full-mouth dental radiographs to diagnose problem areas, then the pet returns in a month or two for extractions.

11.1.3 Pain

Our clients often associate human dentists with pain, and may assume this on behalf of their beloved pets, too. This is an opportunity to explain how your hospital uses multimodal pain management, including pain-relieving preoperative drugs, regional anaesthetic nerve blocks and postoperative pain medications sent home (Holzman, 2006). The client may also be unaware that periodontal disease, a fractured tooth or malocclusion is currently causing their pet discomfort, since animals are skilled at hiding pain (Woodward, 2004).

11.1.4 Fear of extractions

One major client concern rarely recognized or addressed by veterinary professionals is that the pet won't be able to chew or eat if they have a tooth extracted (American Society for the Prevention of Cruelty to Animals (ASPCA), 2015; Bellows, 2015). Many clients don't understand that if a tooth is so diseased as to require removal, the pet is already experiencing pain, having difficulty chewing, or may be chewing on the opposite side of the mouth (Lewis, 2017). They also might not consider the fact that, unlike wild animals, companion animals don't need their teeth to survive (Hale, 2010). Our pets aren't obliged to bring down prey, tear flesh or crack open bones to obtain nourishment. And most commercially prepared diets, even hard kibble, don't require much chewing (Bellows, 2015).

Veterinarians and nurses know from experience that pets will continue to eat even after full-mouth extractions, but a single extraction can nonetheless cause a pet owner a great deal of distress. For this reason, you should always get owner consent for extractions *before* they are performed (Greenfield, 2018). This often requires a phone call to the client once dental radiographs are taken (Beckman, 2007).

If extractions are anticipated based upon the patient's conscious oral examination, let the client know at the time of booking the procedure that their pet will need to eat soft food for at least a week postoperatively, so they can purchase an appropriate canned diet or try out various soft foods prior to oral surgery, if their pet is picky. Showing that you care about their pet's well-being can go a long way towards gaining a client's trust.

11.1.5 Distracted by other health concerns

Dental problems often go unnoticed by clients until their pet presents for a physical examination regarding another health concern (Dominguez, 2016). If another problem is preoccupying the owner, a conversation about dental care may not occur at all (Sorrell, 2019). How do we make clients care about dental disease when they are more concerned about their dog's ear infection, or their cat urinating outside the litterbox? Dental education and treatment may have to wait until the presenting problem is resolved, but should not be forgotten (Sorrell, 2019). A complimentary follow-up appointment with the nurse or a phone call a week or two later can be useful in catching these patients, who might otherwise slip through the net (Byard, 2008).

11.1.6 The absent primary caregiver

The person in the exam room may not be the pet's primary caregiver but rather the client's partner, daughter, pet-sitter, etc., and unable to make major decisions on the pet's behalf (VetCheck, 2021). Even if they are the pet's primary caregiver, they may not be in charge of the household finances, or may be unwilling to commit to a medical decision without first consulting their spouse (Lue *et al.*, 2008). These scenarios all boil down to the same thing: no matter how well you educate the person in front of you, no procedure, however necessary, will be scheduled today. The more time passes after the appointment, the less likely it is that your conversation will be remembered by the person in the exam room; much less correctly conveyed to the decision-maker in the family.

Some veterinary staff handle this situation by asking the person in the exam room to explain everything to the primary caregiver, and to pass on a handout and/or copy of the estimate. This relies on the non-primary caregiver understanding everything that was communicated, and passing on the information clearly. If you choose this method, make a follow-up call to the primary caregiver to ensure they received the information, and ask if they have any questions or want to schedule the procedure.

A more expedient method is to request that the person in the exam room call the primary caregiver and have them on speakerphone or video call (Veterinary Clinics of America (VCA), 2021) while you explain/show the pet's condition, treatment options and costs. This way, you only have to go over the information once, the primary caregiver has the opportunity to ask questions, and a decision may be immediately forthcoming. However, this is feasible only if the primary caregiver can be contacted during the appointment.

Another option is to email the primary caregiver after the appointment with a summary of their pet's condition and treatment required, and digital photos of their pet's oral cavity (Myers, 2007a; VetCheck, 2021). The client can read the email at their leisure, you can attach information about the condition and a copy of the estimate to the email, and the client can reply with any questions or concerns they may have.

11.2 Dental Estimates: the Treatment Plan

Every veterinary hospital estimates and charges for dental procedures differently, based on their preferences, experience with treating various dental pathologies, and hospital policies. If your hospital currently charges a flat rate for dental procedures (Eisner, 2004), consider listing the prices of each item separately. Items may include preanaesthetic lab testing, anaesthesia depending upon time and/or a patient's anaesthetic risk status, intravenous fluid administration, dental cleaning, dental radiographs, regional dental nerve blocks, extractions, other oral surgery such as gingivectomies, oral biopsies, surgical pack fees, medications administered, etc. (Canadian Veterinary Medical Association (CVMA), 2020). Flat fees can be confusing to clients, because they do not outline exactly what value the client is receiving for the amount they are paying (Dowdy, 2010c; Buzhardt, 2021).

A more accurate term for an estimate in veterinary medicine is 'treatment plan' (Berg, 2020). A treatment plan focuses on the required medical procedures rather than their costs (Myers, 2007b; Sorrell, 2019). Nurses, not veterinarians, should present treatment plans (Woodward, 2004; Myers, 2007c), as clients are more likely to consent to treatment if they associate the veterinarian with medicine, not money (Myers, 2013b).

Do not quote dental prices over the phone (Bellows, 2007; Dowdy, 2010a). It is difficult enough to accurately gauge which dental treatments need to be performed based upon conscious oral exam-room findings; much less based solely upon a pet owner's verbal description (Berg, 2007). Explain that dental disease varies widely from patient to patient, and that without an examination it is impossible to create an accurate treatment plan (Bellows, 2007; Dowdy, 2010a). If this isn't your hospital's policy, talk with the practice owner or office manager about better managing your clients' expectations. What type of clients does your hospital want to cultivate: those who understand the complexities of veterinary medicine and are willing to listen to your recommendations, or 'phone-shoppers' interested only in the cheapest option (Lue *et al.*, 2008)?

11.2.1 Treatment plan templates

Even though flat fees and 'one size fits all' estimates are discouraged, customizable itemized treatment templates should be available (Bellows, 2007; Dowdy, 2010c) for easy reference, printing and emailing to clients once a physical examination is complete (Myers, 2017). The templates your hospital will have on hand depends upon which procedures the veterinarians are willing and qualified to perform. Dental treatment-plan templates for a general practice are often based upon the severity of periodontal disease and/or time required to complete a procedure (Myers, 2017), and may include:

- routine COHAT including full-mouth dental radiographs (30–45 minutes)
- advanced COHAT including full-mouth dental radiographs (45–60 minutes)
- add-on 30 minutes' oral surgery
- add-on 45 minutes' oral surgery
- add-on 1 hour oral surgery

- oral surgery with no dental cleaning (e.g. for younger patients with no calculus and a fractured tooth/teeth)
- deciduous canine tooth extraction (for fractured or persistent deciduous teeth)
- X-rays and biopsy of an oral mass
- feline full-mouth extractions.

The 'add-on' items can be added to any other treatment plan as necessary. For example, the owner of a 10-year-old Chihuahua with heavy calculus, severe gingivitis and several suspected extractions might receive a treatment plan for an advanced COHAT including full-mouth radiographs with add-on 45 minutes' oral surgery, while the owner of a 5-year-old cat with mild calculus and gingivitis and no other obvious dental pathology might receive a treatment plan for a routine COHAT including full-mouth radiographs (Myers, 2007c).

In all cases, advise the owners that the treatment plan is based upon a conscious oral examination, and that once probing and dental radiographs have been done, additional dental pathology may be discovered (Berg, 2007, 2020).

COHAT treatment plans may include the following items: preanaesthetic blood testing, intravenous fluids, anaesthesia, monitoring, a complete oral examination, dental cleaning, polishing, dental charting, full-mouth dental radiographs and hospitalization (Myers, 2007a).

The add-on oral surgery treatment plan may include the following items: a surgical pack fee, regional dental nerve blocks, additional anaesthetic time, oral surgery time (extractions, open root planing, alveolar curettage, suturing, gingivectomy, etc. can all be categorized as oral surgery for ease of estimating), pain medications administered in hospital, and medications sent home (Eisner, 2004). If the veterinarian anticipates that a patient will need more than 1 hour of oral surgery, modify the plan as required.

A time-based approach to oral surgery has several advantages over estimating for extractions of individual teeth types (e.g. carnassial extractions cost X, canine tooth extractions cost Y, and premolar extractions cost Z) (Niemiec, 2012). When creating a treatment plan, we often do not know exactly which teeth will need to be extracted, and it can be easier to give the client a plan based on a general impression of the severity of their pet's periodontal disease. Clients who are given a time-based treatment plan may be more flexible about accepting how many teeth need to be extracted than clients who are given a plan that includes two extractions, when radiographs later indicate that five teeth need to be extracted. Extracting an otherwise healthy fractured or non-vital tooth can also take more time and effort than extracting a periodontally compromised tooth of the same type (Lemmons and Carmichael, 2008; Bellows, 2021).

The treatment plan for X-rays and biopsy of an oral mass may include preanaesthetic blood testing, intravenous fluids, anaesthesia, monitoring, a complete oral examination, dental charting, full-mouth dental radiographs, a surgical pack fee, a regional dental nerve block, 15 minutes of oral surgery (biopsy), pain medications administered in hospital, hospitalization, pain medications sent home, and histopathology.

The treatment plan for feline full-mouth extractions may include preanaesthetic blood testing, intravenous fluids, anaesthesia, monitoring, a complete oral examination, dental charting, full-mouth dental radiographs, a surgical pack fee, full-mouth regional dental blocks, 2 or more hours of oral surgery, placement of a feeding tube, pain medications administered in hospital, hospitalization, pain medications to be sent home, and a case of canned food for tube feeding.

For any of the above treatment plans, procedures such as preoperative chest radiographs, skin mass removal, microchipping, etc. may be added to fit a patient's needs.

Adding 15–20% to the total cost (Walsh, 2017) gives the client a price range rather than a single cost. This allows some 'wriggle room' for unforeseen dental problems, additional medications, a longer-than-anticipated time spent performing dental hygiene, etc. (Sorrell, 2019). For example, instead of quoting a total cost of £500, you would estimate £500–£600. This creates a win–win scenario. If your hospital is able to perform the procedure for the price at the lower end of the treatment plan, the client is happy that the cost is less than it could have been, and if the total is near the high end, the client was already prepared to pay this amount (Berg, 2020).

For hospitals performing advanced dental procedures, some examples of treatment plans include: standard root canal therapy (single-rooted vs multiple-rooted tooth, add-on metal crown, sedation and 6-month recheck X-rays), crown reduction with vital pulpotomy (one tooth vs two teeth, add-on palatal defect repair, sedation and 6-month recheck X-rays), jaw fracture repair (interfragmentary wiring with splint, recheck X-rays and splint removal), hemimandibulectomy, orthodontic movement with incline plane, etc.

Itemization is the key to quick, accurate, clear and fair estimating for veterinary dental services (Dowdy, 2010c). Your hospital may choose to prepare treatment plans differently from those outlined above, but as long as they are prepared consistently by everyone in the hospital, easily explained to clients (Buzhardt, 2021), and based upon prices that are fair for the amount of work performed and similar to the costs of the same procedures at other practices in your region (Moreau, 2008), then they are a good tool for increasing client compliance.

11.3   Presenting Treatment Plans

The best place to present a treatment plan is in an exam room, not a busy lobby or reception counter (Myers, 2007d). This allows you and the client to converse without distractions (Dominguez, 2016).

Often, the veterinarian leaves the exam room and asks the nurse to prepare a treatment plan. When you walk in, smile and introduce yourself to the client (Bellows, 2007; Dowdy, 2010a), giving your name and title. Make sure to know both the client's and pet's names, and use them (Myers, 2007b). Ask for the names of any other family members or children in the room. Your demeanour should be friendly, caring and competent; not rushed or timid. Walk to the same side of the exam table as the client and stand or sit beside them (Myers, 2007b, 2017). This removes any physical barriers between you and the client, which sets the stage for a collaborative conversation about what's best for their pet, as opposed to a confrontation. Say something complimentary about their pet (Beckman, 2007). Luckily, making a fuss over pets comes naturally to most nurses!

Explain that the veterinarian has asked you to discuss their pet's needed dental treatment. Saying 'needed' treatment helps to increase client compliance by emphasizing the medical need for the procedure, while saying 'recommended' implies that the treatment is only a suggestion (Berg, 2020).

Review the treatment plan item by item, explaining why each is necessary in language that a layperson can understand (Myers, 2007a; Berg, 2020). Describe how the treatment will benefit the client, i.e. their pet will have fresh breath, less dental pain, better overall health and live longer (Myers, 2007a).

Once you've reviewed the treatment plan, ask the client whether they have any questions or concerns (Myers, 2007a). Briefly describe what will happen on the day of the procedure, including how long their pet is likely to remain in the clinic and what their options are if dental radiology uncovers additional pathology. Having this information up front can help relieve clients' anxieties, making them more receptive to accepting needed treatment.

Offer to schedule the procedure (Myers, 2017). If the client declines, probe for further concerns and allay them if possible. If the client does book the procedure, discuss preanaesthetic fasting and what to expect after the procedure, including potential diet changes, duration of recovery and rechecks.

11.3.1 Visual aids

Many people are visual learners (Beckman, 2008), and it is often easier to explain medical conditions and procedures using videos, models and other visual aids (Berg, 2020). The better a client is able to understand their pet's dental problems, the more likely they are to accept the treatment plan. Examples of visual aids include the following:

- Videos showing dental diseases and treatments (Dowdy, 2010d; Berg, 2020). These are available from in-clinic digital advertising companies and platforms like YouTube, but you must ensure they are from a reputable source. If you're the creative type, you can even film educational videos yourself. These videos can be displayed on a computer screen or tablet in the exam room.

- Skull models (Berg, 2020). Clear models that allow clients to see tooth roots are particularly useful.
- Websites (Dominguez, 2016). Organizations including the American Veterinary Dental College (AVDC, 2021a), the American Animal Hospital Association (AAHA, 2021b) and the British Veterinary Dental Association (BVDA, 2021) contain photos and descriptions of pathologies and treatments for everything from periodontal disease and fractured teeth to stomatitis and oral tumours. Show these to clients and/or email them links.
- Handouts (Dowdy, 2010d). Create your own or obtain from online libraries such as https://veterinarypartner.vin.com, https://www.life-learn.com and https://wwwbvdacouk/indexphp/bvda-articles.
- Photos (Dowdy, 2010d). These can include digital photos of the pet's oral cavity, so the owner can appreciate the exam findings better than they could on their squirming pet, photos and X-rays of dental pathologies from previous patients, and photos and X-rays in veterinary dental textbooks (like this one!).
- Promotional materials (Eisner, 2008). Veterinary dental equipment, supplies and food companies have developed an astonishing amount of dental-related literature, posters, etc. If you're not sure what's available, contact your local representatives or visit company websites.

11.4 What if They Don't Book Treatment?

If a client chooses not to book treatment but seems open to the idea (e.g. they need to check their schedule or check with their spouse, their pet has another health condition that needs to be treated first, or they are noncommittal but do not refuse outright), most veterinary software programs can generate a reminder in 7 days or any appropriate time interval (Myers, 2017). A reminder makes sure that our patients' dental care isn't lost in the shuffle of our clients' busy lives. Reminders can be phone calls, emails, text messages or mailed reminder cards (Walsh, 2019).

The script for phone or personal email reminders might go as follows. 'Hello, this is Nurse Awesome from the Best Pet Hospital. Dr Caring asked me to follow up with you to schedule Fluffy's needed Comprehensive Oral Health Assessment and Treatment, including an oral exam, dental cleaning and dental X-rays. We have availability this Friday or next Monday. Would either of these days work for you?' (Communication Solutions for Veterinarians (CSV), 2021). If emailing or leaving a message, you can add: 'Please contact us with any questions or to book this appointment.'

For a mailed reminder card, mass email or text message, the script would be slightly different: 'Our records show that it's time for Fluffy's Comprehensive Oral Health Assessment and Treatment. This includes an oral exam, dental cleaning and dental X-rays. Untreated dental disease can lead to bad breath, pain and chronic infection. Please call us to book this appointment.' (Myers, 2007d).

No veterinary practice ever achieves 100% compliance, not even for simpler and less costly care like vaccinations (Sanchez-Vizcaino *et al.*, 2018). All that veterinary nurses can be expected to do is educate the pet owner and thoroughly explain the treatment options. If necessary, the veterinarian may return to the exam room or call the client later to address any questions you were unable to answer. But the final decision rests with the client.

11.5 Lessons from Human Dentists

Our own dentists have educated us as to the need for routine professional cleanings every 6–12 months, and we already brush our teeth multiple times per day. Since fewer than 8% of pet owners currently brush their pets' teeth even once a day (Ipsos, 2016), shouldn't our companion animals' routine professional dental care be at least as frequent?

How do dentists get such excellent compliance from their patients? We can borrow several of their methods.

- Reminders (Walsh, 2019). Dentists send emails or cards to remind us that it is time for our dental hygiene. Most veterinary clinics already send their clients reminders for annual examinations and vaccinations, so why not send every client whose pet previously had a COHAT an annual reminder? Some patients, especially those with small, crowded mouths, or who have had tooth-salvaging procedures, should return for COHATs at least this frequently (Myers, 2007d).
- Forward booking (Sorrell, 2019). Forward booking means scheduling a pet's next appointment before the client leaves the hospital (Myers, 2017). Most dentists schedule our next dental hygiene appointment 6–12 months in advance, then call us several weeks prior to the appointment to confirm or rebook. This ensures that even if the pre-scheduled date or time is no longer convenient, we have the expectation that we will be returning for routine dental care, and will reschedule appropriately. This tool is similar to annual reminders but works even better to gain compliance, because in the client's mind they have already committed to the next COHAT.
- Education (Niemiec and Stewart, 2020). The importance of human dental health is well-promoted. Toothbrush advertisements, tooth-whitening systems, desensitizing toothpastes, veneers for a straighter smile ... our clients are more than familiar with dental care. The reason people take

such good care of their teeth is often vanity: we don't want crooked, yellow teeth or bad breath. Cosmetic considerations are not an issue for pets, but what we want our clients to learn from the human side of dental health is that dental disease negatively affects quality and length of life (Niemiec and Stewart, 2020). Start this education early by letting your clients know the permanent-tooth eruption times for puppies and kittens, so they begin looking in their pets' mouths (AVDC, 2021b). Initiate dental homecare programmes when these patients are young (Myers, 2007d). Explain to clients that even with homecare, annual COHATs are still required, just as they are for people (Roark, 2013). A daily dental homecare routine along with professional cleanings will reduce the need for more expensive periodontal treatment later on (Guthrie Pet Hospital (GPH), 2014), as well as sparing the pet potential pain and infection (Bellows, 2013).

11.6   Delivering on Your Promises

The last step in gaining client compliance in veterinary dentistry is making sure you deliver excellent care. Obtain proper dental equipment and instruments, and learn how to use and maintain them (Berg, 2007) (see Chapter 2, this volume). Follow your local veterinary association's guidelines for current standards of pet dental care (Bellows, 2007). Find a local veterinary dental specialist to whom your hospital can refer patients requiring advanced dental treatments, and whom your veterinarians can call to get advice about cases (AVDC, 2021c).

Educate yourself and your co-workers (Berg, 2007; Dominguez, 2016). Sign up for dental continuing education, and consider giving in-clinic training about what you've learned to your fellow staff members (Myers, 2007b). Obviously, not all staff members need to know the ins and outs of every dental pathology and procedure, but they should know the benefits of oral health to both pets and owners, the problems associated with poor oral health, and the services and products your hospital offers (Berg, 2007; Eisner, 2008).

Recommend Veterinary Oral Health Council (VOHC)-approved dental diets and treats (Berg, 2007) (see Chapter 15, this volume), and display them prominently on your retail shelves. Start a dental homecare programme for your own pets, so you can advise clients on practical techniques and how to avoid common pitfalls (Myers, 2007c).

If you can deliver on your promise to make their pet comfortable and safe during and after treatment, your clients will be impressed and reassured, and will tell their friends, relatives and social media community how well their pet did after a dental procedure at your hospital (Prendergast, 2016).

11.7 Anaesthesia-free Dentistry

As mentioned in Section 11.1.1, this volume, pet owners are often concerned when the word 'anaesthesia' comes up. Some clients assume that the 'anaesthesia-free dental scaling' their groomer offers is the same service that your veterinary hospital performs, except that you endanger their pet with anaesthesia and charge more. Again, educating the client about periodontal disease and what must be done to treat it is the best way of ensuring the dental health of their pet.

In most countries, only licensed veterinarians or properly supervised and trained nurses can legally practice veterinary medicine, including veterinary dentistry (AVDC, 2004). Groomers or other untrained individuals who perform dental scaling can be charged with a criminal offence (AVDC, 2004). Would you trust your hairdresser with your dental health? Not only are groomers and other laypeople completely unable to treat periodontal disease beneath the gumline, they are also incapable of performing a complete oral examination. They are not trained to recognize oral pathology, and are physically unable to see areas such as tooth surfaces facing the tongue or oral mucosa far back in the mouth, which can only be evaluated properly while the pet is anaesthetized or sedated (AVDC, 2004). They cannot probe periodontal pockets, recognize problems such as oral masses, tooth resorption or gum recession, or take dental X-rays. Even worse, they give the pet owner the false sense that their pet's mouth is healthy when in fact only the crowns of the teeth are clean, while periodontal disease may be raging beneath the gumline (AVDC, 2021d). Often, anaesthesia-free dentistry only serves to make a pet wary of having their mouth touched or examined.

11.7.1 Why veterinarians and nurses shouldn't practice anaesthesia-free dentistry

You might be thinking: 'But I'm a trained professional, just like a human dental hygienist. Why shouldn't I or my veterinarian offer anaesthesia-free dentistry?'

The answer is that because human patients cooperate (and very few of them bite!), scaling of human teeth performed by a professional dental hygienist can be successfully completed without anaesthesia (AVDC, 2004). However, access to areas below the gumline is impossible in an awake dog or cat. These areas are often sore, and even a slight head movement could result in damage to the oral tissues of the pet (AVDC, 2004; Bellows *et al.*, 2019). The lingual and caudal tooth surfaces cannot be properly visualized, and areas of disease are likely to be missed. A complete oral examination, including measuring periodontal pockets and taking dental radiographs, is not possible in awake patients, even by trained veterinary staff (AVDC, 2004). Anaesthesia-free dentistry is not recommended by the

American Veterinary Dental College, the American Veterinary Medical Association, the Canadian Veterinary Medical Association or the British Veterinary Dental Association, and position statements warning of its dangers can be found on their websites (AVDC, 2004; BVDA, 2013; CVMA, 2018; AVMA, 2021).

References

AAHA (2021a) Considering when to refer. American Animal Hospital Association. Available at: https://www.aaha.org/aaha-guidelines/dental-care/methods-of-evaluating-oral-health/when-to-refer/ (accessed 4 March 2021).

AAHA (2021b) Essential steps of dental cleaning and therapy. American Animal Hospital Association. Available at: https://www.aaha.org/aaha-guidelines/dental-care/essentials-steps/essential-steps/ (accessed 4 March 2021).

ASPCA (2015) Untreated dental issues can lead to major pain for pets. American Society for the Prevention of Cruelty to Animals. Available at: https://www.aspca.org/news/untreated-dental-issues-can-lead-major-pain-pets (accessed 4 March 2021).

AVDC (2004) Companion animal scaling without anesthesia. American Veterinary Dental College. Available at: https://avdc.org/about/#pos-stmts (accessed 7 December 2020).

AVDC (2021a) Primary care practice resources. American Veterinary Dental College. Available at: https://avdc.org/primary-care-practice/ (accessed 4 March 2021).

AVDC (2021b) AVDC nomenclature. American Veterinary Dental College. Available at: https://avdc.org/avdc-nomenclature/ (accessed 12 February 2021).

AVDC (2021c) Find a board certified veterinary dentist. American Veterinary Dental College. Available at: https://avdc.org/find-a-veterinary-specialist/ (accessed 5 March 2021).

AVDC (2021d) Are anesthesia free dental cleanings really cheaper? American Veterinary Dental College. Available at: https://afd.avdc.org/are-anesthesia-free-dental-cleanings-really-cheaper/ (accessed 5 March 2021).

AVMA (2021) Veterinary dentistry. American Veterinary Medical Association. Available at: https://www.avma.org/resources-tools/avma-policies/veterinary-dentistry (accessed 5 March 2021).

Beckman, B. (2007) Exam room to discharge – a case oriented approach to periodontal disease. In: *Proceedings of the 21st Annual Veterinary Dental Forum.* Omnipress, Madison, Wisconsin, pp. 181–182.

Beckman, B. (2008) Increasing client compliance for veterinary dentistry. Dvm360. Available at: https://www.dvm360.com/view/increasing-client-compliance-veterinary-dentistry-proceedings (accessed 4 March 2021).

Bellows, J. (2007) Creating the five star dental practice. In: *Proceedings of the 21st Annual Veterinary Dental Forum.* Omnipress, Madison, Wisconsin, pp. 301–305.

Bellows, J. (2013) Brushing your dog's teeth. Veterinary partner. Available at: https://veterinarypartner.vin.com/default.aspx?pid=19239&id=4951297 (accessed 5 March 2021).

Bellows, J. (2015) Dental extractions: Leave 'em, take 'em, hold 'em or fold 'em? Dvm360. Available at: https://www.dvm360.com/view/dental-extractions-leave-em-take-em-hold-em-or-fold-em (accessed 4 March 2021).

Bellows, J. (2021) Fractured teeth in dogs. VCA. Available at: https://vcahospitals.com/know-your-pet/fractured-teeth-in-dogs (accessed 4 March 2021).

Bellows, J., Berg, M., Dennis, S., Harvey, R., Lobprise, H.B. *et al.* (2019) 2019 AAHA dental care guidelines for dogs and cats. *Journal of the American Animal Hospital Association* 55(2), 49–69. Available at: https://www.aaha.org/globalassets/02-guidelines/dental/aaha_dental_guidelines.pdf (accessed 10 September 2020).

Berg, M. (2007) One form at a time – client communications. In: *Proceedings of the 21st Annual Veterinary Dental Forum.* Omnipress, Madison, Wisconsin, pp. 313–317.

Berg, M. (2020) The examination room and the dental patient. In: Perrone, J. (ed.) *Small Animal Dental Procedures for Veterinary Technicians and Nurses.* Wiley Blackwell, Hoboken, New Jersey, pp. 21–28.

Buzhardt, L. (2021) Why does my veterinarian charge so much? VCA. Available at: https://vcahospitals.com/know-your-pet/why-does-my-veterinarian-charge-so-much (accessed 4 March 2021).

BVDA (2013) A statement on 'Anesthesia-free dental procedures' for cats and dogs. British Veterinary Dental Association. Available at: https://www.bvda.co.uk/images/pdf/Anaesthesia-Free%20Dental%20Procedures.pdf (accessed 5 March 2021).

BVDA (2021) Dental articles. British Veterinary Dental Association. Available at: https://www.bvda.co.uk/index.php/bvda-articles (accessed 4 March 2021).

Byard, V. (2008) Brushing up on dentistry: Promoting dentistry in the veterinary practice. VetFolio. Available at: https://www.vetfolio.com/learn/article/brushing-up-on-dentistry-promoting-dentistry-in-the-veterinary-practice (accessed 7 December 2020).

Camilo, P.G. (2008) Jump-start your prevention with oral ATP. In: *Proceedings of the 22nd Annual Veterinary Dental Forum.* Omnipress, Madison, Wisconsin, pp. 357–359.

CSV (2021) Make dental callbacks when clients don't schedule. Communication Solutions for Veterinarians. Available at: https://csvets.com/2019/02/08/make-dental-callbacks-when-clients-dont-schedule/ (accessed 5 March 2021).

CVMA (2018) Veterinary dentistry – position statement. Canadian Veterinary Medical Association. Available at: https://www.canadianveterinarians.net/documents/veterinary-dentistry-position-statement (accessed 5 March 2021).

CVMA (2020) The Canadian Veterinary Medical Association suggested fee guide for small animal procedures 2020. Canadian Veterinary Medical Association. Available at: https://www.canadianveterinarians.net/uploads/userfiles/files/suggested%20fee%20guides%20for%20small%20animals/2020/ab%20 20%20sm%20fee%20guide.pdf (accessed 4 March 2021).

Dominguez, P.M. (2016) Increasing clients' – and your own – dental awareness: From the exam room to the dental suite. Today's Veterinary Nurse. Available at: https://todaysveterinarynurse.com/articles/increasing-clients-and-your-own-dental-awareness-from-the-exam-room-to-the-dental-suite/ (accessed 7 December 2020).

Dowdy, T. (2010a) Involve your team in dentistry. In: *Proceedings of the 24th Annual Veterinary Dental Forum.* Omnipress, Madison, Wisconsin (CD Rom).

Dowdy, T. (2010b) Creating awareness of your dental services. In: *Proceedings of the 24th Annual Veterinary Dental Forum.* Omnipress, Madison, Wisconsin (CD Rom).

Dowdy, T. (2010c) Developing a successful fee schedule and return on investment. In: *Proceedings of the 24th Annual Veterinary Dental Forum.* Omnipress, Madison, Wisconsin (CD Rom).

Dowdy, T. (2010d) Marketing to expand your dental service. In: *Proceedings of the 24th Annual Veterinary Dental Forum.* Omnipress, Madison, Wisconsin (CD Rom).

Eisner, C. (2004) Price for success: Developing a fee schedule that pays dividends. In: *Proceedings of the 18th Annual Veterinary Dental Forum.* Omnipress, Madison, Wisconsin, pp. 237–241.

Eisner, C. (2008) It takes a team! In: *Proceedings of the 22nd Annual Veterinary Dental Forum.* Omnipress, Madison, Wisconsin, pp. 345–349.

GPH (2014) Dental cleaning in pets: Why is it so expensive? Guthrie Pet Hospital. Available at: https://www.guthriepet.net/blog/dental-cleaning/ (accessed 5 March 2021).

Greenfield, B. (2018) Avoid surprising clients after dental procedures. Dvm360. Available at: https://www.dvm360.com/view/avoid-surprising-clients-after-dental-procedures (accessed 4 March 2021).

Hale, F.A. (2010) Things I tell our clients. Hale Veterinary Clinic. Available at: http://www.toothvet.ca/PDFfiles/Things_I_tell_clients.pdf (accessed 4 March 2021).

Hale, F.A. (2011) Periodontal disease is hidden. Hale Veterinary Clinic. Available at: http://www.toothvet.ca/PDFfiles/perio.pdf (accessed 4 March 2021).

Hauser, W. (2020) Let's talk money. Today's Veterinary Business. Available at: https://todaysveterinarybusiness.com/lets-talk-money-recommendations/ (accessed 7 December, 2020).

Holzman, G. (2006) Dental analgesic techniques. In: *Proceedings of the 20th Annual Veterinary Dental Forum.* Omnipress, Madison, Wisconsin, pp. 403–409.

Ipsos (2016) Most (95%) pet owners brush their own teeth daily, but few brush their dog's (8%) or cat's (4%) teeth on a daily basis. Ipsos. Available at: https://www.ipsos.com/en-ca/news-polls/most-95-pet-owners-brush-their-own-teeth-daily-few-brush-their-dogs-8-or-cats-4-teeth-daily-basis (accessed 19 October 2020).

Lemmons, M. and Carmichael, D.T. (2008) Dental corner: Dental fracture treatment options in dogs and cats. Dvm360. Available at: https://www.dvm360.com/view/dental-corner-dental-fracture-treatment-options-dogs-and-cats (accessed 16 February 2021).

Lewis, J. (2017) How to spot signs of oral pain in your pet patients. Veterinary Practice News. Available at: https://www.veterinarypracticenews.com/how-to-spot-signs-of-oral-pain-in-your-pet-patients/ (accessed 27 January 2021).

Lue, T.W., Pantenburg, D.P. and Crawford, P.M. (2008) Impact of the owner-pet and client-veterinarian bond on the care that pets receive. *Journal of the American Veterinary Medical Association* 232(4), 531–540. Available at: https://avmajournals.avma.org/doi/pdf/10.2460/javma.232.4.531 (accessed 4 March 2021).

Moreau, P. (2008) Pricing and fees in veterinary practices. In: *World Small Animal Veterinary Association World Congress Proceedings, 2008.* Available at: https://www.

vin.com/apputil/content/defaultadv1.aspx?id=3866558&pid=11268 (accessed 4 March 2021).

Myers, W.S. (2007a) Creating awareness of dental services. In: *Proceedings of the 21st Annual Veterinary Dental Forum.* Omnipress, Madison, Wisconsin, pp. 337–342.

Myers, W.S. (2007b) Ways to wow! Your clients with exceptional service. In: *Proceedings of the 21st Annual Veterinary Dental Forum.* Omnipress, Madison, Wisconsin, pp. 325–335.

Myers, W.S. (2007c) Grow dentistry to 5% of revenue. In: *Proceedings of the 21st Annual Veterinary Dental Forum.* Omnipress, Madison, Wisconsin, pp. 343–347.

Myers, W.S. (2007d) How to promote your dental services year-round. In: *Proceedings of the 21st Annual Veterinary Dental Forum.* Omnipress, Madison, Wisconsin, pp. 349–354.

Myers, W.S. (2013a) Creating the client experience for dentistry. Veterinary Practice News. Available at: https://www.veterinarypracticenews.com/creating-the-client-experience-for-dentistry/ (accessed 7 December, 2020).

Myers, W.S. (2013b) Explaining finances with confidence. Veterinary Practice News. Available at: https://www.veterinarypracticenews.com/explaining-finances-with-confidence/ (accessed 4 March 2021).

Myers, W.S. (2017) How to get to YES for dentistry. Communication Solutions for Veterinarians. Available at: https://www.isvma.org/wp-content/uploads/2017/10/How-to-get_YES_for_dentistry.pdf (accessed 7 December, 2020).

Niemiec, B.A. (2012) Dental extractions: Five steps to improve client education, surgical procedures, and patient care. Today's Veterinary Practice. Available at: https://todaysveterinarypractice.com/practical-dentistry-dental-extractions/ (accessed 16 February 2021).

Niemiec, B.A. and Stewart, K. (2020) Current concepts in periodontal disease. Today's Veterinary Practice. Available at: https://todaysveterinarypractice.com/current-concepts-in-periodontal-disease/ (accessed 5 March 2021).

Prendergast, H. (2016) Tips and tricks to rev up your client customer service. Today's Veterinary Nurse. Available at: https://todaysveterinarynurse.com/articles/tips-and-tricks-to-rev-up-your-client-service-game/ (accessed 5 March 2021).

Roark, A. (2013) Veterinarian confession: 'I don't brush my dog's teeth.' Vet Street. Available at: http://www.vetstreet.com/our-pet-experts/veterinarian-confession-i-dont-brush-my-dogs-teeth (accessed 5 March 2021).

Sanchez-Vizcaino, F., Muniesa, A., Singleton, D.A., Jones, P.H., Noble, P.J. *et al.* (2018) Use of vaccines and factors associated with their uptake variability in dogs, cats and rabbits attending a large sentinel network of veterinary practices across Great Britain. *Epidemiology and Infection* 146(7), 895–903. Available at: https://www.ncbi.nlm.nih.gov/pmc/articles/PMC5960348/ (accessed 5 March 2021).

Sorrell, K. (2019) Dental compliance: Here's how to help your clients say yes to the vet. Vetsuccess.com blog, 15 October. VetSuccess. Available at: https://vetsuccess.com/blog/dental-compliance-say-yes-to-the-vet/ (accessed 4 March 2021).

VCA (2021) Your telehealth options. Veterinary Clinics of America. Available at: https://vcahospitals.com/telemedicine (accessed 4 March 2021).

VetCheck (2021) Why good communication is key to good veterinary practice. VetCheck. Available at: http://vetcheck.it/communication/ (accessed 4 March 2021).

Walsh, S. (2017) Craft a treatment plan game plan. Today's Veterinary Business. Available at: https://todaysveterinarybusiness.com/craft-treatment-plan-game-plan/ (accessed 4 March 2021).

Walsh, S. (2019) Veterinary client reminders: 5 effective ways to reach your clients. Practice Life. Available at: https://www.practicelife.com/en/latest/veterinary-client-reminders-5-effective-ways-to-reach-your-clients/ (accessed 5 March 2021).

Woodward, T.M. (2004) Blowing the top off your dental department: A guide for the general practitioner. In: *Proceedings of the 18th Annual Veterinary Dental Forum*. Omnipress, Madison, Wisconsin, pp. 225–236.

Admitting, Preparing and Recovering Dental Patients; a Day in the Life of a Pet Receiving a COHAT

12

Although a Comprehensive Oral Health Assessment and Treatment (COHAT) is a matter of routine to veterinary staff, it can cause upheavals in the lives of both our clients and patients. Your client may be stressed and anxious the night before the procedure, the pet's routine is thrown out by missing their breakfast (Grubb *et al.*, 2020), and your client may have to reschedule their day to accommodate pet drop-off and pick-up. While some upheaval is unavoidable, veterinary nurses can play a large role in minimizing these stressors.

The first part of this chapter provides a comprehensive review of a nurse's role in preparing, performing, assisting in, recording and billing for dental procedures, while the second part recounts an example of a day in the life of a client and their pet having a COHAT. This chapter can be used as a guide to refine a hospital's current dental protocol, and/or to give to clients to read in order to help them understand the preparation and skill that goes into a COHAT; what occurs during a COHAT, including the discovery of unforeseen dental pathology; and to allay any fears or concerns about the procedure.

12.1 Preanaesthetic Fasting

Withholding food and water prior to anaesthesia (in non-emergency situations) is done to prevent complications from gastric reflux during anaesthesia, including oesophageal inflammation; oesophageal stricture; or death due to pulmonary aspiration of gastric contents (Heskin, 2018). In the past, it was commonly recommended to withhold food and water for up to 12 hours (O'Dwyer, 2016) prior to anaesthetic induction of healthy patients. Recent research has shown that preanaesthetic fasting beyond 10 hours is associated with an increased risk of gastric reflux and oesophageal injury (Heskin, 2018). The current American Animal Hospital Association (AAHA) preanaesthetic fasting guidelines for dogs and cats are as follows (Grubb *et al.*, 2020).

DOI: 10.1079/9781789248869.0012

- Healthy patients: withhold food for 4–6 hours; allow free access to water.
- Patients <8 weeks of age or <2 kg: due to the risk of hypoglycaemia, withhold food for no longer than 1–2 hours; allow free access to water. Blood glucose should be monitored before, during and after anaesthesia. These patients' procedures should be performed as the first case of the day.
- Diabetic patients: withhold food for 2–4 hours; allow free access to water; give ½ the patient's usual dose of insulin 2–4 hours prior to anaesthesia. Blood glucose should be monitored before, during and after anaesthesia. These patients' procedures should be performed as the first case of the day.
- Patients with a history of regurgitation or who are at risk for regurgitation: withhold food and water for 6–12 hours, and give preoperative anti-emetic, antacid and promotility medications.
- Emergency patients: withhold food and water as soon as possible, and give preoperative anti-emetic, antacid and promotility medications.

In practical terms, these suggested fasting times may be difficult to achieve (O'Dwyer, 2016): we certainly don't want our clients to have to wake up to feed their pets at 3 o'clock in the morning because their COHAT is scheduled for 9 o'clock! An overnight fast is acceptable in healthy, non-paediatric patients (Heskin, 2018). However, most patients who are undergoing anaesthesia later in the day may be safely given ½–2 tablespoons (depending upon patient size) of soft food in-clinic several hours prior to their procedure (O'Dwyer, 2016).

For patients receiving chronic oral medications, most can be administered as usual prior to anaesthesia with 1–2 tablespoons of canned food (Grubb *et al.*, 2020). Thyroid medications, cardiac medications, antibiotics, steroids and most behavioural and analgesic medications may be continued as usual prior to anaesthesia. Discontinue antihypertensive medications such as angiotensin-converting enzyme (ACE) inhibitors on the day of anaesthesia. Anticoagulants may need to be discontinued 2 weeks prior to surgery based upon the risk of bleeding (Grubb *et al.*, 2020).

For preanaesthetic instructions for rabbits, rodents and ferrets, see Chapter 10, this volume.

12.2   The Intake Appointment: Informed Consent

Informed consent doesn't begin on the morning of admission: it begins when the pet is first diagnosed with a dental problem that needs treatment. At that time, the procedure, risks, options, what will be done in the event that the procedure fails, and fees should be discussed with the client by the veterinarian and nurse, before the client even schedules a dental procedure (Berg, 2020). By the time they come in for their pet's dental procedure intake appointment, the client should already have a good understanding of what they're signing for.

The veterinary nurse, not the front-office staff, should perform dental intake appointments (Bellows, 2006). As in the case of presenting treatment plans (see Chapter 11, this volume), this discussion should take place in a quiet exam room, not in the hospital lobby (Myers, 2007). The variables including anaesthetic risk, treatment options, procedure in the event of treatment failure, and fees must be explained to and consented to by the pet owner (Grubb *et al.*, 2020). Intakes should be scheduled as true appointments, giving each client a specific time to arrive, with the expectation that they will be in the clinic for approximately 10 minutes to revisit the treatment plan and sign consent forms (Myers, 2004).

A consent form signed by the client prior to a procedure not only gives the veterinary practice legal protection in case of a client complaint (Ashall *et al.*, 2018) but also gives the nurse an opportunity to make sure the client understands the procedure(s) that will be performed, address client concerns, verify that the pet has been fasted appropriately, and discover if there are any new health concerns or medications, etc. (Rothstein, 2010). Consent forms can also be signed electronically on a tablet and uploaded directly into the patient's medical record.

12.2.1   Components to include on a dental consent form

1. **Authority to consent** (Gray, 2020). A declaration that the signatory is the pet owner or has the authority to consent to treatment on behalf of the owner.
2. **Treatment plan and associated fees** (Myers, 2004). An itemized list of the procedures to be done, with associated fees for each and the total estimated cost.
3. **Options available** (Gray, 2020). May include treatment options such as endodontic treatment vs extraction of a fractured tooth, or add-on services such as nail trimming, microchipping, etc.
4. **Emergency treatment authorization** (Ohio State University (OSU), 2018). Informs the client that their pet will be undergoing general anaesthetic, outlines the risks involved, and asks whether they consent to or decline emergency treatments such as cardiopulmonary resuscitation (CPR) in the event of cardiopulmonary arrest.
5. **Food and medication questionnaire** (Rothstein, 2010; AAHA, 2020a). The client records what and when the pet was last fed, any food/ medication allergies, and the name, dosage and timing of any current medications.
6. **Other health concerns** (Rothstein, 2010; AAHA, 2020a). The client records any other health concerns. These may be new issues such as vomiting or an ear infection, or information like a previous adverse drug reaction.

7. **Contact information** (Hale, 2009). Phone numbers of the client and/or other pet guardians.
8. **Consent for additional services** (Myers, 2004). This section allows the client to decide beforehand that, in the event they cannot be contacted to discuss any unanticipated dental problems, they authorize the veterinarian to: a) perform all necessary dental procedures, b) perform only the dental procedures listed on the treatment plan, or c) perform any necessary dental procedures up to an additional cost of X.

The veterinarian or hospital manager may have other components they wish to include, such as a list of belongings left with the pet, behavioural concerns, etc.

Some clients express a desire to speak with the veterinarian prior to the procedure. If the veterinarian is unavailable at the time of the intake appointment, ask the client to sign the form with the proviso that the veterinarian will call them prior to performing the procedure. If the client is not comfortable enough to sign the consent form once you have thoroughly explained it, then they are not comfortable enough to leave their pet for treatment today. Reschedule the procedure after the veterinarian is able to speak with them.

12.3   The Preanaesthetic Examination

This examination is performed by the nurse in the exam room with the client present, or in the treatment area (Bellows *et al.*, 2019; McMahon, 2020). Assess and record the patient's body weight, temperature, heart rate, respiration rate, mucous-membrane colour and capillary refill time (Grubb *et al.*, 2020; Mills, 2020). Examine the patient's head, face and oral cavity to check for any dental problems that may have occurred since the initial examination, such as new swellings, fractured teeth, etc. (McMahon, 2020). If preanaesthetic labwork was not previously done, collect blood and urine to be analysed (Grubb *et al.*, 2020) by in-house laboratory equipment. Perform any other required testing such as chest X-rays.

Consult with the veterinarian and record the following upon the patient's anaesthetic chart: pre-existing medical conditions, ASA score (an anaesthetic risk score developed by the American Society of Anesthesiologists – see Chapter 2, this volume), intravenous (IV) fluid type and rate, preanaesthetic and induction drugs and dosages (base calculations upon lean body weight) (Grubb *et al.*, 2020), and any desired intraoperative medications, including dental regional nerve blocks, continuous rate infusions (CRIs) of pain medications, injectable antibiotics, etc. (Stepaniuk, 2007a). Calculate drug volumes and draw them up in syringes labelled with the drug and patient's name (Stein, 2004; University of Bristol (UOB), 2017).

12.4 Preparing the Dental Operatory

12.4.1 Anaesthetic and monitoring equipment

Fill the anaesthetic machine vaporizer with inhalant, ensure that the oxygen tank pressure is at least 500 psi, turn on the scavenging system, and check that the CO_2 absorbing granules are fresh (Zeltzman, 2017a; Sonopath, 2020). Determine whether the patient will be placed on a rebreathing system (patient >5 kg) or non-rebreathing system (patient <5 kg) (AAHA, 2020b), attach the required anaesthetic hoses and select an appropriately sized reservoir bag. The bag should be six times the patient's tidal volume (10–20 ml/kg), allowing the patient to take a deep breath without emptying the bag (Hunyady, 2019). A quick rule of thumb is 1 l per 10kg of body weight, rounding up to the nearest size bag. For instance, for a patient weighing 15 kg, use a 2-l bag.

Check the reservoir bags, breathing hoses, one-way valves and domes, and CO_2 canisters for any visible wear, cracks, loose connections or holes (Mills, 2020). Test the anaesthetic system for leaks by closing the pop-off valve and occluding the end of the anaesthetic hose with your thumb or palm, then turn on the oxygen flow meter or press the oxygen flush valve until the manometer registers a pressure of 20–30 cmH_2O (Grubb *et al.*, 2020). Turn off the flow meter or release the oxygen flush valve. If no leaks are present, the manometer pressure indicator should remain steady for at least 15 seconds (Palmer, 2020). Some non-rebreathing systems have no manometer. In this case, fill the reservoir bag completely (Palmer, 2020). It should remain full for at least 15 seconds. If a leak is suspected, spray soapy water solution onto the hose, connections, and reservoir bag, then perform the leak test again. Bubbles will form at the source of the leak (Palmer, 2020). Replace or repair any leaky equipment, then re-test. Do not forget to open the pop-off valve after testing (Zeltzman, 2017a).

Choose three endotracheal tube sizes for the patient: one based upon the lean body weight of the patient, one half a size smaller and another half a size larger, to allow for individual variation (Mills, 2020). There are many charts in textbooks and online that can guide endotracheal tube size selection, or you can palpate the trachea or measure the width between the nares to estimate tube diameter (Sonopath, 2013). Keep in mind that brachycephalic breeds often have smaller tracheas than mesocephalic patients of similar body weight (Hunyady, 2019). Inflate the cuffs of all three tubes to check for leaks (Hunyady, 2019).

Prepare all materials needed for intravenous catheter placement and anaesthetic induction, including tape, gauze squares, IV catheters, PRN (*pro re nata* – 'as needed') adapters, saline flush, IV fluid bag, IV extension set, IV pump, laryngoscope with appropriately sized blade, lubricant for the endotracheal tube, lidocaine spray or liquid, endotracheal tube tie, and syringe to inflate the endotracheal tube cuff (Bellows, 2006; Hunyady, 2019; Altier, 2020).

Turn on the multiparameter monitoring machine and ensure that it is working properly (Mills, 2020). Gather all associated materials including electrocardiogram (ECG) clips, ultrasonic gel, SPO_2 (oxygen saturation) sensor, CO_2 sensor, thermometer probe covers and blood-pressure cuffs.

Attach a clean blanket, pad or mattress to the patient-warming device to prevent hypothermia (Mills, 2020), which is of particular concern in smaller patients or patients undergoing longer procedures. Electric heating pads are not advised, as they can cause thermal burns (Stepaniuk, 2007b).

Have an emergency drug kit and emergency drug dosage chart on hand for all anaesthetized patients (Jones, 2014).

12.4.2   Dental equipment

Turn on all dental machines to ensure they are fully operational, including the dental radiography unit and computer (and check the software). Fill the dental unit bottles with distilled water and add a daily waterline treatment product; turn on the compressor; and test the ultrasonic scaler, high- and low-speed handpieces (make sure to place a bur or blank in the high-speed handpiece before testing) and suction (if available). Gather all accessories such as X-ray sensor or phosphor-plate covers, ultrasonic scaler tips, prophy angles, polish cups, and high- and low-volume suction tips (Bellows, 2006; Bellows *et al.*, 2019; Altier, 2020).

Prepare materials and instruments for the anticipated dental procedure, such as chlorhexidine rinse, flexible mouth gags, a pharyngeal gauze pack (Stepaniuk, 2007a), and a periodontal instrument tray stocked with a sterilized periodontal probe, dental explorer, dental mirror, calculus-removal forceps, hand scalers and curettes (Altier, 2020; McMahon, 2020). If oral surgery is anticipated, prepare a surgery tray (Bellows, 2006) including sterilized thumb forceps, scalpel handle and blade, periosteal elevators, needle drivers, scissors, luxators, extraction forceps, root-tip forceps, suture material and a selection of high-speed burs.

Other materials you may need to prepare include an electrocautery unit and tips; CO_2 laser; formalin jars for biopsy samples; endodontic instruments and materials including hand or rotary files, gutta percha and paper points, restorative materials, etc.; or stainless steel wire, wire cutters and acrylic for jaw fracture repairs.

Ensure the overhead lights in the dental operatory are functional and bright. Gloves, masks and protective eyewear should be available for everyone in the dental area, including the anaesthesia nurse and any other assistants (Altier, 2020). Surgical caps and gowns may also be required, depending upon hospital policy.

12.5 Premedication, Anaesthetic Induction and Monitoring

After you have tested and prepared all anaesthetic and dental machines and materials, the patient can receive their premedication injection (Grubb *et al.*, 2020). Record the method, location and time of administration on the patient's chart (Stepaniuk, 2007a). Monitor the patient closely for vomiting or any other adverse effects while the drugs take effect (Grubb *et al.*, 2020). Patients with brachycephalic syndrome are particularly at risk for airway obstruction after sedation (Lucero, 2019). Depending upon the drugs chosen for the patient, intramuscular premedication usually takes 15–20 minutes to reach peak effect (Stein, 2004; Grubb *et al.*, 2020). If administered intravenously, premedication generally takes effect within 2–5 minutes (Grubb *et al.*, 2020).

Once the pet is sufficiently sedate, record the pre-induction heart rate and place an IV catheter (McMahon, 2020) if not already placed. Pre-oxygenate the patient with 100% oxygen (Grubb *et al.*, 2020) for at least 5 minutes prior to induction (patients with airway or breathing dysfunction such as brachycephalics or asthmatics should be pre-oxygenated for 10–15 minutes) (McNerney, 2017). Pre-oxygenation delays the onset of arterial hypoxemia by increasing the body's oxygen stores (Grubb *et al.*, 2020). Pre-oxygenation is usually done by mask, though if the patient struggles against the mask, this decreases pre-oxygenation efficacy, and flow-by oxygen 2.5 cm from the nares should be provided instead (Carrozzo, 2018).

Induce anaesthesia as directed for the drug(s) chosen. In most cases, a bolus of ¼ –⅓ of the calculated induction dose is given slowly, then repeated as necessary, titrating to effect (Grubb *et al.*, 2020) until the patient's jaw tone has sufficiently decreased to allow intubation (Hunyady, 2019). Cats should receive a spray or drops of liquid lidocaine onto either side of the larynx to prevent laryngospasm (Stein, 2004). Apply lubricant to the chosen endotracheal tube and cuff and intubate the patient, checking that the tube has been placed into the trachea by visualizing condensation in clear tubes as the animal breathes, feeling at the exposed end of the tube for exhaled breaths, or attaching a CO_2 monitor to the endotracheal tube and visualizing the capnograph tracing (Grubb *et al.*, 2020).

Tie the endotracheal tube in place, attach the endotracheal tube to the anaesthetic hose and set the oxygen flow rate and vaporizer percentage (Mills, 2020). Check the animal's breathing, pulse rate and quality. Determine whether the endotracheal tube cuff needs to be inflated by pressing the safety pop-off occlusion valve and squeezing the reservoir bag until the manometer reaches 20 cmH$_2$0 while listening at the patient's mouth for any hissing sound that would indicate air leakage around an under-inflated cuff (Grubb *et al.*, 2020). If you hear escaping air, slowly inflate the cuff with a small amount of air and retest.

Attach the multiparameter monitoring equipment and record initial readings of the patient's heart rate, respiration rate, SPO_2, end tidal CO_2, blood pressure and temperature on the anaesthetic chart (Mills, 2020). The SPO_2 probe of most machines is designed to be placed upon the tongue, but in dental patients this may get in the way of performing procedures or become dislodged. Alternate areas for SPO_2 probe placement are the pinna, toe, prepuce or vulva (Mills, 2020). Apply eye lubricant after induction and every 2–4 hours thereafter (Grubb *et al.*, 2020). Turn on the warming device and place it on the patient, adjusting the temperature as required to prevent hypothermia (Stein, 2004). Begin intravenous fluid administration (Grubb *et al.*, 2020).

Adjust the vaporizer settings and oxygen flow rate as necessary to maintain a surgical plane of anaesthesia. The patient should have no voluntary movement, no palpebral reflex, and a relaxed jaw (Grubb *et al.*, 2020). A nurse dedicated to anaesthesia should continue monitoring the patient's parameters, recording them every 5 minutes (Mills, 2020), adjusting the depth of anaesthesia as necessary, and alerting the veterinarian immediately if any parameters begin to stray from the normal range.

When changing the patient's head or body position, for example when taking dental radiographs, disconnect the endotracheal tube from the breathing hose prior to moving the patient to prevent tube rotation within the trachea, which may cause tracheal tears (Stein, 2004).

12.6 The Dental Procedure

The most common dental procedure in general practice is a COHAT (see Chapter 2, this volume), including dental hygiene, oral examination and charting, and dental X-rays (Bellows *et al.*, 2019). This is done by the nurse under the supervision of a veterinarian (McMahon, 2020), just as a human dental hygienist performs dental cleanings and takes radiographs under the supervision of a dentist. In most veterinary practices, this entails the nurse performing an oral examination, cleaning the pet's teeth both supra- and subgingivally using ultrasonic and hand instruments, polishing the teeth, rinsing the mouth, charting oral or dental pathology (McMahon, 2020) and taking full-mouth X-rays (Bird, 2020), after which the veterinarian assesses the patient, reviews the charting and X-rays, and performs any surgical procedures including extractions, biopsy, endodontics, etc. (Perrone *et al.*, 2020). Take photographs of the patient's oral cavity prior to and after the COHAT to show the client (Lewis, 2013). Either the nurse or the veterinarian may place dental regional nerve blocks prior to a painful procedure (Mills, 2020).

12.6.1 Four-handed dentistry

'Four-handed dentistry' is common in human dental practices (Finkbeiner, 2000). The 'four hands' referred to are an assistant's hands aiding the dentist's hands (Square Practice, 2020), to increase efficiency, ensure the ergonomic comfort of the dentist, and decrease the time required for the procedure. For veterinary patients, this is particularly important, since decreasing procedure time means less time spent under general anaesthesia.

The goal of four-handed dentistry is to ensure the dentist must never or only rarely turn away from the patient's oral cavity during a procedure (Square Practice, 2020). The veterinarian asks for what they require and the nurse brings it within easy reach (Finkbeiner, 2000). This could mean changing burs, passing instruments directly into the veterinarian's hand or onto the dental tray, providing suction, preparing restorative materials, using light-curing guns, etc. (DeForge, 2009). In time, nurses should be able to anticipate which instruments and materials are required for common dental procedures and get them ready without the veterinarian having to ask (Finkbeiner, 2000; DeForge, 2009). The veterinarian can also dictate any observed pathology and treatments performed while the nurse records them on the dental chart (Hernandez, 2007).

12.7   Recovery

Monitoring patients during recovery from general anaesthesia is crucial to a successful outcome (Grubb *et al.*, 2020). After the dental procedure is complete, remove any packing material and debris from the patient's mouth, checking the back of the throat and beneath the tongue (McMahon, 2020). Bloody gauze can be difficult to discern from oral tissues, so check well! Suction or wipe excess fluid from the oral cavity. Because dental procedures often involve drilling teeth and bone, using water spray, and oral bleeding, the patient's head and face may be wet and bloody (Dominguez, 2020). Clean blood and debris from the fur with saline, dry the pet's head and face with a towel, and comb out any matts.

Discontinue inhalant anaesthesia while keeping the patient on 100% oxygen for several minutes until their reflexes begin to return (McMahon, 2020). Continue to monitor physiologic parameters including SPO_2, CO_2, heart rate, respiratory rate and body temperature until the patient is awake and able to move around on their own (Grubb *et al.*, 2020). Hypothermia can cause delayed drug metabolism, slowing recovery, so continue the use of warming devices throughout the recovery period (Grubb *et al.*, 2020).

Recover dental patients (except brachycephalic breeds: see below) with their head slightly lower than the rest of their body, to keep fluid and debris from being aspirated (Grubb *et al.*, 2020). Extubate the patient when their respiration rate and SPO_2 are within normal limits and their swallowing reflex has returned (McMahon, 2020). Deflate the cuff just prior to removing the endotracheal tube (Grubb *et al.*, 2020).

Recover brachycephalic patients in sternal recumbency with their head extended, slightly elevated, and their tongue pulled out (Lucero, 2019).

Keep the endotracheal tube in place until the patient is almost completely awake (McMahon, 2020), since these animals have a high risk of airway swelling and obstruction during the postoperative period, and may also have abnormalities of the gastrointestinal tract that can cause regurgitation or vomiting (O'Dwyer, 2017). Patients who begin to chew the tube will require extubation sooner.

After extubation, disconnect the patient from monitoring equipment and place them in a warm, comfortable, padded kennel to complete their recovery (McMahon, 2020). Place larger patients on a foam mat or thickly folded blankets. Recovery should take place in a highly visible area where patients can be readily observed by the nurse and veterinarian (Stepaniuk, 2007a).

Keep the patient's IV catheter in place until the patient is completely recovered, so pain or emergency drugs can be quickly given if necessary (Grubb *et al.*, 2020). Discontinue IV fluids unless the patient is debilitated, dehydrated or has renal disease (AAHA, 2020c). Some patients may express their anal sacs or have loose stool during recovery, which will require cleaning.

Thrashing during recovery can be due to either emergence delirium or dysphoria (Grubb *et al.*, 2020). Emergence delirium occurs when the patient wakes up from anaesthesia very quickly, while dysphoria may be due to uncontrolled pain (Grubb *et al.*, 2020). If pain is suspected, an analgesic should be administered intravenously, so that it can take effect quickly. If emergence delirium is suspected, a small dose of sedative such as dexmedetomidine should be administered intravenously (Grubb *et al.*, 2020).

Measure and record heart and respiration rate, temperature, mucousmembrane colour and capillary refill time at least hourly while the patient recovers (McMahon, 2020). Perform pain scoring (see Chapter 3, this volume) to ensure pain control remains adequate throughout recovery (Grubb *et al.*, 2020). If necessary, CRI's may be continued, initiated, or additional pain medication given (McMahon, 2020).

Monitor blood glucose periodically for all postoperative tiny, neonatal or diabetic patients (Grubb *et al.*, 2020). Intravenous or oral dextrose solutions may be administered if blood glucose drops too low. Offer small amounts of highly palatable, canned food to patients once they are ambulatory (Cox, 2019; McMahon, 2020). The patient's bladder may be full, especially if the procedure was lengthy. Take dogs outside if possible to relieve themselves, and offer cats a litterbox (McMahon, 2020).

12.8 Billing, Arranging Discharge, and Medical Records

After the patient has recovered, the nurse is usually responsible for billing for the procedure (YTI, 2020). Many veterinary computer programs will allow a previously created estimate to be transferred to an invoice (IDEXX

Laboratories, 2015). Any additional procedures that were performed but not initially estimated for must be added to the invoice, along with all drugs given in hospital and medications, food or dental homecare products being sent home. Log any controlled drugs used (Walsh, 2017).

Call or text the owner to let them know that their pet is out of anaesthesia and doing well. Many owners appreciate a texted photo of their pet awake, clean and pain-free after a dental procedure. If a discharge time has not already been arranged, do this now. If additional procedures were performed that were not on the initial treatment plan, advise the owner of the final total of the invoice.

Transfer the signed consent form, anaesthetic chart and dental chart into the patient's computer or paper file (Alberta Veterinary Medical Association (ABVMA), 2013; Zeltzman, 2017b). Record the details of the dental procedure in the patient's medical record. Depending upon your local veterinary regulatory association guidelines, this could include the following (ABVMA, 2013; Zeltzman, 2017b; Catanzaro, 2018):

- the names of the veterinarian(s) and nurse(s) administering treatment
- preanaesthetic exam findings; results of diagnostic tests; ASA score
- premedication and induction drugs, dosages, time(s) and method(s) of administration
- size and location of IV catheter placement; type and total volume of intravenous fluids administered
- endotracheal tube type and size; presence or absence of cuff and whether the cuff was inflated
- rebreathing vs non-rebreathing system; size of anaesthetic reservoir bag; physiologic parameters monitored (e.g. heart rate (HR), respiration rate (RR), SPO_2, end tidal CO_2, blood pressure, ECG, body temperature)
- any problems or complications associated with anaesthesia
- dental pathology findings
- dental treatment(s) performed
- intraoperative medications administered, including location, dosage and volume (include dental regional nerve blocks)
- any other treatment(s) performed, such as mass removals
- time of extubation
- quality of recovery
- postoperative monitoring results, including pain scoring, and postoperative medications administered in hospital
- medications sent home and summary of postoperative instructions
- timing of rechecks and any additional treatment(s) the patient must return to receive.

A computer template for this record may be available or created in a word-processing program where the nurse can simply 'fill in the blanks' for each patient, which standardizes recording by all staff members and ensures no critical information is missed.

Generate reminders to call the client the next day for a postoperative update, as well as reminders to call the client to schedule recheck appointments.

Create a discharge sheet for the owner outlining the procedure(s) performed, potential complications to watch for, medication and feeding instructions, and timing of rechecks (Dominguez, 2020). Print out pre- and postoperative photos and X-rays or have them available to show on a screen at discharge (Lewis, 2013; Dominguez, 2020). Patient discharge is covered in more detail in Chapter 13, this volume.

12.9 A Day in the Life of a Pet Receiving a COHAT

Milo, a 12-year-old, neutered, male shih tzu mix, was brought to the Best Friends Animal Clinic for the first time for a yearly health exam and vaccinations by his owner, Susan, who recently moved into the area. During Milo's examination, Dr Banerjee noted that he had halitosis, heavy calculus deposits on most teeth, moderate gingivitis, crowded premolars, and some loose lower incisors. After Dr Banerjee left the exam room, Emma, the veterinary nurse, came in to present Susan with a treatment plan for Milo, including preanaesthetic bloodwork and chest X-rays, an advanced COHAT with full-mouth radiographs, and 30 minutes of oral surgery. Emma explained that although the oral examination Dr Banerjee had performed provided a good idea of what dental treatment Milo would require, the majority of periodontal disease occurs beneath the gumline, and more disease might be detected once Milo received full-mouth dental X-rays and dental probing under general anaesthesia.

Susan hesitated to schedule this procedure, because she was concerned about anaesthesia at Milo's age, her finances were tight, and she was worried about Milo being in pain after having teeth extracted.

Emma was able to address each of these concerns. She let Susan know that the COHAT would treat the current infection and pain in Milo's mouth and that he would have fresher breath and a better quality of life, and may even live longer. She also explained that although no anaesthetic procedure is 100% risk-free, the preanaesthetic bloodwork and chest X-rays would make anaesthesia safer for Milo by detecting any underlying conditions such as anaemia, kidney or liver disease, or abnormalities of the heart and lungs, allowing Dr Banerjee to tailor his anaesthetic protocol accordingly. She told Susan that during anaesthesia Milo would receive intravenous fluids to keep him hydrated and help regulate his blood pressure, and that the IV catheter would allow access to veins in order to administer any needed drugs and pain medications. A nurse dedicated to his anaesthesia would monitor Milo closely throughout the procedure, and he would be kept warm with a heated air blanket. Multiple methods of pain control, including injectable pain medications, dental nerve blocks ('like the freezing your own dentist uses', Emma explained) and oral pain medications sent home would keep Milo comfortable until his extraction sites healed.

Emma provided Susan with a handout on periodontal disease, information about third-party financing, and links to several reputable websites including the American Veterinary Dental College and the British Veterinary Dental Association. Susan still wanted to think it over before scheduling the procedure, so Emma asked if she could follow up with Susan by phone in a few days.

Once Susan got home, she checked the third-party financing company's website to see if she would qualify for financing. She also visited the veterinary websites, and everything she read confirmed what Dr Banerjee and Emma had explained to her.

When Emma phoned a few days later, Susan agreed to schedule Milo's COHAT. Emma booked the COHAT for the following Monday, and asked Susan to bring Milo in several days beforehand, to have the preanaesthetic bloodwork and chest X-rays done. Emma also told her not to feed Milo breakfast on Monday morning, because he needed to fast prior to anaesthesia. Milo's intake exam was scheduled for 8:30 on Monday morning.

On Saturday, Susan brought Milo back to the clinic for his bloodwork and chest X-rays. His X-rays were clear, but the bloodwork showed that his liver enzymes were mildly elevated. Dr Banerjee explained that Milo's liver was functioning well enough that she wasn't concerned about his anaesthetic risk, but she would recheck his bloodwork in 3 months' time to monitor for any further changes.

Susan didn't sleep very well on Sunday night. Although she knew Dr Banerjee and Emma and the rest of the veterinary staff would do their best to keep Milo safe and comfortable, she couldn't help worrying. And on Monday morning, when Milo begged her for his breakfast, she felt guilty. It didn't help that her other dog, Noodle, kept barking at the empty food dish, since she'd decided it would be easier to fast them both. At 8 o'clock, she put Milo in the car, ran back into the house to feed Noodle, then drove Milo to the hospital.

Once they arrived, the client services representative at the front desk greeted Susan and Milo by name. She weighed Milo on the scale in the lobby, then showed them to an exam room. Emma came in a few minutes later to go over the consent form and to make sure Susan was comfortable with the planned procedure.

The first page of the consent form included the treatment plan Susan had already received. She signed that she agreed to the planned procedure and associated costs. There were boxes to check to say whether she wanted Milo to receive nail trimming or a microchip while under anaesthesia. Milo was already microchipped, but Susan decided to take advantage of the nail trimming, since Milo was not very well behaved for his nail trims at home.

The next section was the emergency treatment authorization. Susan read through the risks of general anaesthetic, and signed her consent to any required emergency treatments, including CPR. Below this were questions regarding what time Milo last ate, what type of food he ate, whether he had any allergies, and if he was currently receiving medications. Susan filled this out, noting that he had food allergies to beef and chicken. There was also a section asking if Milo had any recent health problems including vomiting, diarrhoea, coughing, sneezing, or any other health concerns. Susan happily checked 'no' to all of these. On the following page, Susan filled out her contact information, including her mobile and work phone numbers.

The last question was titled 'consent for additional services'. Emma explained that if Dr Banerjee discovered any additional dental problems once Milo was under general anaesthesia, she would try to contact Susan, but if Susan couldn't be reached, the doctor needed to know beforehand what Susan's wishes would be regarding further treatment. Susan initialled beside the option that in the event she could not be contacted, she authorized the veterinarian to perform any necessary procedures up to an additional cost. Susan wrote down £100, which she thought she could afford, as the high end of the estimate.

After Susan hugged and kissed Milo goodbye, Emma took him to the treatment area to perform his preanaesthetic exam. She noted his heart and respiration rate and listened for any abnormalities, took his temperature, checked his gum colour, and examined his mouth to make sure there were no new dental problems since his initial oral exam. She placed him on a blanket in a heated kennel in the treatment area, where he could be readily observed while she prepared for his COHAT.

Dr Banerjee had already assigned Milo an ASA score of 2, meaning that anaesthesia for Milo was considered a slight risk because of mild systemic disease or age. She had also recorded the drugs he was to receive both pre- and intraoperatively, and their dosages in milligrams per kilogram. Emma calculated the drug volumes based on Milo's current body weight and drew them up, carefully labelling the syringes. She printed an emergency drug dosage chart to refer to in case of any problems while he was under anaesthesia. She also calculated his intravenous fluid volume per hour and put a new fluid bag on the IV pump. She then set up the anaesthetic machine in the dental operatory with the appropriate sizes of anaesthetic hoses, bags and endotracheal tubes for Milo, inspecting each for leaks. She turned on the ultrasonic dental unit and compressor, filled the unit's water bottles, and inserted a sterilized ultrasonic scaler tip. She placed a new prophy angle on the low-speed handpiece for polishing, a dental bur onto the high-speed handpiece, and tested these along with the air-water syringe. She set out a periodontal tray of instruments she would use to clean Milo's teeth, and a surgery tray with instruments for Dr Banerjee to use to perform extractions. She entered Milo's information into the veterinary X-ray software, turned on the multiparameter monitor, connected the necessary clips to monitor Milo's vital signs under anaesthesia, and attached a clean blanket to the hose of the patient-warming system. Then, the client services representative paged her to let her know that the next patient had arrived for their intake appointment. Emma went into the exam room to admit the next patient just as she had done for Milo.

Dr Banerjee had several examination appointments booked before Milo's scheduled COHAT. While Dr Banerjee was seeing her last appointment, Emma administered Milo's premedication drugs. These consisted of a sedative and an opioid for pain relief. After 15 minutes, Milo was sleepy and Dr Banerjee was available to supervise the COHAT.

Emma and another veterinary nurse took Milo into the dental operatory, placed an IV catheter into one of his leg veins, and gave him oxygen by mask for 5 minutes to increase his body's oxygen stores before starting anaesthesia. Emma administered an injectable anaesthetic drug through his IV catheter, which caused Milo to become very sleepy, allowing her to place a cuffed endotracheal tube into his throat. The endotracheal tube would deliver oxygen and gas anaesthesia and protect his airway from fluid and debris during the dental procedure.

Next, they placed Milo on his back into a V-shaped trough padded with blankets, angling him so his head was slightly lower than his chest to allow fluids and debris to drain from his mouth. They connected his endotracheal tube to the anaesthetic machine, and began administering gas anaesthetic and oxygen. The nurse monitoring Milo's anaesthesia connected the clips and sensors of the multiparameter monitor, which would monitor his ECG, heart rate, oxygen saturation, respiration rate, end tidal carbon dioxide levels, blood pressure and temperature. She placed the warm air-heated blanket on Milo, started his IV fluids, and began recording his vital signs.

Meanwhile, Emma placed lubricating gel into Milo's eyes to keep them moist and protect them from debris. She put on a new pair of gloves, a mask, a cap, and magnifying loupes to protect her eyes and allow her to better see Milo's teeth. She reminded the anaesthesia nurse to wear a pair of goggles and a mask too, as protection from any aerosolized debris.

Emma checked Milo's eye position, jaw tone and reflexes, and determined that he was in a good plane of anaesthesia to begin the dental cleaning. She took preoperative photographs of Milo's mouth to show Susan the condition of his teeth, then rinsed his mouth with a chlorhexidine gluconate solution to kill surface bacteria, thereby reducing the number of bacteria that could enter his bloodstream during the procedure while also reducing contamination of the dental operatory from bacterial aerosolization.

Next, Emma used calculus-removal forceps to gently remove the larger chunks of tartar, then removed the remaining tartar and plaque from the teeth both above and below the gumline with an ultrasonic scaler, hand scalers and curettes. She dried Milo's teeth with the air-water syringe to detect any areas of plaque she might have missed.

After Milo's teeth were clean, Emma examined his face, throat, tongue, cheeks and gums, checking for any lesions, swellings or other abnormalities. She recorded on his dental chart that he had small chewing lesions on the inside of both cheeks, moderate gingivitis throughout most of his mouth, and severe gingivitis around his lower incisors and his right lower first molar. She used a dental probe to measure for any periodontal pockets (areas where the gum tissue has become detached from the tooth due to infection) and gingival recession (loss of gum tissue due to infection), by moving the probe around each tooth and recording the measurements at each site. She discovered deep pockets of 5–7 mm around most of Milo's lower incisors, pockets of 4 mm around both lower canine teeth, 4-mm pockets and crowding between his left and right upper second and third premolars, and a 6-mm pocket on the distal (back) root of his right lower first molar. There was also gingival recession of 4 mm around his right lower first molar. There was gingival hyperplasia (overgrowth of the gums) over both of his upper fourth premolars. All of his lower incisors were mobile and there was a fracture of his left upper canine tooth, which did not extend into the pulp, and abrasion of his right upper canine tooth. His right upper first premolar and both of his lower third molars appeared to be missing.

Once Emma had finished charting Milo's oral pathology, she polished his teeth to smooth their surfaces, reducing any microabrasions that could attract plaque. She flushed his teeth above and below the gumline with water to remove any debris and polishing paste, suctioned out his mouth, then took dental X-rays of all of his teeth.

Dr Banerjee studied the X-rays, making notes of any subgingival pathology on Milo's dental chart, including severe bone loss around all of the lower incisors and along the distal root of his right lower first molar, moderate bone loss around both lower canine teeth and the left and right upper second and third premolars, and a retained root tip belonging to Milo's 'missing' right upper first premolar. There was a dark area on the X-ray around the tip of the retained root, which was a sign of bone loss in that area, possibly due to infection. She confirmed Emma's dental charting with a thorough oral examination, and determined that she would need to extract Milo's lower incisors, his right lower first molar, the retained tooth root, and his crowded left and right upper second and third premolars. Emma would then perform closed root planing and subgingival curettage, and apply a perioceutic (antibiotic gel) into the periodontal pockets around both of Milo's lower canine teeth. These treatments would alleviate Milo's oral pain and infection; prevent further bone loss in his lower right jaw, which could lead to potential jaw fracture; and reduce the pocket depths of his lower canine teeth, hopefully halting or slowing further progression of periodontal disease in those areas.

Dr Banerjee thought she could accomplish the extractions within 45 minutes. Emma updated Milo's treatment plan, adding the extra surgery time and the perioceutic application. The total would come to £200 over Susan's initial estimate.

While Dr Banerjee called Susan to explain Milo's dental pathology and the treatment he needed, Emma administered regional nerve blocks to stop pain transmission at the extraction sites, allowing the use of a lower concentration of inhalant anaesthetic during the procedure. The dental nerve blocks would also make him more comfortable upon recovery from anaesthesia. Next, she gave him an injection of a non-steroidal anti-inflammatory drug to relieve pain and inflammation both intra- and post-operatively. She lubricated his eyes again and swapped the periodontal tray for the surgery tray she had already prepared.

Susan wasn't happy to learn that Milo had more dental problems than Dr Banerjee had been able to see during his conscious exam, but, since Emma had already prepared her for the possibility, she wasn't surprised. She certainly didn't want his periodontal disease to progress to the point that his jaw might fracture. She decided she would stretch her budget to have all of Milo's necessary dental work done today, while he was already under anaesthesia and doing well.

Dr Banerjee returned to the dental operatory and put on her magnifying loupes, a mask, cap, and surgical gown. Emma handed her dental instruments while she extracted Milo's teeth, sectioning multi-rooted teeth and carefully luxating each root from its socket. She smoothed the bone of each tooth socket, curetted away any infected tissue, and flushed the extraction sites with water. Then she closed the gum tissue with absorbable suture.

Emma took postoperative X-rays to ensure there were no retained tooth roots or other complications following the extractions. Next, she curetted the exposed surfaces of the roots of both lower canine teeth within their periodontal pockets, creating a smooth root surface to encourage gingival attachment. She also removed diseased tissue and debris from the soft tissue lining the periodontal pockets. She mixed the perioceutic gel and instilled it into each periodontal pocket.

Emma dried Milo's teeth, then applied fluoride to help prevent tooth sensitivity and to strengthen Milo's teeth by encouraging enamel remineralization. After 1 minute, she wiped the fluoride away with gauze. She suctioned Milo's oral cavity a final time and made sure there was no debris, gauze or other foreign material left in his mouth or throat. She took postoperative photographs of his teeth and the extraction sites, cleaned his face, combed out his beard, trimmed his nails, and lubricated his eyes a final time.

The anaesthesia nurse discontinued Milo's gas anaesthetic, and Emma turned him gently onto his side to wake up. He continued to receive 100% oxygen through the endotracheal tube until his swallowing reflex returned. At this point, Emma deflated the cuff and removed the tube. Once Milo started lifting his head and trying to stand up, she removed his monitoring clips and sensors, and stopped his IV fluids. She carried him out of the dental operatory and placed him back into the heated kennel in the treatment area, where he would be closely monitored during recovery from anaesthesia. She periodically checked his vital signs and used a canine pain scoring chart to assess any postoperative discomfort.

Once Milo was fully awake, Emma called Susan to let her know that Milo was recovering well and confirmed his discharge time later in the afternoon. She also texted Susan a photo of Milo sitting up in his kennel.

Dr Banerjee told Emma which postoperative medications she wanted Milo sent home with, and Emma got the prescriptions ready. She completed his bill, entered procedure notes into his computer medical records, and set up reminders for a postoperative follow-up call the following day, a recheck appointment in 14 days, and another COHAT and radiographs in 6 months, as Dr Banerjee had requested. She printed out Milo's dental photographs and X-rays, created a discharge sheet listing all of his postoperative instructions, and put everything into a bag. She offered Milo a small amount of hypoallergenic canned food, and he took a few licks. She took him outside to allow him to urinate. Then it was time to premedicate the next patient.

After work, Susan came to pick Milo up, and Emma met her in the exam room. Emma showed her Milo's dental chart, photographs and X-rays. She advised Susan that Milo would be a bit groggy tonight, and to monitor him carefully, especially around stairs to make sure he didn't take a tumble. She told Susan not to take him on any long walks for the next couple of days, although short walks to relieve himself would be fine. She discussed his postoperative care, including feeding only soft food until his recheck, and not allowing Milo access to hard treats or toys. Since Susan's other dog, Noodle, would still be eating his regular kibble, Susan decided to feed them in separate rooms. Emma also explained how and when to give Milo's postoperative pain medications, and told Susan to discontinue them and call the clinic should he develop vomiting or diarrhoea. She also told her that a small amount of blood-tinged saliva is normal for the first day or two following oral surgery, and that she might notice a slight cough if Milo's throat was dry or irritated from the endotracheal tube. If Milo had any profuse oral bleeding or severe coughing, Emma instructed Susan to bring him for a recheck as soon as possible.

Susan asked if she should start brushing Milo's teeth. Emma instructed her to wait until after the recheck appointment, because Milo's mouth would be sore until his extraction sites healed, and brushing might dislodge the perioceutic gel instilled into the pockets of his lower canine teeth. She gave Susan a small bottle of chlorhexidine oral rinse to use twice daily to kill plaque bacteria until his recheck appointment, at which time Emma would demonstrate how to start brushing Milo's teeth, and discuss using other dental homecare products. She also told Susan that Milo would need another COHAT and full-mouth X-rays in 6 months' time to prevent worsening of his periodontal disease and to monitor the health of his lower canine teeth.

Susan didn't have any other questions, so Emma led her to the reception area. Susan had arranged third-party financing, and while she was signing the paperwork for this with the client services representative, Emma returned to the treatment area, checked Milo's vital signs again, removed his IV catheter, and placed a bandage over the area. When she brought him to the lobby, Milo perked up as soon as he saw Susan. Emma told Susan to remove the bandage when she got home.

At home, Milo was more subdued than usual. He ate a little bit of canned food and cuddled quietly beside Susan on the sofa. Noodle sniffed him, then wandered off. Later that evening, it was time for Milo's first dose of oral pain medication. Susan was nervous about opening his mouth to give it to him. She drew up the liquid in the syringe like Emma had shown her, and although Milo wriggled around a bit when she put the end of the syringe into his mouth, it was easier to administer than she'd thought.

In the morning, Milo seemed more like his usual hungry, perky, barky self. Susan fed him some canned food for breakfast, gave him his second dose of pain medication, and rinsed his mouth with the chlorhexidine solution. She supervised closely while he relieved himself in the garden, to make sure he didn't chew any sticks or rocks. As she left for work, Susan felt confident that Milo would be fine, and was glad she'd gone ahead and treated his dental disease.

References

AAHA (2020a) Questions to ask prior to a pet's anesthesia. American Animal Hospital Association. Available at: https://www.aaha.org/globalassets/02-guidelines/2020-anesthesia/pre-anesthesia-client-questionnaire.pdf (accessed 5 March 2021).

AAHA (2020b) Step 2: Equipment preparation. American Animal Hospital Association. Available at: https://www.aaha.org/aaha-guidelines/2020-aaha-anesthesia-and-monitoring-guidelines-for-dogs-and-cats/phase-2-day-of-anesthesia/step-2-equipment-preparation/ (accessed 9 November 2020).

AAHA (2020c) Fluids and Anesthesia. American Animal Hospital Association. Available at: https://www.aaha.org/aaha-guidelines/fluid-therapy/fluids-and-anesthesia/ (accessed 5 March 2021).

ABVMA (2013) Alberta Veterinary Medical Association Medical Records Handbook. Alberta Veterinary Medical Association. Available at: https://www.easav.ca/upload/files/MedicalRecordsHandbookFullColor%20(1).pdf (accessed 11 November 2020).

Altier, B. (2020) Components of the Dental Operatory. In: Perrone, J. (ed.) *Small Animal Dental Procedures for Veterinary Technicians and Nurses.* Wiley Blackwell, Hoboken, New Jersey, pp. 29–49.

Ashall, V., Millar, K. and Hubson-West, P. (2018) Informed consent in veterinary medicine: Ethical implications for the profession and the animal 'patient'. *Food Ethics* 1(3), 247–258. Available at: https://link.springer.com/article/10.1007/s41055-017-0016-2 (accessed 5 March 2021).

Bellows, J. (2006) Let technicians polish dental practice success. Dvm360. Available at: https://www.dvm360.com/view/let-technicians-polish-dental-practice-success (accessed 5 March 2021).

Bellows, J., Berg, M., Dennis, S., Harvey, R., Lobprise, H.B. *et al.* (2019) 2019 AAHA dental care guidelines for dogs and cats. *Journal of the American Animal Hospital Association* 55(2), 49–69. Available at: https://www.aaha.org/globalassets/02-guidelines/dental/aaha_dental_guidelines.pdf (accessed 10 September 2020).

Berg, M. (2020) The examination room and the dental patient. In: Perrone, J. (ed.) *Small Animal Dental Procedures for Veterinary Technicians and Nurses.* Wiley Blackwell, Hoboken, New Jersey, pp. 21–28.

Bird, L. (2020) Dental radiology. In: Perrone, J. (ed.) *Small Animal Dental Procedures for Veterinary Technicians and Nurses.* Wiley Blackwell, Hoboken, New Jersey, pp. 93–130.

Carrozzo, A.B. (2018) Desaturation times between dogs preoxygenated via face mask or flow-by technique before induction of anesthesia. Alfaxan Multidose. Available at: https://www.alfaxan.co.uk/news/preoxygenation-study-highlights (accessed 5 March 2021).

Catanzaro, T.E. (2018) Team support by the medical records. The practice success prescription: Team-based veterinary healthcare delivery by Drs. Leak. Morris Humphries. Available at: https://www.vin.com/apputil/content/defaultadv1.aspx?id=3862726&pid=11227 (accessed 9 November 2020).

Cox, A. (2019) Nutritional support of dogs and cats after surgery. Today's Veterinary Nurse. Available at: https://todaysveterinarynurse.com/articles/nutritional-support-of-dogs-and-cats-after-surgery/ (accessed 9 November 2020).

DeForge, D.H. (2009) Pain management and the dental tech. Veterinary Practice News. Available at: https://www.veterinarypracticenews.com/pain-management-and-the-dental-tech/ (accessed 5 March 2021).

Dominguez, P. (2020) Discharging the dental patient. In: Perrone, J. (ed.) *Small Animal Dental Procedures for Veterinary Technicians and Nurses.* Wiley Blackwell, Hoboken, New Jersey, pp. 213–222.

Finkbeiner, B.L. (2000) Four-handed dentistry revisited. *Journal of Contemporary Dental Practice* 1(4), 1–9. DOI: 10.5005/jcdp-1-4-25.

Gray, C. (2020) Role of the consent form in UK veterinary practice. *Veterinary Record* 187(8), 318–318. Available at: https://bvajournals.onlinelibrary.wiley.com/doi/full/10.1136/vr.105762 (accessed 10 November 2020).

Grubb, T., Sager, J., Gaynor, J.S., Montgomery, E. and Parker, J.A. (2020) 2020 AAHA anesthesia and monitoring guidelines for dogs and cats. American Animal Hospital Association. *Journal of the American Animal Hospital Association* 56, 59–82. Available at: https://www.aaha.org/globalassets/02-guidelines/2020-anesthesia/anesthesia_and_monitoring-guidelines_final.pdf (accessed 15 April 2020).

Hale, F.A. (2009) Informed owner consent. The College of Veterinarians of Ontario. Available at: http://www.toothvet.ca/PDFfiles/CVO_Informed_Owner_Consent.pdf (accessed 5 March 2021).

Hernandez, M. (2007) Identification of oral pathology and dental chart-ing. In: *World Small Animal Veterinary Association World Congress Proceedings, 2007.* Available at: https://www.vin.com/apputil/content/defaultadv1.aspx?id=3860804&pid=11242 (accessed 5 March 2021).

Heskin, K. (2018) Food for thought: Pre-anesthetic fasting. Alfaxan Multidose. Available at: https://www.alfaxan.co.uk/news/pre-anaesthetic-fasting (accessed 9 November 2020).

Hunyady, K. (2019) Anesthesia cheat sheet. University of Wisconsin-Madison School of Veterinary Medicine. Available at: https://www.vetmed.wisc.edu/wp-content/uploads/2019/07/Anesthesia-1.pdf (accessed 9 November 2020).

IDEXX (2015) IDEXX Cornerstone user's manual. IDEXX Laboratories. Available at: https://www.idexx.com/files/cornerstone-users-manual-en.pdf (accessed 5 March 2021).

Jones, N. (2014) CPR for dogs and cats: The RECOVER guidelines for veterinary resuscitation. Today's Veterinary Practice. Available at: https://todaysveteri-narypractice.com/cardiopulmonary-resuscitation-the-recover-guidelines/ (accessed 5 March 2021).

Lewis, J. (2013) 9 steps of a professional pet dental cleaning. Veterinary Practice News. Available at: https://www.veterinarypracticenews.com/a-professional-pet-dental-cleaning-in-9-steps/ (accessed 5 March 2021).

Lucero, R. (2019) Brachycephalic breeds and anesthesia. VetFolio. Available at: https://www.vetfolio.com/learn/article/brachycephalic-breeds-and-anesthesia (accessed 5 March 2021).

McMahon, J. (2020) The dental cleaning. In: Perrone, J. (ed.) *Small Animal Dental Procedures for Veterinary Technicians and Nurses.* Wiley Blackwell, Hoboken, New Jersey, pp. 65–91.

McNerney, T. (2017) Anesthetic consideration in brachycephalic dogs. Veterinary Team Brief. Available at: https://files.brief.vet/migration/article/36376/anesthetic-considerations-in-brachycephalic-dogs-36376-article.pdf (accessed 5 March 2021).

Mills, A. (2020) Anesthesia and the dental patient. In: Perrone, J. (ed.) *Small Animal Dental Procedures for Veterinary Technicians and Nurses.* Wiley Blackwell, Hoboken, New Jersey, pp. 51–63.

Myers, W.S. (2004) Involve your team in veterinary dentistry. In: *Proceedings of the 18th Annual Veterinary Dental Forum.* Omnipress, Madison, Wisconsin, pp. 198–205.

Myers, W.S. (2007) How to promote your dental services year-round. In: *Proceedings of the 21st Annual Veterinary Dental Forum.* Omnipress, Madison, Wisconsin, pp. 349–354.

O'Dwyer, L. (2016) Nursing notes: pre-surgery fasting and anaesthesia. Vet Times. Available at: https://www.vettimes.co.uk/app/uploads/wp-post-to-pdf-en-hanced-cache/1/nursing-notes-pre-surgery-fasting-and-anaesthesia.pdf (accessed 9 November 2020).

O'Dwyer, L. (2017) Anesthesia for the bracycephalic patient. In: *World Small Animal Veterinary Association Congress Proceedings, 2017.* Available at: https://www.vin.com/apputil/content/defaultadv1.aspx?id=8506297&pid=20539 (accessed 5 March 2021).

OSU (2018) General consent form. The Ohio State University Veterinary Medical Center. Available at: https://vet.osu.edu/vmc/sites/default/files/files/companion/behavior/Registration%20Form%20and%20Consent%20Form.pdf (accessed 5 March 2021).

Palmer, D. (2020) How to test an anesthesia machine for leaks. *Firstline* 16(3), 8–16.

Perrone, J., Sharp, S. and March, P. (2020) Common dental conditions and treatments. In: Perrone, J. (ed.) *Small Animal Dental Procedures for Veterinary Technicians and Nurses*. Wiley Blackwell, Hoboken, New Jersey, pp. 131–168.

Rothstein, J. (2010) Anesthesia/surgery/treatment consent form. Dvm360. Available at: https://www.dvm360.com/view/anesthesia-surgery-and-treatment-consent-form (accessed 5 March 2021).

Sonopath (2013) Endotracheal intubation. SonoPath. Available at: https://sonopath.com/articles/endotracheal-intubation (accessed 5 March 2021).

Sonopath (2020) Basic anesthesia machine checklist. SonoPath. Available at: https://sonopath.com/articles/basic-anesthesia-machine-checklist (accessed 9 November 2020).

Square Practice (2020) The importance of 4-handed dentistry. Square Practice. Blog, 17 August. Available at: https://blog.squarepractice.com/the-importance-of-4-handed-dentistry (accessed 10 November 2020).

Stein, B. (2004) Small animal anesthesia guide. Veterinary Anesthesia & Analgesia Support Group. Available at: http://www.vasg.org/word_docs/Anesthesia_Guide_VASG_12_4_04.doc (accessed 9 November 2020).

Stepaniuk, K. (2007a) General anesthesia for the canine and feline dental patient part 1. In: *Proceedings of the 21st Annual Veterinary Dental Forum*. Omnipress, Madison, Wisconsin, pp. 205–208.

Stepaniuk, K. (2007b) General anesthesia for the canine and feline dental patient part 2. In: *Proceedings of the 21st Annual Veterinary Dental Forum*. Omnipress, Madison, Wisconsin, pp. 209–210.

UOB (2017) Calculating and drawing up anaesthetic drugs. University of Bristol. Available at: https://www.bristol.ac.uk/media-library/sites/vetscience/documents/clinical-skills/Calculating%20and%20Drawing%20Up%20Anaesthetic%20Drugs.pdf (accessed 5 March 2021).

Walsh, S. (2017) Learn drug security basics. Today's Veterinary Business. Available at: https://todaysveterinarybusiness.com/learn-drug-security-basics/ (accessed 5 March 2021).

YTI (2020) What's a career where I can work with animals? YTI Career Institute. Blog, 9 March. Available at: https://yti.edu/blog/whats-career-where-i-can-work-animals (accessed 5 March 2021).

Zeltzman, P. (2017a) 10 Secrets of veterinary anesthesia machines. Veterinary Practice News. Available at: https://www.veterinarypracticenews.com/10-secrets-of-veterinary-anesthesia-machines/ (accessed 9 November 2020).

Zeltzman, P. (2017b) Could your veterinary records get you in trouble? Veterinary Practice News. Available at: https://www.veterinarypracticenews.com/could-your-veterinary-records-get-you-in-trouble/ (accessed 5 March 2021).

Sending them Home: Postoperative Care

13

Like intake appointments, discharge appointments should be performed in the examination room (Dominguez, 2020). To prevent distraction for the client, the pet shouldn't be present until after all information has been conveyed. Visual aids are especially useful in explaining oral pathology and treatment. These can include skull models, dental charts, photos, handouts explaining oral pathology, and videos showing how to brush teeth.

If the pet has received a routine COHAT without oral surgery or perioceutic placement, talk to the client about starting a dental homecare programme and demonstrate tooth brushing. If the pet has had oral surgery and/or perioceutic placement, the discharge appointment should focus on the treatments performed and postoperative instructions, including soft diets, pain medications, rechecks, etc. (Dominguez, 2020), to avoid information overload (Bellows *et al.*, 2019). Inform the client that their pet will need a dental homecare programme to prevent periodontal disease, which will be discussed during the recheck appointment (Myers, 2007a; Bellows *et al.*, 2019).

13.1 Discharge Materials for Clients

- **Discharge sheet** (Dominguez, 2020; Perrone, 2020) (further details in the following section). Include a description of any oral pathology found, treatments performed, potential complications, what to expect after anaesthesia and oral surgery, feeding instructions, medication instructions and potential side effects, timing and frequency of rechecks, when dental homecare can begin, when to schedule the next COHAT, hospital contact information, and/or phone numbers of local emergency clinics in case of concerns after regular clinic hours.
- **Pre- and postoperative dental photos and X-rays** (Perrone, 2020). Print out or show to the client on a screen during the discharge appointment.

DOI: 10.1079/9781789248869.0013

- **Medications** (if necessary) (Perrone *et al.*, 2020). Liquid formulations may be easier for owners to give than capsules or tablets, especially for cats.
- **Dental homecare plan** (Dominguez, 2020). Include instructions on how to brush teeth and information about dental homecare products including oral rinses, water additives, dental diets, dental treats and chew aids. (See Chapters 14 and 15, this volume).
- **Pet toothbrush and toothpaste** (Myers, 2007b). Consider incorporating the cost of these into the COHAT price, to encourage owners to try tooth brushing.
- **Samples of oral rinses, dental treats, etc.** (Myers, 2007b).

Patients who have had advanced procedures such as full-mouth extractions, jaw fracture repairs or mandibulectomies will require lengthier discharges. Include instructions on oesophagostomy tube feeding and maintenance, treatment plans for upcoming procedures including recheck dental radiographs, splint removal, and future extractions or endodontic treatment (Perrone *et al.*, 2020).

13.2 General Dental Discharge Guidelines

Use the postoperative guidelines listed below to create dental discharge sheets for your patients. Further details about homecare can be found in previous chapters covering dental pathologies.

13.2.1 Guidelines for patients recovering from routine COHATs

- You may offer small amounts of food and water to your pet once you arrive home, to reduce the chance of stomach upset following anaesthesia (Perrone, 2020).
- Anaesthesia may cause your pet to be fairly quiet overnight. Older animals may take longer to recover than younger patients (Low *et al.*, 2021). To prevent injuries, monitor your pet around stairs, prevent them jumping on and off furniture, and take them for short walks on a leash only for a day or two following anaesthesia (Low *et al.*, 2021).
- Some pets may develop a slight cough from irritation due to the breathing tube used during anaesthesia. Please call us if this persists for longer than 2 days (American Animal Hospital Association (AAHA), 2020).
- Abstain from brushing the teeth for 2–3 days after cleaning, because there may be areas in your pet's mouth that are sore or sensitive from subgingival curettage or probing (Myers, 2007b). Use oral rinses, water additives, dental diets and dental treats during this time to reduce plaque bacteria.
- The veterinarian may advise a follow-up appointment in 3, 6 or 12 months to evaluate the success of your dental homecare programme (Myers, 2007b).

- Schedule the next COHAT in 12 months or as per the veterinarian's recommended timeline (Myers, 2007b).

13.2.2 Guidelines for patients recovering from closed root planing and perioceutic application, open root planing, or guided tissue regeneration

- Feed soft food only and restrict access to hard toys, ropes, raw hides or bones for 10–14 days postoperatively, to prevent pain and dehiscence of any sutures (Perrone *et al.*, 2020). Soft food can consist of either canned food or your pet's usual dry food soaked in warm water or broth to soften the kibble (Low *et al.*, 2021). You may offer small amounts of food and water to your pet once you arrive home, to reduce the chance of stomach upset following anaesthesia (Perrone, 2020).
- Anaesthesia may cause your pet to be fairly quiet overnight. Older animals may take longer to recover than younger patients (Low *et al.*, 2021). To prevent injuries, monitor your pet around stairs, prevent them jumping on and off furniture, and take them for short walks on a leash only for a day or two following anaesthesia (Low *et al.*, 2021).
- Some pets may develop a slight cough from irritation due to the breathing tube used during anaesthesia. Please call us if this persists for longer than 2 days (AAHA, 2020).
- A blood tinge to the saliva is normal for a day or two after oral surgery. If there is profuse bleeding, return to the clinic or nearest emergency facility immediately (Perrone, 2020).
- Follow all medication instructions (Low *et al.*, 2021). If your pet seems uncomfortable or unwilling to eat, call the hospital (AAHA, 2020).
- Abstain from brushing the teeth for 14 days after the procedure, to prevent dislodging the perioceutic gel and to allow the oral tissues to heal (Zoetis, 2021). Use oral rinses, water additives, dental diets and dental treats during this time to reduce plaque bacteria (Perrone *et al.*, 2020).
- A recheck is required in 14 days, after which daily tooth brushing should begin (Perrone *et al.*, 2020).
- Schedule a COHAT and full-mouth X-rays in 3–6 months or as per the veterinarian's recommended timeline, to evaluate the success of treatment and prevent the progression of periodontal disease (Perrone *et al.*, 2020).

13.2.3 Guidelines for patients recovering from extractions, crown amputations, or other oral surgery including biopsies

- Feed soft food only and restrict access to hard toys, ropes, raw hides or bones for 7–10 days postoperatively to prevent pain and dehiscence of any sutures (Juriga, 2008). Soft food can consist of either canned food or your pet's usual dry food soaked in warm water or broth to soften the kibble (Low *et al.*, 2021). You may offer small amounts of food and water to your pet once you arrive home, to reduce the chance of stomach upset following anaesthesia (Perrone, 2020).

- Anaesthesia may cause your pet to be fairly quiet overnight. Older animals may take longer to recover than younger patients (Low *et al.*, 2021). To prevent injuries, monitor your pet around stairs, prevent them jumping on and off furniture, and take them for short walks on a leash only for a day or two following anaesthesia (Low *et al.*, 2021).
- Some pets may develop a slight cough from irritation due to the breathing tube used during anaesthesia. Please call us if this persists for longer than 2 days (AAHA, 2020).
- A blood tinge to the saliva is normal for a day or two after oral surgery. If there is profuse bleeding, return to the clinic or nearest emergency facility immediately (Perrone, 2020).
- If there is postoperative facial swelling, place an ice pack or bag of frozen vegetables wrapped in a thin towel on the area for up to 15 minutes 2–3 times daily (Zeltzman, 2021).
- Follow all medication instructions (Low *et al.*, 2021). If your pet seems uncomfortable or unwilling to eat, call the hospital (AAHA, 2020).
- Use oral rinses, water additives, dental diets and dental treats while the oral tissues are healing to reduce plaque bacteria (Perrone *et al.*, 2020).
- A recheck is required in 10–14 days, after which daily tooth brushing should begin (Khuly, 2020; Perrone *et al.*, 2020)
- The veterinarian may advise a follow-up appointment in 3, 6 or 12 months to evaluate the success of your dental homecare programme (Perrone *et al.*, 2020).
- Schedule the next COHAT in 12 months or as per the veterinarian's recommended timeline (Myers, 2007b).

13.2.4 Guidelines for patients recovering from standard root canal therapy

- You may offer small amounts of food and water to your pet once you arrive home, to reduce the chance of stomach upset following anaesthesia (Perrone, 2020).
- Anaesthesia may cause your pet to be fairly quiet overnight. Older animals may take longer to recover than younger patients (Low *et al.*, 2021). To prevent injuries, monitor your pet around stairs, prevent them jumping on and off furniture, and take them for short walks on a leash only for a day or two following anaesthesia (Low *et al.*, 2021).
- Some pets may develop a slight cough from irritation due to the breathing tube used during anaesthesia. Please call us if this persists for longer than 2 days (AAHA, 2020).

- Tooth brushing can begin immediately (Hale, 2012).
- Schedule follow-up radiographs in 6 months, then yearly, to monitor the success of treatment and to check the state of the restoration (Perrone *et al.*, 2020).

13.2.5 Guidelines for patients recovering from vital pulp therapy

- You may offer small amounts of food and water to your pet once you arrive home, to reduce the chance of stomach upset following anaesthesia (Perrone, 2020).
- Anaesthesia may cause your pet to be fairly quiet overnight. Older animals may take longer to recover than younger patients (Low *et al.*, 2021). To prevent injuries, monitor your pet around stairs, prevent them jumping on and off furniture, and take them for short walks on a leash only for a day or two following anaesthesia (Low *et al.*, 2021).
- Some pets may develop a slight cough from irritation due to the breathing tube used during anaesthesia. Please call us if this persists for longer than 2 days (AAHA, 2020).
- Tooth brushing can begin immediately (Hale, 2012).
- Schedule follow-up radiographs in 3–6 months, then at least yearly, to monitor for continued tooth vitality (Perrone *et al.*, 2020). If the tooth becomes non-vital, root canal therapy or extraction must be performed (Klima, 2008).

13.2.6 Guidelines for patients recovering from jaw fracture repair

- Feed a very soft, semi-liquid diet until the fracture has completely healed (Legendre, 1998; Stevens, 2006). This can be made by mixing your pet's regular canned food or a high-calorie recovery canned diet with water in a blender. Restrict access to hard kibble, treats and toys until the fracture has completely healed and any appliances removed (Hall and Wiggs, 2005; Stevens, 2006). You may offer small amounts of food and water to your pet once you arrive home, to reduce the chance of stomach upset following anaesthesia (Perrone, 2020).
- Anaesthesia may cause your pet to be fairly quiet overnight. Older animals may take longer to recover than younger patients (Low *et al.*, 2021). To prevent injuries, monitor your pet around stairs, prevent them jumping on and off furniture, and take them for short walks on a leash only for a day or two following anaesthesia (Low *et al.*, 2021).
- Some pets may develop a slight cough from irritation due to the breathing tube used during anaesthesia. Please call us if this persists for longer than 2 days (AAHA, 2020).

- A blood tinge to the saliva is normal for a day or two after oral surgery. If there is profuse bleeding, return to the clinic or nearest emergency facility immediately (Perrone, 2020).
- If there is postoperative facial swelling, place an ice pack or bag of frozen vegetables wrapped in a thin towel on the area for up to 15 minutes 2–3 times daily (Zeltzman, 2021).
- Follow all medication instructions (Low *et al.*, 2021). If your pet seems uncomfortable or unwilling to eat, call the hospital (AAHA, 2020).
- An Elizabethan collar should be worn to prevent pawing at or rubbing of the face and damaging any appliances, wiring or splints (Stevens, 2006).
- Use oral rinses and/or water additives until the jaw has healed to reduce plaque bacteria (Legendre, 2003; Stevens, 2006). Use chlorhexidine oral rinse to clean any appliances twice daily (Legendre, 2003).
- Return to the hospital immediately if the appliance becomes dislodged.
- A recheck is required in 7–10 days. Schedule further rechecks as per the veterinarian's directions (Perrone *et al.*, 2020).
- Recheck X-rays are required in 4–8 weeks to assess bone healing (Perrone *et al.*, 2020). Once the fracture has healed, any appliances will be removed, the teeth cleaned, and any compromised teeth must be extracted or receive endodontic treatment (Lantz, 2010; Perrone *et al.*, 2020).

13.2.7 Guidelines for patients recovering from full-mouth extractions due to stomatitis

- Feed soft food only and restrict access to hard toys until directed otherwise, to prevent pain and dehiscence of any sutures (Crawford and Losey, 2020). Soft food can consist of either canned food or your pet's usual dry food soaked in warm water or broth to soften the kibble (Low *et al.*, 2021). You may offer small amounts of food and water to your pet once you arrive home, to reduce the chance of stomach upset following anaesthesia (Perrone, 2020).
- If a feeding tube has been placed, additional instructions will be given outlining its use, including appropriate feeding volumes and frequency, maintenance and rechecks (Crawford and Losey, 2020).
- Anaesthesia may cause your pet to be fairly quiet overnight. Older animals may take longer to recover than younger patients (Low *et al.*, 2021). To prevent injuries, monitor your pet around stairs and prevent them jumping on and off furniture (Low *et al.*, 2021). Keep cats indoors until all oral inflammation resolves, unless directed otherwise by the veterinarian.
- Some pets may develop a slight cough from irritation due to the breathing tube used during anaesthesia. Please call us if this persists for longer than 2 days (AAHA, 2020).

- A blood tinge to the saliva is normal for a day or two after oral surgery. If there is profuse bleeding, return to the clinic or nearest emergency facility immediately (Perrone, 2020).
- If there is postoperative facial swelling, place an ice pack or bag of frozen vegetables wrapped in a thin towel on the area for up to 15 minutes 2–3 times daily (Zeltzman, 2021).
- Follow all medication instructions (Low *et al.*, 2021). If your pet seems uncomfortable or unwilling to eat, call the hospital (AAHA, 2020).
- Schedule postoperative rechecks every 2 weeks until the inflammation subsides (Rochette, 2012). Additional treatment may be required in some cases (Lewis, 2014).

References

AAHA (2020) Phase 3: Return home. American Animal Hospital Association. Available at: https://www.aaha.org/aaha-guidelines/2020-aaha-anesthesia-and-monitoring-guidelines-for-dogs-and-cats/phase-3-return-home/ (accessed 6 March 2021).

Bellows, J., Berg, M.L., Dennis, S., Harvey, R., Lobprise, H.B. *et al.* (2019) 2019 AAHA dental care guidelines for dogs and cats. *Journal of the American Animal Hospital Association* 55(2), 49–69. Available at: https://www.aaha.org/globalassets/02-guidelines/dental/aaha_dental_guidelines.pdf (accessed 10 September 2020).

Crawford, J. and Losey, B.J. (2020) Feline dentistry. In: Perrone, J. (ed.) *Small Animal Dental Procedures for Veterinary Technicians and Nurses.* Wiley Blackwell, Hoboken, New Jersey, pp. 169–186.

Dominguez, P. (2020) Discharging the dental patient. In: Perrone, J. (ed.) *Small Animal Dental Procedures for Veterinary Technicians and Nurses.* Wiley Blackwell, Hoboken, New Jersey, pp. 213–222.

Hale, F.A. (2012) What is root canal treatment? Hale Veterinary Clinic. Available at: http://www.toothvet.ca/PDFfiles/root_canal_treatment.pdf (accessed 16 February 2021).

Hall, B.P. and Wiggs, R.B. (2005) Acrylic splint and circumferential mandibular wire for mandibular fracture repair in a dog. *Journal of Veterinary Dentistry* 22(3), 170–175. DOI: 10.1177/089875640502200304.

Juriga, S. (2008) Surgical extraction techniques. In: *Proceedings of the 22nd Annual Veterinary Dental Forum.* Omnipress, Madison, Wisconsin, pp. 257–261.

Khuly, P. (2020) Tooth extractions in dogs: Causes, procedures, recovery and prevention. Hill's. Available at: https://www.hillspet.com/dog-care/healthcare/dog-tooth-extractions (accessed 16 February 2021).

Klima, L. (2008) Addressing uncomplicated (no pulp exposure) and complicated (pulp exposure) crown fractures. In: *Proceedings of the 22nd Annual Veterinary Dental Forum.* Omnipress, Madison, Wisconsin, pp. 265–267.

Lantz, G.C. (2010) Management of facial fractures. In: *Proceedings of the 24th Annual Veterinary Dental Forum.* Omnipress, Madison, Wisconsin (CD Rom).

Legendre, L. (1998) Use of maxillary and mandibular splints for restoration of normal occlusion following jaw trauma in a cat: A case report. *Journal of Veterinary Dentistry* 15(4), 179–181. DOI: 10.1177/089875649801500406.

Legendre, L. (2003) Intraoral acrylic splints for maxillofacial fracture repair. *Journal of Veterinary Dentistry* 20(2), 70–78. DOI: 10.1177/089875640302000201.

Lewis, J. (2014) Feline stomatitis: Medical therapy for refractory cases. Veterinary Practice News. Available at: https://www.veterinarypracticenews.com/Feline-Stomatitis-Medical-Therapy-for-Refractory-Cases/ (accessed 26 October 2020).

Low, R., Grubb, T., Kochis, S. and Brannon, R. (2021) Anesthesia essentials for pet owners. VCA Animal Hospitals. Available at: https://vcahospitals.com/northwest-veterinary-specialists/-/media/vca/documents/hospitals/oregon/northwest-veterinary-specialists/anesthesia-essentials_qref.pdf?la=en&hash=D3AA1BD16E33EA3D1A0638485364C7DF (accessed 6 March 2021).

Myers, W.S. (2007a) Grow dentistry to 5% of revenue. In: *Proceedings of the 21st Annual Veterinary Dental Forum*. Omnipress, Madison, Wisconsin, pp. 343–347.

Myers, W.S. (2007b) Involving your team in dentistry. In: *Proceedings of the 21st Annual Veterinary Dental Forum*. Omnipress, Madison, Wisconsin, pp. 355–362.

Perrone, J. (2020) Appendices. In: Perrone, J. (ed.) *Small Animal Dental Procedures for Veterinary Technicians and Nurses*. Wiley Blackwell, Hoboken, New Jersey, pp. 223–243.

Perrone, J., Sharp, S. and March, P. (2020) Common dental conditions and treatments. In: Perrone, J. (ed.) *Small Animal Dental Procedures for Veterinary Technicians and Nurses*. Wiley Blackwell, Hoboken, New Jersey, pp. 131–168.

Rochette, J. (2012) Feline stomatitis. Clinician's Brief. Available at: https://www.cliniciansbrief.com/article/feline-stomatitis (accessed 1 March 2021).

Stevens, A.G. (2006) Acrylic for repair of mandibular fractures. Clinician's Brief. Available at: https://www.cliniciansbrief.com/article/acrylic-repair-mandibular-fractures (accessed 25 January 2021).

Zeltzman, P. (2021) Using cold therapy for dogs. Pet Health Network. Available at: https://www.pethealthnetwork.com/dog-health/dog-diseases-conditions-a-z/using-cold-therapy-dogs (accessed 16 February 2021).

Zoetis (2021) Doxirobe gel. Zoetis. Available at: https://www.zoetisus.com/_locale-assets/mcm-portal-assets/msds_pi/pi/doxirobe-gel-marketing-package-insert.pdf (accessed 10 February 2021).

14

Developing Dental Homecare Programmes; How to Brush the Teeth of Dogs and Cats

Before we can help pet owners to develop an effective dental homecare routine, we must step into their shoes. How difficult is it to do something on a daily basis that your pet actively dislikes, at least at the beginning? How difficult is it to make this dislikeable activity part of your daily routine? And how easy is it to slip back into your previous low-maintenance, happier-pet lifestyle?

You may be personally familiar with these difficulties. Many veterinarians and veterinary nurses, like the vast majority of pet owners, don't brush their pets' teeth (Preventive Vet, 2018). A 2016 Canadian survey (Ipsos, 2016) found that only 8% of dog owners brush their pets' teeth daily. The statistics for feline dental care are even worse: only 4% of surveyed cat owners brush their pets' teeth daily. Nearly three-quarters of pet owners never brush their pets' teeth. A 2020 American survey (Bark, 2020) found that 47% of dog owners who don't brush their pets' teeth believe that dental chews are as effective as tooth brushing. The top reasons owners gave for not brushing their pets' teeth were that the pet doesn't sit still, they are afraid they are going to hurt the pet while brushing their teeth, and that tooth brushing is difficult and inconvenient. One-quarter of surveyed dog owners who do brush their dogs' teeth said that tooth brushing is the worst part of having a dog.

With such daunting numbers, it might seem as though getting our clients to implement dental homecare is an impossible task. But with proper education and encouragement, we can motivate our clients to begin (and stick with) a dental homecare programme. Less than a decade ago, only 1% of owners brushed their pets' teeth (Niemiec, 2015), so our efforts in promoting pet dental homecare have already shown improvement. There's nowhere to go but up!

14.1 What Dental Homecare Can Do, and What it Can't

Tooth brushing is the most effective method of plaque and calculus prevention (Roudebush *et al.*, 2005). That's why our own dentists have us brush

© CAB International 2022. *An Introduction to Pet Dental Care: For Veterinary Technicians and Nurses* (K. Istace)
DOI: 10.1079/9781789248869.0014

our teeth daily (Kim, 2012). Mouthwash, oral rinses and plaque-inhibiting chewing gum are adjuncts, not replacements, to tooth brushing (Marsh, 2019). This is also true for our veterinary patients. While passive dental homecare methods such as dental diets, treats, chews, oral rinses and water additives are the easiest (and in some cases, the only) option, they are not as effective at disrupting the plaque biofilm as the active mechanical action of a toothbrush (Roudebush *et al.*, 2005; McMahon, 2020). Daily tooth brushing has been shown to be more than three times as effective at controlling plaque accumulation in dogs than using a daily dental chew or dental diet (Allan *et al.*, 2018). Dental diets and chews can clean only the surfaces of teeth directly involved in chewing, so the incisors and canine teeth don't benefit from these products (Hale, 2020). Oral rinses and water additives may be better able to reach all teeth surfaces, but they can't clean beneath the gumline (Hale, 2020).

Even the best dental homecare programme cannot reverse attachment loss (Hale, 2012). No product, including the bristles of a toothbrush, can reach more than a couple of millimetres beneath the gumline, so even diligent dental homecare cannot clean deep periodontal pockets (Hale, 2020). Brushing the teeth of an animal with sore gums, tooth resorption or mobile teeth will cause them pain, and they may resist having their teeth brushed ever again, even after professional treatment of their periodontal disease (Hale, 2020).

Dental homecare can prevent, or at least slow, the progression of periodontal disease (McMahon, 2020). In order to do this, it must occur before periodontal disease develops (this state usually exists only in pets less than 1 year of age) or after any existing periodontal disease has been treated and the oral tissues have healed (Hale, 2020). However, even diligent daily dental homecare cannot completely eliminate plaque formation on every tooth surface, so the pet will still need regular COHATs – just as humans receive professional dental cleanings despite daily tooth brushing (Hale, 2012). Homecare can lengthen the time interval between needed professional dental cleanings (Vetstreet, 2014), resulting in fewer anaesthetic experiences for the pet and less expense for the pet owner.

Dental homecare is essential to the successful outcome of any COHAT (Hale, 2020). Without daily homecare, the tooth's crown can become recolonized with plaque bacteria within 24 hours of professional dental hygiene, and periodontal pockets can become recolonized with plaque bacteria within 2 weeks (Niemiec, 2015).

14.2 Creating Dental Homecare Programmes

A successful dental homecare programme consists of the following:

- Method(s) of plaque control: only methods and products that have been scientifically proven to reduce plaque should be recommended (Canadian Veterinary Medical Association (CVMA), 2015; Hale, 2020).
- Consistency: the method must be performed or the product used at least once daily (CVMA, 2015).
- Monitoring: the pet should receive an oral examination at least once yearly (more often in pets who have been previously diagnosed with periodontal disease), to evaluate the success of the homecare programme (CVMA, 2015; McMahon, 2020).

The best way to learn how to create a dental homecare programme is to start (or re-start) your own pet's homecare programme (Myers, 2007a). Developing a programme that works for your pet and your family will help you better develop plans for your clients, because you will become familiar with common products, pitfalls, useful tips and techniques.

14.2.1   Method(s) of plaque control

Tooth brushing is the most effective method of plaque control, so should be strongly encouraged unless the pet has existing periodontal disease, is healing from oral surgery, or is aggressive (McMahon, 2020). Clients with mobility issues or conditions such as arthritis may not be able to brush their pet's teeth.

Have a frank discussion with the client about the realities of periodontal disease progression, their own expectations and abilities, and their pet's temperament, to determine which method of plaque control they're most likely to stick with (Berg, 2010). And don't send them away to find dental homecare products on their own (Hale, 2020)! Pet dental products sold in-store and online have little to no regulation, and their labels often carry false claims (CVMA, 2015). Seek out reputable, tested products that you can trust (see Chapter 15, this volume) and have your manager stock them in your hospital for purchase. The more methods of plaque control you can offer your clients, the better (Myers, 2007b).

Veterinary staff usually discuss starting dental homecare programmes with their clients after the pet receives a COHAT (Hale, 2020), but this can be likened to closing the stable door after the horse has already bolted. Start a dental homecare programme when your patients are puppies and kittens. The younger the patient is when tooth brushing begins, the more compliant they will be for the process (Myers, 2007b). Another benefit is that your clients will be examining their pet's growing mouth daily, allowing them to identify any tooth eruption problems, fractures of deciduous teeth, malocclusions, etc. If dental homecare has not been addressed during the pet's first few health examinations, an excellent time to discuss this with clients is during the discharge appointment at spay or neuter (Hale, 2020). At this age, most pets have just finished erupting their permanent teeth.

If the client is able to try tooth brushing, have them start slowly (Hale, 2020). Pets who have rarely had their mouths handled before are understandably resistant to the sudden presence of an unwanted foreign object in their mouth. The type of toothbrush matters, too. The small rubber or plastic protrusions on a fingerbrush don't provide the same abrasiveness as a standard toothbrush; nor are they able to reach beneath the gumline, where periodontal disease begins, so should only be used in the initial stage of getting a pet used to tooth brushing (McMahon, 2020). Encourage graduating to a regular toothbrush as soon as possible. Soft-bristled human toothbrushes (Niemiec, 2015) work just as well as pet toothbrushes, and are often less expensive. Adult toothbrushes fit into the mouths of larger dogs, while toothbrushes made for toddlers (Hale, 2020) can serve to clean the teeth of small dogs and cats. Some dogs even learn to love electric toothbrushes (Carmichael, 2007)!

Despite what you may have seen on toothpaste advertisements, toothpaste is not nearly as critical for plaque control as the bristles of a toothbrush (Roudebush *et al.*, 2005; University of Utah Hospitals and Clinics (UOU), 2019). Brushing with plain water will disrupt the plaque biofilm at no added expense. However, pet toothpaste can be useful in increasing brushing compliance, because it is available in many pet-friendly flavours such as poultry, beef, malt and peanut butter, and tastes like a treat (Hale, 2020). Only use veterinary toothpastes, because the detergents, flavourings and fluoride contained in human toothpastes cannot be spit out by our patients and may cause gastrointestinal (GI) upset or toxicity (McMahon, 2020). Likewise, brushing with baking soda can cause GI upset (CVMA, 2015). Some veterinary toothpastes contain enzymes or antimicrobials that reduce plaque formation. Pets who have previously been treated for periodontal disease may benefit from using a chlorhexidine oral solution rather than toothpaste on the toothbrush (Niemiec *et al.*, 2020).

Clients who are interested in starting a tooth-brushing routine can have the process demonstrated to them on their own pet, a dental model, or a clinic pet (McMahon, 2020). There are also online videos showing how to brush pets' teeth.

Sending home at least two methods of plaque control is preferable in case the pet prefers one over the other, or the owner is more compliant with one than the other (Myers, 2007b). Having multiple methods of plaque control on hand also allows for more flexibility if a pet's or family's normal routine is disrupted. For example, a homecare programme could consist of tooth brushing and a dental diet, or a daily dental chew plus a water additive. If the family member who usually brushes the pet's teeth is out of town, the remaining family members can still feed the pet the dental diet; or, if the client runs out of dental chews, the pet still receives plaque control via their water additive until more chews are purchased.

Patients recovering from oral surgery should receive oral rinses and/or water additives to control plaque until the recheck appointment, at which time tooth brushing should be demonstrated (Khuly, 2020).

14.2.2 Consistency

Plaque control must be performed or administered daily (CVMA, 2015) or, even better, twice daily (Niemiec *et al.*, 2020), to effectively prevent plaque build-up. This is easier when one person in the household is responsible for brushing the pet's teeth (McMahon, 2020). Have a discussion with the client about their schedule. Is it more likely that they will be able to brush the pet's teeth in the morning before work? After they get home from the gym? At bedtime when the family's children are brushing their teeth, too? Link the pet's homecare to something the client does every day, so it becomes a habit. This could be something like brushing during the first commercial of the evening news.

14.2.3 Monitoring

All clients given pet dental homecare recommendations should receive a follow-up call approximately 1 week later to see if they have had any difficulties in implementing the programme (Dominguez, 2016). At the very least, this follow-up call will remind them about performing regular plaque removal. If they are having any problems or have given up with the programme, give suggestions to increase compliance or recommend alternative methods of plaque control.

Schedule rechecks at regular intervals for either the nurse or veterinarian to examine the patient's oral cavity for plaque build-up and gingivitis, especially if the patient has already had treatment for periodontal disease (Bellows *et al.*, 2019). A dental recheck every 3–6 months is usually sufficient to keep pet owners on track (Myers, 2007a).

Routine oral examination by a veterinarian should already be part of your patients' yearly physical examinations, but other health concerns often overshadow dental disease during these appointments (see Chapter 11, this volume).

14.3 How to Brush the Teeth of Dogs and Cats

1. For the first several days (or longer), gently rub the pet's muzzle while giving praise and treats (Hale, 2020). The pet's head should be at or near the same height as yours. Place smaller pets on a chair, bed or counter, or in your lap (McMahon, 2020). The aim is to make the pet comfortable with having its mouth handled. Gradually increase the time period until the pet is able to sit relatively calmly for about 1 minute. More compliant animals can skip this step and go directly to Step Two.

2. Once the pet will sit quietly while its muzzle is being rubbed, lift its upper lip and gently rub the teeth with your finger (Hale, 2020). If the pet seems upset by this, return to Step One for a few more days. Offer flavoured veterinary toothpaste on your finger for your pet to lick.

3. Wrap your finger with a piece of wet gauze or a rag, or use a finger-brush (Hale, 2020). Some cats more readily accept a cotton-tipped swab (Bellows, 2017). Apply veterinary toothpaste if desired. Massage the teeth and gums for 1–2 minutes. Don't forget to praise and give treats!

4. Once the pet tolerates a gauze or fingerbrush, switch to a soft-bristled toothbrush (Hale, 2020). Pet toothbrushes are available in various sizes and shapes, and human adult or children's toothbrushes also work well. Wet the brush, apply toothpaste if desired, and move the toothbrush in gentle circular motions, brushing every tooth (McMahon, 2020). This should take approximately 2 minutes. Expect that the pet may chew on the brush bristles or move its head around.

5. Immediately after brushing, praise the pet and give it a high-value treat (Hale, 2020), preferably something it doesn't receive at any other time of day. Pets who are not treat-motivated may prefer a few minutes of play with a favourite toy.

6. As the pet's acceptance of tooth brushing increases, perfect your technique by angling the brush at 45 degrees to the teeth surfaces, to allow the bristles to reach beneath the gumline (Hale, 2020; McMahon, 2020).

7. The lingual and palatal surfaces of the teeth are challenging to brush, with pets often biting the brush or pushing it out of their mouth with their tongue. However, some pets will allow brushing of these surfaces, so once the pet is comfortable with having the outside surfaces of their teeth brushed, try brushing the inside surfaces also (Hale, 2020).

References

Allan, R.M., Adams, V.J. and Johnston, N.W. (2018) Prospective randomised blind-ed clinical trial assessing effectiveness of three dental plaque control methods in dogs. *Journal of Small Animal Practice* 60(4), 212–217. Available at: https://onlinelibrary.wiley.com/doi/abs/10.1111/jsap.12964 (accessed 19 October 2020).

Bark (2020) New study: Nearly 70% of dog parents have never brushed their dogs' teeth. Available at: https://bark.co/articles/new-study-nearly-70-of-dog-par-ents-have-never-brushed-their-dogs-teeth/ (accessed 19 October 2020).

Bellows, J. (2017) The ultimate guide to veterinary dental homecare. DVm360. Available at: https://www.dvm360.com/view/ultimate-guide-veterinary-dental-home-care (accessed 8 March 2021).

Bellows, J., Berg, M., Dennis, S., Harvey, R., Lobprise, H.B. *et al.* (2019) 2019 AAHA dental care guidelines for dogs and cats. *Journal of the American Animal Hospital Association* 55(2), 49–69. Available at: https://www.aaha.org/

globalassets/02-guidelines/dental/aaha_dental_guidelines.pdf (accessed 10 September 2020).

Berg, M. (2010) Home dental care and client education. In: *Proceedings of the 24th Annual Veterinary Dental Forum*. Omnipress, Madison, Wisconsin (CD Rom).

Carmichael, D.T. (2007) Dental corner: educate your clients about dental home care for their pets. Dvm360. Available at: https://www.dvm360.com/view/dental-corner-educate-your-clients-about-dental-home-care-their-pets (accessed 8 March 2021).

CVMA (2015) Bad breath can be prevented in pets. Canadian Veterinary Medical Association. Available at: https://www.canadianveterinarians.net/documents/bad-breath-can-be-prevented-in-pets (accessed 8 March 2021).

Dominguez, P.M. (2016) Increasing clients' – and your own – dental awareness: from the exam room to the dental suite. Today's Veterinary Nurse. Available at: https://todaysveterinarynurse.com/articles/increasing-clients-and-your-own-dental-awareness-from-the-exam-room-to-the-dental-suite/ (accessed 7 December 2020).

Hale, F.A. (2012) Reasonable expectations for dental home care. Hale Veterinary Clinic. Available at: http://www.toothvet.ca/PDFfiles/reasonable_expectations.pdf (accessed accessed 19 October 2020).

Hale, F.A. (2020) Home Dental Care. Hale Veterinary Clinic. Available at: http://www.toothvet.ca/PDFfiles/HomeCarePack.pdf (accessed 15 February 2021).

Ipsos (2016) Most (95%) pet owners brush their own teeth daily, but few brush their dog's (8%) or cat's (4%) teeth on a daily basis. Ipsos. Available at: https://www.ipsos.com/en-ca/news-polls/most-95-pet-owners-brush-their-own-teeth-daily-few-brush-their-dogs-8-or-cats-4-teeth-daily-basis (accessed 19 October 2020).

Khuly, P. (2020) Tooth extractions in dogs: Causes, procedures, recovery and prevention. Hill's. Available at: https://www.hillspet.com/dog-care/healthcare/dog-tooth-extractions (accessed 16 February 2021).

Kim, J.H. (2012) A review of mechanical dental plaque control. Perio-Implant Advisory. Available at: https://www.perioimplantadvisory.com/clinical-tips/hygiene-techniques/article/16412146/a-review-of-mechanical-dental-plaque-control (accessed 8 March 2021).

Marsh, L. (2019) Evidence for mouthrinses as adjunctive therapy. *Decisions in Dentistry* 5(5), 40–42. Available at: https://decisionsindentistry.com/article/evidence-for-mouthrinses-as-adjunctive-therapy/ (accessed 8 March 2021).

McMahon, J. (2020) The dental cleaning. In: Perrone, J. (ed.) *Small Animal Dental Procedures for Veterinary Technicians and Nurses*. Wiley Blackwell, Hoboken, New Jersey, pp. 65–91.

Myers, W.S. (2007a) Grow dentistry to 5% of revenue. In: *Proceedings of the 21st Annual Veterinary Dental Forum*. Omnipress, Madison, Wisconsin, pp. 343–347.

Myers, W.S. (2007b) How to promote your dental services year-round. In: *Proceedings of the 21st Annual Veterinary Dental Forum*. Omnipress, Madison, Wisconsin, pp. 349–354.

Niemiec, B.A. (2015) Top 5 tools and techniques for oral home care. Clinician's Brief. Available at: https://cliniciansbrief.com/article/top-5-tools-techniques-oral-home-care (accessed 5 March 2021).

Niemiec, B., Gawor, J., Nemec, A., Clarke, D., McLeod, K. *et al.* (2020) World small animal veterinary association global dental guidelines, 26 July. *Journal of*

Small Animal Practice 61(7). Available at: https://onlinelibrary.wiley.com/doi/ (accessed 21 September 2020).

Preventive Vet (2018) Much ado about brushing: How to keep our pets' teeth clean when we don't brush them regularly. Preventive Vet. Available at: https://www.preventivevet.com/pawsandplay/how-to-clean-your-pets-teeth-when-you-arent-great-at-brushing (accessed 7 March 2021).

Roudebush, P., Logan, E. and Hale, F.A. (2005) Evidence-based veterinary dentistry: A systematic review of homecare for prevention of periodontal disease in dogs and cats. *Journal of Veterinary Dentistry* 22(1), 6–15. DOI: 10.1177/089875640502200101.

UOU (2019) Are there benefits to using fluoride-free toothpaste? University of Utah Hospitals and Clinics. Available at: https://healthcare.utah.edu/the-scope/shows.php?shows=0_bfiah6xp (accessed 7 March 2021).

Vetstreet (2014) Dental cleaning for dogs and cats. Vet Street. Available at: http://www.vetstreet.com/care/dental-cleaning-for-dogs-and-cats (accessed 7 March 2021).

Understanding the Science Behind Dental Homecare Products

15

There are hundreds of dental homecare products on the market, each advertising itself as the best thing ever designed in the history of pet dental care (Holmstrom *et al.*, 2000; Istace, 2019). Every day, more products appear on the market. How are we as veterinary nurses to know which are truly effective? Understanding the science behind common dental homecare ingredients can help.

Regardless of a product's hype, most dental homecare products fall into one (or more) of these categories (Logan and Burns, 2007; Istace, 2019):

1. Mechanical removal of plaque and calculus.
2. Chemical control of calculus formation.
3. Antimicrobial agents.
4. Barriers against plaque attachment.

15.1 Mechanical Removal of Plaque and Calculus

These products mechanically remove or prevent the accumulation of plaque and tartar (Roudebush *et al.*, 2005; Logan and Burns, 2007; Istace, 2019).

15.1.1 Toothbrushes

- Toothbrushes should be soft-bristled (Roudebush *et al.*, 2005), not medium or hard (Istace, 2019).
- They can be designed for pets or humans, as long as the size of the head is appropriate to the patient's mouth (Lobprise and Wiggs, 2000; Istace, 2019). Children's toothbrushes work well (Holmstrom *et al.*, 2000).
- Plastic or nylon fingerbrushes are more useful for training than for actual brushing (McMahon, 2020; Istace, 2019). Try to get owners to graduate to bristled brushes.

© CAB International 2022. *An Introduction to Pet Dental Care: For Veterinary Technicians and Nurses* (K. Istace)
DOI: 10.1079/9781789248869.0015

- Rotating electric brushes are a favourite for many large-breed dogs (Carmichael, 2007; Istace, 2019).
- Small, round-headed brushes are available for cats (Istace, 2019; McMahon, 2020).
- Pets who don't accept toothbrushes may accept the owner's finger wrapped in gauze or a rag (Hale, 2020; Istace, 2019).
- Toothbrushes can be used either with pet toothpastes or only water (Roudebush *et al.*, 2005).

15.1.2 Diets

- Specially tailored food products formulated to scrub plaque and calculus from teeth during chewing (Roudebush *et al.*, 2005; Istace, 2019).
- The large kibble size of these diets ensures that pets chew each piece (Hennet *et al.*, 2007).
- Some diets have a special texture, allowing teeth to sink into the kibble (Lobprise and Wiggs, 2000), thus scrubbing the entire surface of the tooth (though not under the gumline) (Istace, 2019; Hale, 2020).
- They may be coated with a chemical agent (see Section 15.2, this volume) to reduce calculus formation (Roudebush *et al.*, 2005; Hennet *et al.*, 2007; Istace, 2019).
- They can be used as a pet's sole diet or to supplement an existing diet (PetMD, 2021).
- They clean only those teeth that chew; not incisors or canines (Istace, 2019; Hale, 2020).

15.1.3 Treats

- Tooth-cleaning treats use mechanical abrasion from a wide variety of ingredients to scrub plaque and tartar from teeth (Roudebush *et al.*, 2005; Istace, 2019).
- They may also contain antimicrobial agents (Roudebush *et al.*, 2005; Istace, 2019) (see Section 15.3, this volume).
- They are a source of calories, but not the main source of calories, in a pet's diet (Logan and Burns, 2007; Istace, 2019).
- They are designed to be effective while allowing the pet to eat their regular diet (Istace, 2019; Pet Nutrition Alliance (PNA), 2021).
- They clean only those teeth that chew, not incisors or canines (Istace, 2019; Hale, 2020).
- Very hard treats can cause tooth fractures (Istace, 2019).

15.1.4 Chew aids

- Examples of chew aids include rawhide, pig's ears, beef tendons, etc. (Brown and McGenity, 2005).

- They use mechanical abrasion to scrub plaque and tartar from teeth (Roudebush *et al.*, 2005; Brown and McGenity, 2005; Istace, 2019).
- The pet gains psychological satisfaction from chewing (Lobprise and Wiggs, 2000; Istace, 2019).
- Some chew aids may also contain antimicrobial agents (Brown and McGenity, 2005; Istace, 2019) (see Section 15.3, this volume).
- They can cause digestive upset (Texas A&M University Veterinary Medicine & Biomedical Sciences (TAMU), 2019; Istace, 2019).
- They must be used under supervision, as they can cause choking (Istace, 2019; Hale, 2020) or intestinal blockage (Istace, 2019; McMahon, 2020).
- Very hard or compressed chew aids can cause tooth fractures (Roudebush *et al.*, 2005; Istace, 2019).

15.1.5 Chew toys

- Chew toys are non-consumable items, so are not needed in frequent supply (Istace, 2019)
- They come in a wide variety of materials: e.g. rubber, rope or nylon; natural bones; tennis balls (Roudebush *et al.*, 2005; Istace, 2019; Hale, 2020).
- Some can cause tooth fracture (Roudebush *et al.*, 2005; Istace, 2019).
- The fuzz from tennis balls can cause tooth abrasion (Istace, 2019; Hale, 2020).
- They may have grooves or holes to place treats or soft food into, to increase chewing compliance (Istace, 2019).

15.2 Chemical Control of Calculus Formation

The most common chemical compounds for calculus control are polyphosphates (Roudebush *et al.*, 2005). These trap the calcium ions in saliva, decreasing the mineralization of plaque into calculus (Istace, 2019). When sprayed onto the surface of diets, treats or chew aids, they reduce the formation of tartar, even on non-chewing teeth (Roudebush *et al.*, 2005; Istace, 2019). They don't remove plaque, which is the true cause of periodontal disease, but may increase the efficacy of mechanical plaque-removal methods such as tooth brushing (Hennet *et al.*, 2007; Istace, 2019). Look for 'sodium hexametaphosphate' (McMahon, 2020) or 'sodium tripolyphosphate' (Hennet *et al.*, 2007) on ingredient labels.

Another agent which inhibits calcium precipitation into calculus is xylitol, but as it also inhibits the growth of plaque bacteria (Clarke, 2006; Istace, 2019), it is discussed in more detail below (see Section 15.3.5, this volume).

15.3   Antimicrobial Agents

Various antimicrobial agents are used to control plaque (Istace, 2019) by inhibiting bacterial growth.

15.3.1   Chlorhexidine gluconate

- Chlorhexidine gluconate combats both gram-positive and gram-negative bacteria (Istace, 2019) by disrupting their cell membranes (Roudebush *et al.*, 2005).
- It prevents plaque, gingivitis and halitosis (Roudebush *et al.*, 2005; Istace, 2019).
- It binds to tissues in the oral cavity and is released over time (Roudebush *et al.*, 2005; Istace, 2019).
- It can cause tooth staining (Lobprise and Wiggs, 2000; Istace, 2019).
- It is bitter-tasting (Roudebush *et al.*, 2005).
- Products containing chlorhexidine should be kept away from eyes (they can cause corneal ulcers) (Istace, 2019; PubChem, 2021) and ears (can cause deafness at high concentrations) (Igarashi, 1985; Istace, 2019).

15.3.2   Lactoperoxidase and glucose oxidase

- These are enzymes that decrease plaque by killing bacteria (Roudebush *et al.*, 2005).
- They are found in toothpastes and treats (Holmstrom *et al.*, 2000; Istace, 2019).

15.3.3   Zinc

- Zinc has antiseptic activity against both gram-positive and gram-negative bacteria (Clarke, 2001; Roudebush *et al.*, 2005).
- It decreases bacterial growth, plaque formation and gingivitis (Clarke, 2001; Roudebush *et al.*, 2005).
- It is found in oral gels, sprays and drinking-water additives (Roudebush *et al.*, 2005; Bellows, 2017a).

15.3.4 Ascorbic acid (vitamin C)

- Ascorbic acid has antibacterial, antifungal and antiviral properties (Mousavi *et al.*, 2019).
- It is essential for wound healing, collagen production and combating free radicals (Holmstrom *et al.*, 2000; Clarke, 2001; Istace, 2019).
- It is odourless and tasteless (Gawor, 2012).
- It is found in oral gels, oral rinses and drinking-water additives (Istace, 2019).

15.3.5   Xylitol

- Xylitol is a natural sugar alcohol used in human products such as chewing gum to reduce plaque formation and gingivitis (Roudebush *et al.*, 2005; Istace, 2019).
- It inhibits bacterial growth, forms extracellular polysaccharides which make plaque less adhesive to teeth, and decreases the precipitation of calcium into calculus (Clarke, 2006; Istace, 2019).
- Its use is controversial in animals, particularly in dogs, because of concerns about xylitol causing severe hypoglycaemia, liver failure and haemorrhagic gastroenteritis (Istace, 2019; Brutlag, 2021), though it seems to have no ill effects in cats (Clarke, 2006).
- The suggested dental dose is 3.5 mg/kg/day (Anthony *et al.*, 2011); the toxic dose is 100 mg/kg (Brutlag, 2021).
- It is found in drinking-water additives (Istace, 2019).
- It is well accepted by pets, and requires little effort on the part of the owner (Clarke, 2006; Anthony *et al.*, 2011; Istace, 2019).

15.3.6   Chlorine dioxide

- Chlorine dioxide oxidizes the sulphur compounds that contribute to halitosis (Holmstrom *et al.*, 2004; Istace, 2019).
- It has been shown to have antibacterial properties similar to chlorhexidine in humans (Downs *et al.*, 2015).
- It is found in drinking-water additives, toothpastes, gels and sprays.

15.3.7   Citric acid

- Citric acid is an antibacterial agent that inhibits plaque bacteria growth (Al-Sharifi *et al.*, 2019).
- It is found in dental wipes, drinking-water additives and toothpastes.

15.3.8   Essential oils

- These include clove, eucalyptus, thymol, methanol and eugenol (Bellows, 2017a).
- They reduce plaque and gingivitis (Bellows, 2017a).
- They are found in drinking-water additives, gels, sprays and treats.

15.4   Barriers against Plaque Attachment

These are non-toxic waxy or liquid polymers (Bellows, 2016, 2017b) applied to the teeth at the gumline by the nurse or veterinarian after a COHAT (Istace, 2019) or at the time of spay/neuter. Wax barriers prevent plaque bacteria from attaching to the teeth, and are reapplied weekly at home by the owner (Istace, 2019). Liquid polymers seal the gingival sulcus against plaque for 6 months, after which time they are reapplied in-clinic during wellness exams or dental rechecks.

15.5   Miscellaneous Agents

15.5.1 Delmopinol

- This prevents plaque attachment and gingivitis (Bellows, 2017a; Brooks, 2019).
- It is found in dental chews.

15.5.2   Calcium peroxide

- This decreases plaque by dissolving the pellicle (the coating on the teeth formed by saliva) (Bellows, 2017a).
- It is found in toothpastes.

15.5.3   Mutanese and dextranase

- These are enzymes which disrupt the glucan bonds in plaque, making it water-soluble and unable to adhere to teeth (Istace, 2019; Zymox, 2021).
- They are found in oral gels, rinses and drinking-water additives (Istace, 2019).

15.5.4   Bromelain and papain

- These are enzymes which reduce the build-up of salivary glycoproteins in the mouth, reducing plaque formation (Istace, 2019; Scanlan, 2019).
- They are found in oral gels, rinses and drinking-water additives (Istace, 2019).

15.5.5   Acetic acid

- Acetic acid dissolves plaque (Bhat *et al.*, 2014).
- It is found in dental gels and wipes.

15.5.6   Alcohol

- Alcohol is used in human dental products such as mouthwash to reduce plaque (Kulkami *et al.*, 2017; Istace, 2019).
- It has been linked to oral cancers in humans (Kulkami *et al.*, 2017; Istace, 2019).

- It can cause GI irritation (Kulkami *et al.*, 2017; Istace, 2019) and toxicity in animals (Bellows, 2017a).
- It is found in dental sprays and rinses.

15.5.7 Coenzyme Q10

- Coenzyme Q10 is an enzyme that has been shown to improve gingival health when ingested (Istace, 2019; Scanlan, 2019).
- It can decrease blood pressure, so should be used with caution in animals receiving antihypertensive medications (Gollakner, 2021).

15.5.8 Chlorophyll

- This reduces halitosis (Brooks, 2019).
- It has little effect on gingivitis or bacteria (Lowell, 2004).
- It is found in water additives, gels, sprays and treats.

15.6 Veterinary Oral Health Council (VOHC)

The following guidance is according to Istace (2019) and VOHC (2021).

The best way to be sure that a product you are recommending is safe and effective is to look for the Veterinary Oral Health Council seal. The VOHC awards products the VOHC Seal of Acceptance following review of data from trials conducted according to VOHC protocols. VOHC testing is a voluntary, expensive and time-consuming process. A product without a VOHC seal may be effective, but its manufacturers may not have chosen to pursue clinical trials and submission to the VOHC. However, a product with the VOHC seal is known to be effective when used as directed. A list of approved products is available at www.vohc.org.

References

Al-Sharifi, E.A., Alkaisy, N. and Al-Mahmood, A.A. (2019) Efficacy of citric acid on periodontal disease. *Biomedical Research* 30(3). Available at: https://www.allie dacademies.org/articles/efficacy-of-citric-acid-on-periodontal-disease-11334. html (accessed 19 October 2020).

Anthony, J.M.G., Weber, L.P. and Alkemade, S. (2011) Blood glucose and liver function in dogs administered a xylitol drinking water additive at zero, one and five times dosage rates. *Veterinary Science Development* 1(1), 2. Available at: https://www.pagepress.org/journals/index.php/vsd/article/view/vsd.2011.e2/2805 (accessed 19 October, 2020).

Bellows, J. (2016) Go one step beyond in veterinary dental care. Dvm360. Available at: https://www.dvm360.com/view/go-one-step-beyond-veterinary-dental-care (accessed 19 October 2020).

Bellows, J. (2017a) The ultimate guide to veterinary dental homecare. Dvm360. Available at: https://www.dvm360.com/view/ultimate-guide-veterinary-dental-home-care (accessed 8 March 2021).

Bellows, J. (2017b) 10 Veterinary dental products you can recommend with a smile. Dvm360. Available at: https://www.dvm360.com/view/10-veterinary-dental-products-you-can-recommend-with-smile (accessed 19 October 2020).

Bhat, M., Prasad, K.V., Trivedi, D. and Acharya, A.B. (2014) Dental plaque dissolving agents: An in vitro study. *International Journal of Advanced Health Sciences* 1(3). Available at: https://www.researchgate.net/publication/280571976_Dental_Plaque_Dissolving_Agents_An_In_Vitro_Study (accessed 19 October 2020).

Brooks, W. (2019) Dental home care for dogs and cats. Veterinary Partner. Available at: https://www.vin.com/apputil/project/defaultadv1.aspx?pId=17256&SAId=1&catId=93571&id=4951515&ind=1693&objType ID=1007 (accessed 19 October 2020).

Brown, W.Y. and McGenity, P. (2005) Periodontal disease control using dental hygiene chews. *Journal of Veterinary Dentistry* 22(1), 16–19. DOI: 10.1177/089875640502200102.

Brutlag, A. (2021) Xylitol toxicity in dogs. VCA. Available at: https://vcahospitals.com/know-your-pet/xylitol-toxicity-in-dogs (accessed 8 March 2021).

Carmichael, D.T. (2007) Dental corner: Educate your clients about dental home care for their pets. Dvm360. Available at: https://www.dvm360.com/view/dental-corner-educate-your-clients-about-dental-home-care-their-pets (accessed 8 March 2021).

Clarke, D.E. (2001) Clinical and microbiological effects of oral zinc ascorbate gel in cats. *Journal of Veterinary Dentistry* 18(4), 177–183. DOI: 10.1177/089875640101800401.

Clarke, D.E. (2006) Drinking water additive decreases plaque and calculus accumulation in cats. *Journal of Veterinary Dentistry* 23(2), 79–82. DOI: 10.1177/089875640602300203.

Downs, R.D., Banas, J.A. and Zhu, M. (2015) An in vitro study comparing a two-part activated chlorine dioxide oral rinse to chlorhexidine. Perio-Implant Advisory. Available at: https://www.perioimplantadvisory.com/clinical-tips/hygiene-techniques/article/16411500/an-in-vitro-study-comparing-a-twopart-activated-chlorine-dioxide-oral-rinse-to-chlorhexidine (accessed 8 March 2021).

Gawor, J. (2012) Zinc ascorbate oral gel and five major clinical applications in dogs and cats. In: *Proceedings of the 26th Annual Veterinary Dental Forum*. Omnipress, Madison, Wisconsin (CD Rom).

Gollakner, R. (2021) Coenzyme Q-10. VCA. Available at: https://vcahospitals.com/know-your-pet/coenzyme-q-10 (accessed 8 March 2021).

Hale, F.A. (2020) Home dental care. Hale Veterinary Clinic. Available at: http://www.toothvet.ca/PDFfiles/HomeCarePack.pdf (accessed accessed 15 February 2021).

Hennett, P., Ing, S.E., Ing, S.Y. and Biourge, V. (2007) Effect of pellet size and polyphosphates in preventing calculus accumulation in dogs. *Journal of veterinary dentistry* 24(4), 236–239. DOI: 10.1177/089875640702400405.

Holmstrom, S., Holmstrom, L.A., McGrath, C.J., Richey, M.T. and Wiggs, R.B. (2000) Home-care instruction. In: Holmstrom, S. (ed.) *Veterinary Dentistry for the Technician & Office Staff.* Saunders, Philadelphia, Pennsylvania, pp. 183–195.

Holmstrom, S., Frost, P. and Eisner, E. (2004) Dental prophylaxis. In: Eisner, E. (ed.) *Veterinary Dental Techniques for the Small Animal Practitioner.* Saunders, Philadelphia, Pennsylvania, pp. 255–318.

Igarashi, Y. (1985) Cochlear ototoxicity of chlorhexidine gluconate in cats. *Archives of Oto-Rhino-Laryngology* 242(2), 167–176. Available at: https://link.springer.com/article/10.1007/BF00454417 (accessed 8 March 2021).

Istace, K. (2019) The science behind dental homecare products. In: *44th World Small Animal Veterinary Association Congress,* 16–19 July, 2019, Toronto, Canada, pp. 591–592. Available at: https://emdstudio.co.il/ebook/wsava2019/mobile/index.html (accessed 3 May 2021).

Kulkami, P., Singh, D.K., Jalaluddin, M. and Mandal, A. (2017) Comparative evaluation of antiplaque efficacy between essential oils with alcohol-based and chlorhexidine with nonalcohol-based mouthrinses. *Journal of International Society of Preventive and Community Dentistry* 7(7), 36. Available at: https://www.ncbi.nlm.nih.gov/pmc/articles/PMC5502550/ (accessed 8 March 2021).

Lobprise, H.B. and Wiggs, R.B. (2000) Periodontal disease. In: Lobprise, H.B. and Wiggs, R.B. (eds) *The Veterinarian's Companion for Common Dental Procedures.* AAHA Press, Lakewood, Colorado, pp. 39–70.

Logan, E.I. and Burns, K.M. (2007) Improving home care compliance with a team approach. In: *Proceedings of the 21st Annual Veterinary Dental Forum.* Omnipress, Madison, Wisconsin, pp. 455–458.

Lowell, J.A. (2004) Amazing claims for chlorophyll. Quackwatch. Available at: https://quackwatch.org/related/dsh/chlorophyll/ (accessed 27 July 2021).

McMahon, J. (2020) The dental cleaning. In: Perrone, J. (ed.) *Small Animal Dental Procedures for Veterinary Technicians and Nurses.* Wiley Blackwell, Hoboken, New Jersey, pp. 65–91.

Mousavi, S., Bereswill, S. and Hemesaat, M.M. (2019) Immunomodulatory and antimicrobial effects of Vitamin C. *European Journal of Microbiology and Immunology* 9(3), 73–79. Available at: https://www.ncbi.nlm.nih.gov/pmc/articles/PMC6798581/ (accessed 8 March 2021).

PetMD (2021) Dental diets for better oral health. PetMD. Available at: https://www.petmd.com/dog/nutrition/evr_multi_dental_diets (accessed 8 March 2021).

PNA (2021) If dental treats will be part of a pet's diet, how should they be fed? Pet Nutrition Alliance. Available at: https://petnutritionalliance.org/site/pnatool/if-dental-treats-will-be-a-part-of-a-pets-diet-how-should-they-be-fed/ (accessed 8 March 2021).

PubChem (2021) Chlorhexidine. PubChem. Available at: https://pubchem.ncbi.nlm.nih.gov/compound/Chlorhexidine#section=Skin-Eye-and-Respiratory-Irritations (accessed 13 March 2021).

Roudebush, P., Logan, E. and Hale, F.A. (2005) Evidence-based veterinary dentistry, a systematic review of homecare for prevention of periodontal disease in dogs and cats. *Journal of Veterinary Dentistry* 22(1), 6–15. DOI: 10.1177/089875640502200101.

Scanlan, N. (2019) 9 Nutrients for canine dental disease. Animal Wellness. Available at: https://animalwellnessmagazine.com/nutrients-canine-dental-disease/ (accessed 8 March 2021).

TAMU (2019) How to 'chews' the best dog chew toys. Texas A&M University Veterinary Medicine & Biomedical Sciences. Available at: https://vetmed. tamu.edu/news/pet-talk/how-to-chews-the-best-dog-chew-toys/ (accessed 8 March 2021).

VOHC (2021) Veterinary Oral Health Council. Available at: http://www.vohc.org (accessed 8 March 2021).

Zymox (2021) Disruption of biofilm with biofilm reducing enzymes. Zymox. Available at: https://www.zymox.com/lp3-system-2/biofilm-reducing-complex-or-antibiofilm-enzyme-system/ (accessed 8 March 2021).

Advocating for Pet Dental Health   16

Veterinary practices often fail to make pet dental care a priority (Berg, 2007), even though periodontal disease and other oral conditions take a significant toll on the quality of life of our patients. This is especially true in the case of preventive dental care, despite the fact that disease prevention is preferable to treating established disease. Veterinary nurses can play an important role in changing practice culture to better serve our patients' needs (Myers, 2007a).

16.1 Staff Education

Now that you've read this book, share your knowledge about pet dental care. Organize a staff meeting to develop a plan for every patient to receive either a dental homecare programme or a treatment plan for a COHAT, or both (Myers, 2007b). Seek out dental continuing education opportunities and encourage your fellow nurses, veterinarians and support staff to attend (Myers, 2007a). Ask your office manager or practice owner about offering discounted COHATs for staff pets, so front-office staff, nurses' assistants, etc. will see the benefits and be able to sincerely endorse dental care to clients (Myers, 2007c). If everyone in the hospital is on the same page when it comes to the importance of pet dental care, clients will hear a consistent and credible message from each member of your team (Berg, 2007). Not everyone may be excited about veterinary dentistry, but the more colleagues you can get on board, the better for both patient health and the financial health of the practice. Remember: 80% of adult dogs and 70% of adult cats have periodontal disease (Berg, 2007). That's a lot of potentially untapped revenue.

16.2 Client Education

Use the tools described in Chapter 11, this volume, to educate your clients about the importance of treating oral disease; and the techniques outlined

© CAB International 2022. *An Introduction to Pet Dental Care: For Veterinary Technicians and Nurses* (K. Istace)
DOI: 10.1079/9781789248869.0016

in Chapters 14 and 15, this volume, to help your clients implement preventive dental care. Don't wait until a pet has dental disease to begin discussing dental care: start at the pet's first visit to your hospital (Myers, 2007b).

16.3 Financing

Medical need, not a client's ability to pay, should determine a pet's treatment. Research shows that pet owners who have pet health insurance spend more at veterinary visits and are more willing to approve the tests and treatments their veterinarian recommends (Dominguez, 2016). If your practice doesn't routinely promote pet health insurance, approach your manager about changing this. Invite representatives from pet insurance companies to discuss their dental care policies, find out if they offer free trials for new patients, ask colleagues at other local veterinary hospitals which insurance companies they recommend, and actively encourage your clients to sign up.

Offer third-party financing options (Myers, 2017) for clients who do not have pet insurance, or whose pets have pre-existing health issues or conditions not covered by insurance. The practice can enrol with payment plan or loan companies. Your clients can then apply for financing, usually online (McKinney, 2017). Approval is often quick, and the client can use the financing for any medical services within an approved limit.

16.4 Pain Management

Dental diseases and their treatments are often painful (Mills, 2020). Veterinary nurses often have the most contact with hospitalized patients, so are in an excellent position to be on alert for signs of pain (Tabor, 2016). Don't be afraid to bring any concerns to the veterinarian's attention and/or make suggestions to improve patient comfort. In addition to pain-management protocols including medications and nerve blocks, ensuring that patients are warm, clean, given the opportunity to relieve themselves and are closely monitored during the perioperative period (Lee, 2020) will go a long way to improving patient well-being.

16.5 Referrals

Most general practices don't have the ability to offer all available dental treatments, including endodontics, prosthodontics, maxillofacial surgery, treatment of oral cancers, etc. That doesn't mean that these treatment options shouldn't be accessible to your clients. For example, instead of automatically recommending the extraction of fractured teeth, clients should be given the option of referral for potential root canal therapy

(DeBowes, 2005). If the veterinarians at your hospital aren't in the habit of referring patients who could benefit from advanced dental procedures to veterinary dental specialists, initiate a discussion to advocate this. Seek out veterinary dental specialists in your area (American Veterinary Dental College (AVDC), 2021a). Many have online forms to make the referral process easy, and can give ballpark cost estimates for their procedures. They often welcome phone calls or emails to discuss difficult cases and puzzling radiographs (AVDC, 2021b).

If a patient presents with an oral condition beyond your hospital's ability or desire to treat, it's best to refer them as soon as possible. Most veterinary specialists prefer taking their own dental radiographs, so the referring practice is not obliged to have radiographs prior to referral. Do send along a complete medical history including recent lab results, current medications and/or medication reactions, previous dental charts and anaesthetic records, allergies and vaccination status. If a patient is suspected of having a serious medical condition that could cause complications under general anaesthesia, this should be addressed prior to referral.

Clients will appreciate the fact that your practice cares enough about their pet's health to refer them elsewhere to receive the best treatment (DeBowes, 2005).

By advocating for pet dental health, veterinary nurses can increase both the quality and length of our patient's lives, improve the human–animal bond between our clients and their pets, boost practice income, and become invaluable members of the veterinary team (Smith, 2012).

References

AVDC (2021a) Find a board certified veterinary dentist. American Veterinary Dental College. Available at: https://avdc.org/find-a-veterinary-specialist/ (accessed 5 March 2021).

AVDC (2021b) Primary care practice resources. American Veterinary Dental College. Available at: https://avdc.org/primary-care-practice/ (accessed 4 March 2021).

Berg, M. (2007) One form at a time – client communications. In: *Proceedings of the 21st Annual Veterinary Dental Forum*. Omnipress, Madison, Wisconsin, pp. 313–317.

DeBowes, L.J. (2005) When to refer? Dvm360. Available at: https://www.dvm360. com/view/when-refer (accessed 9 March 2021).

Dominguez, P.M. (2016) Increasing clients' – and your own – dental awareness: From the exam room to the dental suite. Today's Veterinary Nurse. Available at: https://todaysveterinarynurse.com/articles/increasing-clients-and-your-own-dental-awareness-from-the-exam-room-to-the-dental-suite/ (accessed 7 December 2020).

Lee, L. (2020) Perioperative pain management. Western University of Health Sciences. Available at: https://www.westernu.edu/mediafiles/veterinary/vet-anesthesia-analgesia/perioperative-pain-management.pdf (accessed 9 March 2021).

McKinney, M. (2017) The benefits of third-party financing. Dvm360. Available at: https://www.dvm360.com/view/the-benefits-of-thirdparty-financing (accessed 9 March 2021).

Mills, A. (2020) Anesthesia and the dental patient. In: Perrone, J. (ed.) *Small Animal Dental Procedures for Veterinary Technicians and Nurses.* Wiley Blackwell, Hoboken, New Jersey, pp. 51–63.

Myers, W.S. (2007a) Involving your team in dentistry. In: *Proceedings of the 21st Annual Veterinary Dental Forum.* Omnipress, Madison, Wisconsin, pp. 355–362.

Myers, W.S. (2007b) How to promote your dental services year-round. In: *Proceedings of the 21st Annual Veterinary Dental Forum.* Omnipress, Madison, Wisconsin, pp. 349–354.

Myers, W.S. (2007c) Grow dentistry to 5% of revenue. In: *Proceedings of the 21st Annual Veterinary Dental Forum.* Omnipress, Madison, Wisconsin, pp. 343–347.

Myers, W.S. (2017) How to get to YES for dentistry. Communication solutions for veterinarians. Available at: https://www.isvma.org/wp-content/uploads/2017/10/How-to-get_YES_for_dentistry.pdf (accessed 7 December, 2020).

Smith, N. (2012) Dental technicians: filling a vital role in veterinary medicine. Dvm360. Available at: https://www.dvm360.com/view/dental-technicians-filling-vital-role-veterinary-medicine (accessed 9 March 2021).

Tabor, B. (2016) Pain recognition and management in critical care patients. Today's Veterinary Nurse. Available at: https://todaysveterinarynurse.com/articles/pain-recognition-and-management-in-critical-care-patients/ (accessed 15 February 2021).

Index

Note: Page numbers in **bold** type refer to **figures.**

CABI – who we are and what we do

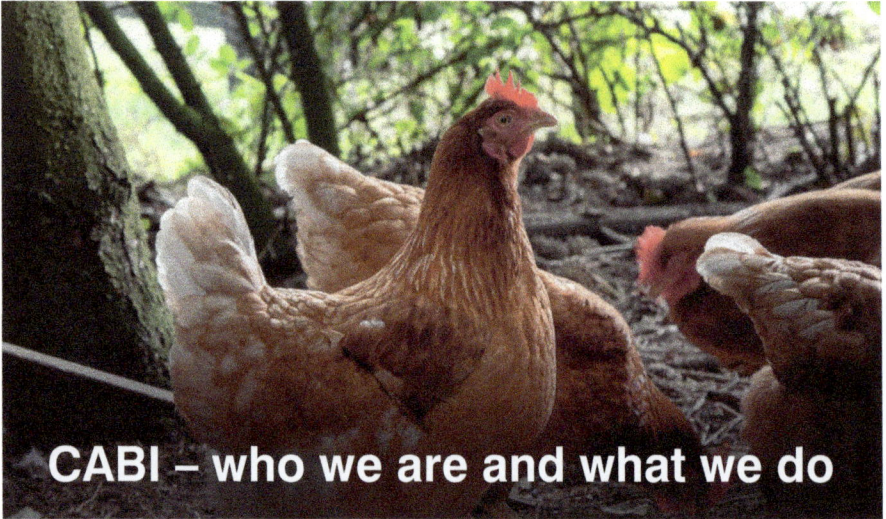

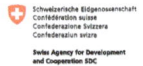

Discover more

To read more about CABI's work, please visit: **www.cabi.org**

Browse our books at: **www.cabi.org/bookshop**,
or explore our online products at: **www.cabi.org/publishing-products**

Interested in writing for CABI? Find our author guidelines here:
www.cabi.org/publishing-products/information-for-authors/